MEDICAL RADIOLOGY

Radiation Oncology

Springer-Verlag Berlin Heidelberg GmbH

W. E. Alberti · G. Richard · R. H. Sagerman (Eds.)

Age-Related Macular Degeneration

Current Treatment Concepts

With Contributions by

W. E. Alberti · K.-G. Au Eong · C. Bellmann · G. J. Bergink · P. Bischoff · P. Blacharski
L.W. Brady · G. Brown · U. Chakravarthy · R. Coquard · P. Crossmann · J. Debus
E. de Juan, Jr. · A.F. Deutmann · E. Egger · K. Engelmann · R. Engenhart-Cabillic · P. T. Finger
J. Freire · G.Y. Fujii · J.-P. Gerard · H. Gerding · G. Goitein · S. Gorty · A. Hassenstein
K. Heimann · U. Höller · F. G. Holz · C. B. Hoyng · I. Immonen · S. B. Klein · M. Kocher
N. Kovács · G. Kovács · K. Krause · R. Krott · J. E. Lahaniatis · S.Y. Lee · D. M. Marcus
P. Martin · M. Mauget-Faÿsee · B. Micaily · C. T. Miyamoto · R.-P. Müller · H. Niederberger
P. Niehoff · D. J. Pieramici · G. Richard · G. Ries · R. H. Sagerman · A. Schalenbourg · F. Schütt
R. Schwartz · W.C. Sheils · J.D. Slater · J. M. Slater · S. Staar · S. Taneri · C. E. Uhlig · K. Unnebrink
C. Valmaggia · M. Valtink · W.A.J. van Daal · R.W. M. van der Maazen · J. R. Vingerling
M. Wannenmacher · J. Weichel · T. E. Yaeger · L. T. Yonemoto · L. Zografos · J. Zurdel

Foreword by

L. W. Brady, H.-P. Heilmann and M. Molls

With 117 Figures in 150 Separate Illustrations, 46 in Color and 33 Tables

Springer

Winfried E. Alberti, MD
Professor, Department of Radiotherapy and Radiooncology
University Hospital Eppendorf
Martinistr. 52
20246 Hamburg
Germany

Gisbert Richard, MD
Professor, Department of Ophthalmology
University Hospital Eppendorf
Martinistr. 52
20246 Hamburg
Germany

Robert H. Sagerman, MD, FACR
Professor, Department of Radiation Oncology
State University of New York
Upstate Medical University
750 East Adams Street
Syracuse, NY 13210
USA

Medical Radiology · Diagnostic Imaging and Radiation Oncology
Continuation of
Handbuch der medizinischen Radiologie
Encyclopedia of Medical Radiology

ISBN 978-3-642-63071-2

Library of Congress Cataloging-in-Publication Data
Age-related macular degeneration : current treatment concepts / W.E. Alberti, G. Richard, R.H. Sagerman (eds.) ; with contributions by W.E. Alberti ... [et al.] ; foreword by L.W. Brady, H.-P. Heilmann and M. Molls
p. ; cm. -- (Medical radiology)
Includes bibliographical references and index.
ISBN 978-3-642-63071-2 ISBN 978-3-642-56439-0 (eBook)
DOI 10.1007/978-3-642-56439-0
1. Retinal degeneration. I. Alberti, W. II. Richard, G. (Gisbert), 1949- III. Sagerman, Robert H., 1930- IV. Series.
[DNLM: 1. Macular Degeneration--radiotherapy. 2. Macular Degeneration--surgery. WW 270 A26495 2000]
RE661.D3 A33 2000
617.7'3506--dc21 00-055661

Originally published by Springer-Verlag Berlin Heidelberg New York in 2001
Softcover reprint of the hardcover 1st edition 2001

Cover-Design and Typesetting: Verlagsservice Teichmann, 69256 Mauer

SPIN: 107 393 34 21/3130 – 5 4 3 2 1 0 – Printed on acid-free paper

Dedicated to

GABRIELE, CLAUDIA and MALYNE

whose intelligence, humor, and support
sustained us throughout this project.

Foreword

This volume, edited by Professors Alberti, Richard and Sagerman, presents relevant and contemporary data on age-related macular degeneration. Age-related macular degeneration is the leading cause of severe blindness today in both the United States and Europe. The incidence increases with age, affecting 11% of those individuals between the ages of 65 and 74 years with rates rising to 28% of patients older than 75 years. Exudative or wet type macular degeneration occurs when the choroidal vessels penetrate Bruch's membrane, causing proliferation beneath the retinal pigment epithelium which leads to choroidal neovascularization, subretinal hemorrhage, serous retinal detachment, and, ultimately, sclerosis and fibriosis. Approximately 10% of patients with age-related macular degeneration develop the wet form and these patients account for the majority of those who become legally blind.

When the choroidal neovascular membrane is subfoveal in character, prognosis is poor, with severe visual loss in more than 75% of the patients at 2 years following its development. Laser photocoagulation is the only available treatment in selected cases and many patients are deemed ineligible for laser photocoagulation by the strict criteria put forth by the Macular Photocoagulation Study. In those patients treated by laser ablation, there is a significant immediate decline in visual acuity and a permanent scotoma. At 2 years, however, only 20% of those treated had a visual acuity loss of six or more lines, compared with 37% of the untreated eyes. More than 51% of the treated eyes had persistent or recurrent choroidal neovascular membrane at 24 months after treatment.

Many treatment techniques have been pursued in the management of wet type macular degeneration. These have included steroids, aspirin, antioxidants, laser photocoagulation, macular translocation, and local radiation. With almost all studies, the outcome has been disappointing. However, preliminary results from the radiation therapy programs have shown subjective visual improvement as well as documented objective improvement.

This volume deals with the various issues in age-related macular degeneration, not only in its evolution and development, but also discusses the various treatment programs and complications thereof. The contributions from this volume represent an important baseline against which future studies can be measured.

Philadelphia
Hamburg
Munich

L. W. Brady
H.-P. Heilmann
M. Molls

Preface

Among the five senses, loss of vision would be most devastating. Age-related macular degeneration (ARMD) is the most common cause of severe visual loss and of legal blindness for those older than 64 years, and the second most common cause for those aged 45–64, in Western societies. Increasing longevity is lending growing urgency to the search for a way to prevent, or at least treat, macular degeneration. Interventions have included laser therapy, hyperthermia, photodynamic therapy, submacular surgery, external beam and plaque radiotherapy, corticosteroid and interferon intravitreal injection, antioxidant vitamins, trace minerals, and antiangiogenic agents such as thalidomide, isoretinoin and interferon-α and -β.

The Macular Photocoagulation Study Group in the United States, and other groups in Europe, have studied macular degeneration for years. Despite all efforts, the only accepted therapy for neovascular ARMD is laser treatment. However, only about 15–20% of patients meet the criteria for laser therapy, and when the lesion is subfoveal there is an immediate decrease in vision.

For almost a decade low doses of irradiation have been employed in an attempt at reducing the damage secondary to the neovascularization and preserving useful vision. Despite the publication of numerous institutional studies, and a few small, randomized, prospective studies (from Heidelberg, Nijmegen, Zurich, St. Gallen and San Francisco), controversy reigns and radiotherapy has not been established as beneficial. Only the results of larger, well-controlled studies now in progress can settle this debate.

The lively discussions at an international conference held in Hamburg in February 1999 prompted the editors to gather up-to-date reports reflecting current views and techniques from experts around the world to serve as a concise, handy reference of research in progress and of the state of the art in management of macular degeneration.

Hamburg	W. E. Alberti
Hamburg	G. Richard
Syracuse	R. H. Sagerman

Contents

Diagnosis and Clinical Features

1 Age-Related Macular Degeneration: Current Concepts of Pathogenesis and Risk Factors

FLORIAN SCHÜTT and FRANK G. HOLZ

CONTENTS

1.1 Introduction

Age-related macular degeneration (ARMD) is now the most common cause of registrable blindness in Western nations for persons above 50 years of age (KAHN et al. 1973; WORMALD 1995; BIRD 1996; HOLZ, PAULEIKHOFF 1997). While early manifestations with funduscopically visible focal drusen are usually associated with only minor visual complaints, late stages of the disease with choroidal neovascularization and/or geographic atrophy result in severe visual loss. The pathogenesis of age-related macular disease is incompletely understood. Several lines of evidence indicate that ARMD represents a complex disease with various genetic and environmental factors. Age is by far the strongest risk factor. On the cellular and molecular levels, various changes due to aging have been identified in the outer retina. It is thought that changes in the retinal pigment epithelium and Bruch's membrane play a key role in the pathogenetic cascade. However, phenotypically similar manifestations in the macular area with late onset lumped under the heading ARMD may turn out to represent heterogeneous disorders on a molecular level.

F. SCHÜTT, MD; F.G. HOLZ, MD
Department of Ophthalmology, University of Heidelberg, Im Neuenheimer Feld 400, 69120 Heidelberg, Germany

1.2 The Retina–Pigment Epithelium Complex

The retinal pigment epithelium (RPE) represents a cellular monolayer between the retina and the vascular choroid (SCHRAERMEYER, HEIMANN 1999). It has various functions which are essential for normal vision. These include maintenance of the blood–retinal barrier, participation in the vitamin A cycle, permanent phagocytosis of shed outer segments, synthesis of extracellular matrix, and active transport of molecules to and from the interphotoreceptor matrix. Primary RPE dysfunction is associated with a variety of retinal diseases, including Best's macular dystrophy (mutations in the VMD-2 gene) and Leber's congenital amaurosis (RPE65 mutations) (MORIMURA et al. 1998), as well as retinal degeneration in an RCS rat model (D'CRUZ et al. 2000).

Apical (adjacent to photoreceptors) and basal (facing the Bruch's membrane) portions of each RPE cell can be distinguished (Fig. 1.1). The apical side has long microvilli which reach up between the outer segments, partially enveloping them (SPITZNAS, HOGAN 1970; ZINN, MARMOR 1979; BOK 1993). Phagocytosis of shed outer segment discs, enzymatic degradation within the lysosomal system and following release of resulting metabolic waste at the basal cell side, and transport via choriocapillaris into the bloodstream continue throughout life. Lysosomes are specialized organelles responsible for intracellular degradation of metabolic debris. They contain hydrolytic enzymes used for almost complete degradation of biomolecules. For optimal activity they require an acidic environment, and the lysosome provides this by maintaining a pH of about 5 in its interior.

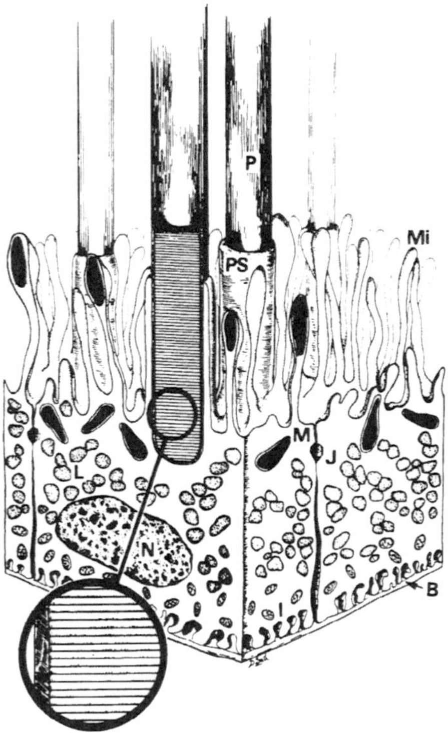

Fig. 1.1. Retinal pigment epithelial cell. *Mi* Microvilli, *M* melanosomes, *L* lipofuscin granules, *PS* adjacent photoreceptor outer segments, *B* Bruch's membrane

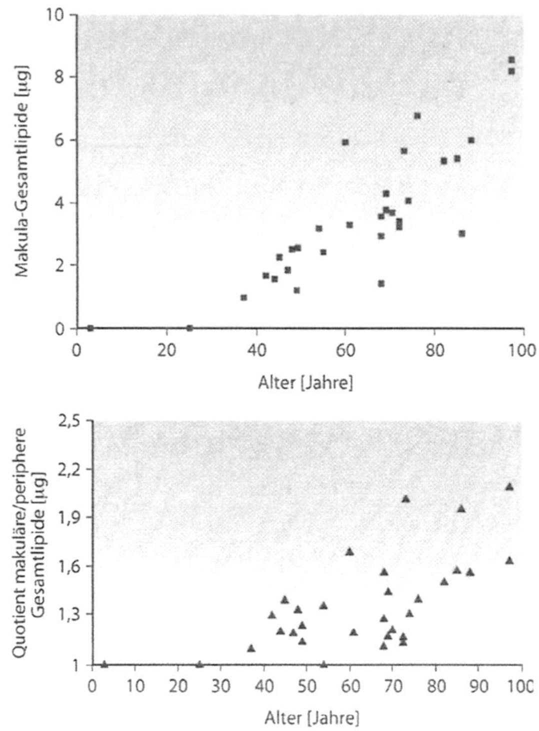

Fig. 1.2. Correlation between total lipid content of Bruch's membrane and age of donor eye (Holz et al. 1994)

Extracellular metabolic products are transported to the lysosome by multiple pathways. Endocytosed macromolecules form intracellular vesicles (endosomes) which convert into lysosomes. Larger particles including shed outer segment discs from the extracellular space can be transported to lysosomes by phagocytosis. In this process, stacks of shed discs are engulfed in the outer retina to form a phagosome which is then converted into a lysosome. A balance between photoreceptor disc shedding, phagocytosis, lysosomal degradation, and secretion into the choriocapillaris via Bruch's membrane is important to normal photoreceptor function. Any disturbance in this process may lead to an accumulation of incompletely degraded material into Bruch's membrane, i.e., focal and diffuse drusen, which are a hallmark of early ARMD (Fig. 1.2).

1.3 Aging Changes Relevant to the Pathogenesis of ARMD

1.3.1 Retinal Pigment Epithelium

Various changes occur in the RPE with age, some of which are thought to be of importance in the pathogenesis of ARMD. A continuous decrease in the melanin content of RPE cells occurs with age. Up to 8% of the cytoplasm of young RPE cells is comprised of melanin granules (Feeney 1978; Weiter et al. 1986). Melanin protects light-sensitive structures within the posterior pole and absorbs free radicals. Therefore, a decrease in melanin may impair protection against damaging short wavelength light and toxic free radicals.

In contrast to melanin, lipofuscin granules accumulate with age in the lysosomal compartments of RPE cells (Fig. 1.3). Lipofuscin accumulation is mainly a by-product of the constant phagocytosis of shed photoreceptor outer segment discs (Feeney-Burns, Eldred 1983; Kennedy et al. 1995; Katz

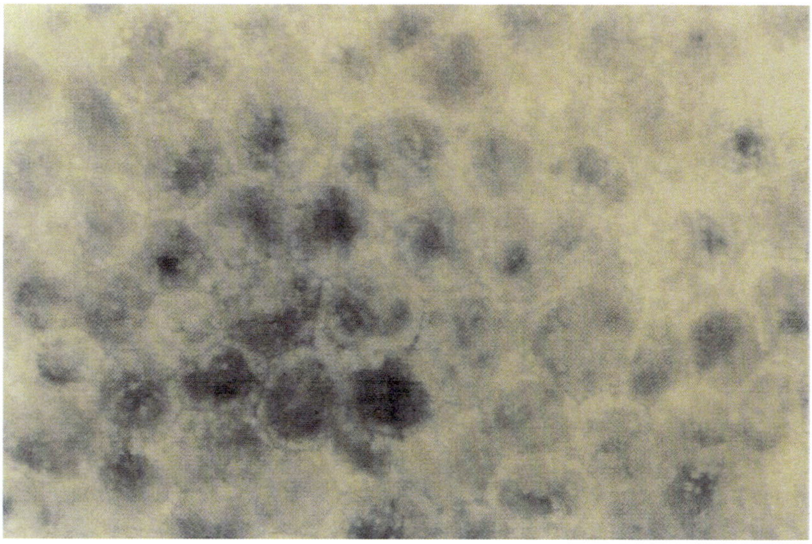

Fig. 1.3. Yellowish lipofuscin granules in human RPE cells

et al. 1996). Detection of lipofuscin is facilitated by its autofluorescent properties. When stimulated with 366 nm light, lipofuscin granules emit a characteristic golden yellow fluorescence; at least ten different fluorophores contribute to this autofluorescent phenomenon (KATZ et al. 1987). The mechanisms of lipofuscinogenesis are not completely understood. Lipid oxidation has been thought to play a role (ELDRED, KATZ 1991). The pigments may arise as a consequence of antioxidant deficiency or under pro-oxidant conditions (HANDELMAN, DRATZ 1986; ANDERSON et al. 1994). Electron microscopic studies have shown a stepwise conversion of lysosomal structures to lipofuscin granula (SAMORAJSKI et al. 1964). Experiments in RCS rats, the RPE of which, due to a genetic defect, cannot phagocytose photoreceptor outer segment (POS) discs, showed a significant reduction in lipofuscin (KATZ et al. 1987). Likewise, a reduction in lipofuscin can be achieved experimentally by destroying the neurosensory retina, indicating that the phagocytosis of POS discs is the main origin of lipofuscin.

Once formed, RPE cells apparently have no means of degrading lipofuscin material and granules or transporting them into the extracellular space via exocytosis. Consequently, these granules are trapped in the cytoplasm (BRIZZEE, ORDY 1981; BOULTON, MARSHALL 1986).

Controversial views have evolved on whether or not lipofuscin accumulation is detrimental to normal RPE cell function. It has been postulated that excessive levels of lipofuscin contribute to the pathogenesis of age-related macular degeneration (DOREY et al. 1989; DELORI et al. 1995; HOLZ et al. 1999a). Several findings support the concept of a pathophysiologic role: genetically determined macular degeneration, including Stargardt's disease and Best's macular dystrophy, is associated with faster accumulation of lipofuscin in the RPE (WEINGEIST et al. 1982). In Stargardt's disease, the RPE contains up to seven times more lipofuscin than normal and this is associated with retinal degeneration. Interestingly, both diseases manifest primarily in the macular region of the retina. Histopathological investigations have demonstrated an association of abnormal accumulation of lipofuscin with degeneration of RPE cells and adjacent photoreceptors in an inherited retinal dystrophy of dogs (AGUIRRE, LATIES 1976). In humans, photoreceptor density was found to correlate with the lipofuscin concentration of the apposing RPE cells (WING et al. 1978). In vivo investigations using scanning laser ophthalmoscopy have demonstrated excessive lipofuscin accumulation in association with various manifestations of age-related macular degeneration (RÜCKMANN et al 1997; HOLZ et al. 1999a). Direct evidence that an individual component of lipofuscin interferes with metabolic functions of RPE cells was not demonstrated until recently (HOLZ et al. 1999b). The major fluorescent compound of lipofuscin, A2-E, initially identified by ELDRED and LASKY (1993), is a strong inhibitor of lysosomal protein and glycosaminoglycan degradation (Fig. 1.4). The mechanism of action is most likely an increase in intralysosomal pH,

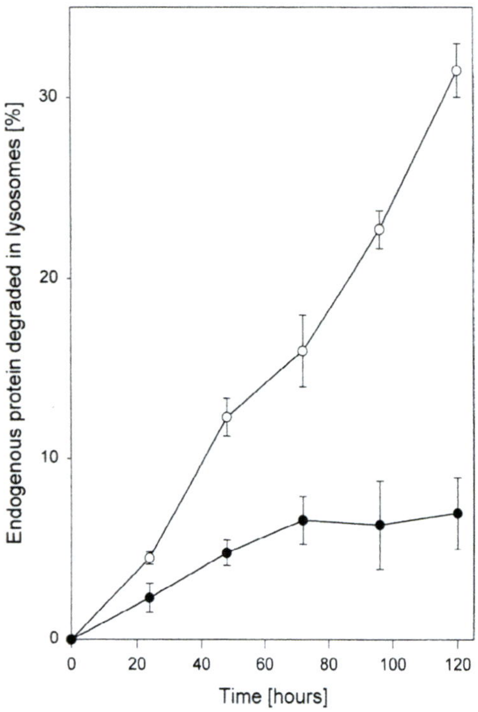

Fig. 1.4. Lysosomal degradation of endogenous protein in cultured human RPE cells is significantly inhibited by A2-E, a major lipofuscin fluorophore. • A2-E-treated cells, o controls (Holz, Schütt et al. 1992)

disturbing the normal acidic intralysosomal milieu required for proper enzyme function (Fig. 1.5). In addition, the lipofuscin component A2-E has been shown to possess phototoxic (Schütt et al. 2000) and detergent properties, the latter causing rupture of the lysosomal membranes when reaching a critical concentration (Bellmann et al. 2000).

1.3.2 Bruch's Membrane and the Choriocapillaris

Various age-dependent histological, ultrastructural, and biochemical changes have been identified in Bruch's membrane. This is an acellular membrane beneath the retinal pigment epithelium composed of five different layers (Killingsworth 1987; Pauleikhoff et al. 1990; Ramrattan 1994). Nutrients and oxygen diffuse from the choriocapillaris through Bruch's membrane to the RPE and retina, whereas metabolic waste is voided in the opposite direction into the choroid. This exchange of metabolites emphasizes the porous structure of this membrane. Age-dependent changes include thickening, calcification, degeneration of collagen and elastic fibers, and splitting. Accumulation of various metabolic products includes lipid-rich material which may impair normal fluid and molecule transport between the biochemically highly active retina, pigment epithelium, and choroid (Fig. 1.2). Electron microscopic studies show granular, vesicular, and amorphous material accumulating in Bruch's membrane with age. The particular biochemical composition points to the RPE as the source of this material (Holz et al. 1994). Age-dependent changes in the choriocapillaris layer of Bruch's membrane may further contribute to an incomplete clearance of material with age (Young 1987). The intercapillary spaces have been shown to become wider, while the number and diameter of capillaries decreases with age. The total thickness of the elderly choroid is reduced, and phlebosclerosis occurs.

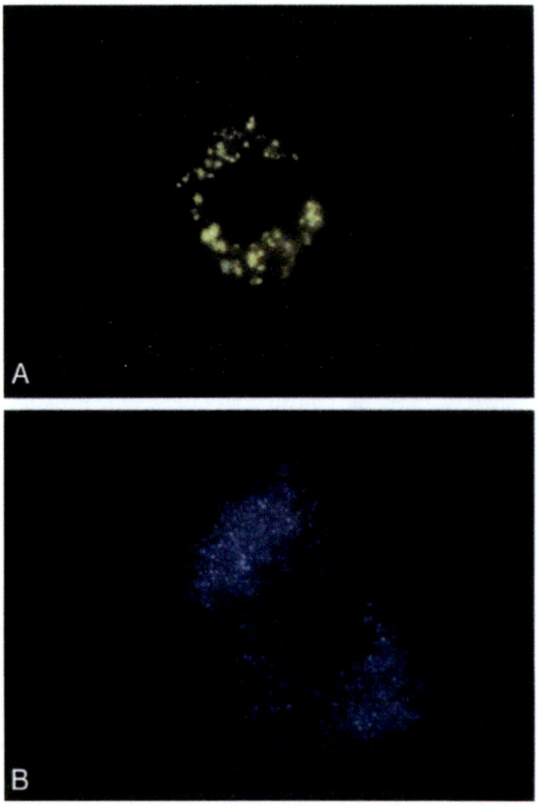

Fig. 1.5. Measurement of intralysosomal pH using a lysosensor, *yellow* indicating acidic pH in the absence and *blue* indicating roughly neutral pH in the presence of the lipofuscin fluorophore A2-E (×1000). Elevation of intralysosomal pH is a mechanism by which A2-E inhibits lysosomal enzymes (Holz et al. 1999)

1.4 Early Manifestations of Disease: Drusen

Funduscopically visible focal drusen in the macular area are the hallmark of early age-related macular disease. Drusen are deposits of extracellular material beneath the RPE in inner aspects of Bruch's membrane (Sarks et al. 1994). The overlying RPE detaches locally and becomes thinned and hypopigmented. During ophthalmoscopic examination, drusen are visible as gray or yellow punctate nodules (hard drusen) or large, pale placoid structures (soft drusen) (Fig. 1.6). Size, shape, distribution, and color vary during the natural course. While the majority of patients show an increase in the number of drusen, partial regression is sometimes observed. Patients with drusen usually have excellent visual acuity. However, they may complain about prolonged dark adaptation or problems when reading in dim light. With advanced confluence of central soft drusen and drusenoid RPE detachments, mild metamorphopsia may occur. Until now, the exact biogenesis of drusen is unknown. Whereas in young individuals the phagocytic degradation of photoreceptor discs results in almost complete catabolism with breakdown products that can be either recirculated to the photoreceptor cells or voided at the basal surface of the RPE and cleared by the choroid, incomplete degradation occurs in the elderly due to impaired degradative capacity of the lysosomes. In addition, structural changes of the macromolecules to be degraded occur, e.g., photochemical damage of lipid-rich outer segment discs (Rozanowska et al. 1995; Gaillard et al. 1995). Therefore, the lysosomal compartment is thought to play an essential role in the biogenesis of drusen material, which is a prerequisite for the development of lesions associated with advanced AMD.

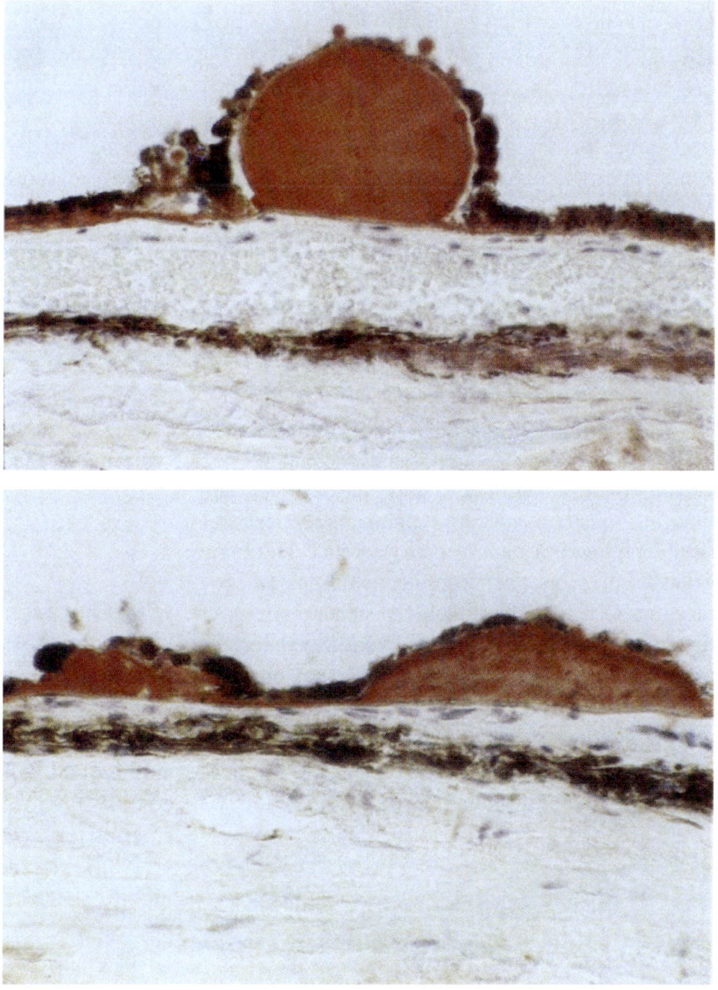

A

B

Fig. 1.6. Light micrograph of a single hard druse (*A*) and two soft drusen (*B*) located at the posterior pole. (Oil red O×400) (Pauleikhoff et al. 1990)

1.5 Late Manifestations of Disease

1.5.1 Choroidal Neovascularization and Retinal Pigment Epithelial Detachment

The growth of new vessels from the choriocapillaris through Bruch's membrane, resulting in degeneration of the overlying neurosensory retina, i.e., choroidal neovascularization (CNV), is the most common cause of severe visual loss in late stages of ARMD (YOUNG 1987; BRESSLER et al. 1988). The growth of new vessels has been attributed to reactive stereotypic processes secondary to abnormal focal and diffuse deposits (drusen) in Bruch's membrane. Contributing factors may involve relative hypoxia, age-dependent breaks in Bruch's membrane, and inflammatory processes. Besides vascular elements, cellular components of the neovascular tissue include macrophages, lymphocytes, and fibroblasts (PENFOLD et al. 1985). Several signaling molecules including VEGF have been identified as involved in the formation of CNV (ADAMIS et al. 1993). The precise cascade of events is, however, incompletely understood. The fine balance of angiogenetic and antiangiogenetic factors appears to be disturbed by the aging changes described above. These factors may originate from various cells including endothelial cells of the choriocapillaris, inflammatory cells, RPE cells, and neuronal or glial cells. Typically, once a feeding vessel has grown through Bruch's membrane, the neovascular net spreads horizontally beneath or above the RPE. Enlargement is usually associated with leakage and bleeding into the extracellular space. The formation of new vessels may or may not be associated with detachment of the RPE. The latter has a typical funduscopic appearance, with a dome-shaped elevation of the RPE and the neurosensory retina. The repair of neovascular lesions by connective tissue and proliferating RPE is followed by the occurrence of a fibrotic, poorly vascularized scar, with degeneration of the overlying neurosensory retina as the end stage of the disease process. These scars are typically confined to the posterior pole. Remaining visual function depends on the size of the scar and the subsequent eccentricity of the new retinal fixation locus.

1.5.2 Geographic Atrophy

Geographic atrophy is a less common cause of severe visual loss in late-stage ARMD (SUNNESS et al. 1997, 1999). Funduscopically, atrophy of the outer retina appears as a well-demarcated area with less pigmentation and fewer visible large choroidal vessels. Histologically, the area of geographic atrophy is not confined to the RPE but also includes outer layers of the neurosensory retina (retinal photoreceptors) and the choriocapillaris. In contrast to CNV, geographic atrophy more frequently occurs initially outside the fovea. Typically, several foci of atrophy enlarge over time and cause a paracentral scotoma which, despite good central vision, may impair reading. Finally the fovea is also involved, due to further spread of the atrophy. The pathogenesis of the atrophy is poorly understood. It is thought that cell death occurs initially at the level of the RPE cells as a result of diffuse and focal deposits in Bruch's membrane. Since choriocapillaris vessels and retinal photoreceptors are both dependent on the presence of vital RPE, cell death subsequently occurs at these levels as well.

In vivo investigations using scanning laser ophthalmoscopy have recently demonstrated excessive lipofuscin accumulation in RPE cells in the junctional zone of areas with geographic atrophy (RÜCKMANN et al. 1997). Development of new atrophic patches and enlargement of existing atrophy has been observed to occur solely in areas with increased lipofuscin-associated fundus autofluorescence in longitudinal studies (HOLZ et al. 1999a) (Fig. 1.7). These in vivo observations suggest that abnormal lipofuscin accumulation in the RPE may be of pathophysiological relevance in the pathogenesis of geographic atrophy.

1.6 Risk Factors

Age is the most important risk factor for ARMD. Several studies indicate a genetic factor in the pathogenesis of the disease. These include twin studies, sibling studies, and comparison of various races (MEYERS et al. 1988; PIGUET et al. 1993; SILVESTRI et al. 1994; KLEIN et al. 1994; SEDDON et al. 1997; KLAVER et al. 1998). The identification of disease-causing gene mutations is particularly difficult in ARMD because of the late onset of the disease and because parents of affected patients are usually not available for clinical examination and molecular biological investigation.

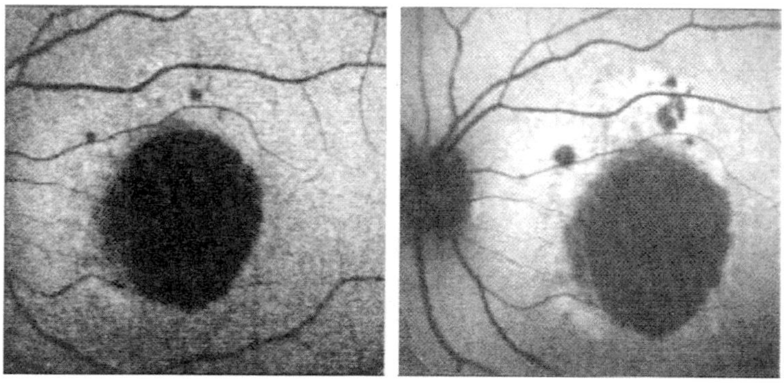

Fig. 1.7. Fundus autofluorescence image in a patient with geographic atrophy secondary to ARMD. Over 3 years, there was enlargement of atrophic areas and occurrence of new atrophic patches confined to areas with increased fundus autofluorescence at baseline

In addition, a monogenetic cause appears unlikely. Rather, there are several genes involved in addition to modulating environmental factors. To date, mutations of only one gene, the ABCR gene (from the ATP-binding cassette family), have been identified as conferring an increased risk for the development of ARMD. However, this appears to apply in only 3% of all ARMD patients (ALLIKMETS et al. 1997). Several large-scale efforts are currently underway to elucidate further the possible genetic causes.

Controversies exist in various epidemiologic studies with regard to other risk factors (reviewed by KLEIN 1999). Some investigations suggest a possible but weak influence of arterial hypertension, light exposure, and light iris color. There is concordance in these studies with regard to smoking as an important risk factor; the underlying mechanism, however, is unclear. It has been speculated that generation of free radicals with oxidative stress and subsequent oxidation of unsaturated fatty acids of phospholipids may play a role.

References

Adamis AP, Shima DT, Yeo KT, Yeo TK, Brown LF, Berse B, D'Amore PA, Folkman J (1993) Synthesis and secretion of vascular permeability factor/vascular endothelial growth factor by human retinal pigment epithelial cells. Biochem Biophys Res Commun 15;193(2):631-638

Aguirre GD, Laties A (1976) Pigment epithelial dystrophy in the dog. Exp Eye Res 23:247-256

Allikmets R, Shroyer NF, Singh N, Seddon JM, Lewis RA, Bernstein PS, Pfeiffer A, Zabriskie NA, Li Y, Hutchinson A, Dean M, Lupski JR, Leppert M (1997) Mutation of the Stargardt's disease gene (ABCR) in age-related macular degeneration. Science 277:1805-1807

Anderson RE, Kretzer FL, Rapp LM (1994) Free radicals and ocular disease. Adv Exp Med Biol 366:73-86

Bellmann C, Bergmann M, Schütt F, Kopitz J, Holz FG (2000) Isolation of intact lysosomes from human RPE cells and effect of A2-E on the integrity of the lysosomal membrane. Invest Ophthalmol Vis Sci 41:S145

Bird AC (1996) Age-related macular disease. Br J Ophthalmol 80:1-2

Bok D (1993) The retinal pigment epithelium: A versatile partner in vision. J Cell Suppl 17:189-95

Boulton M, Marshall J (1986) Effects of increasing numbers of phagocytic inclusions on human retinal pigment epithelial cells in culture: A model for aging. Br J Ophthalmol 70:808-815

Bressler NM, Frost LA, Bressler SB, Murphy RP, Fine SL (1988) Natural course of poorly defined choroidal neovascularization associated with macular degeneration. Arch Ophthalmol 106:1537-42

Brizzee KR, Ordy JM (1981) Cellular features, regional accumulation, and prospects of modification of age pigments in mammals. In: Sohal RS (ed) Age pigments. Elsevier, Amsterdam, pp 101-154

D'Cruz PM, Yasumura D, Weir J, Matthes MT, Abderrahim H, LaVail MM, Vollrath D (2000) Mutation of the receptor tyrosine kinase gene Mertk in the retinal dystrophic RCS rat. Hum Mol Genet 1;9:645-651

Delori FC, Dorey CK, Staurenghi G, Arend O, Goger DG, Weiter JJ (1995) In vivo fluorescence of the ocular fundus exhibits RPE lipofuscin characteristics. Invest Ophthalmol Vis Sci 36:718-729

Dorey CK, Wu G, Ebenstein D, Garsd A, Weiter JJ. (1989) Cell loss in the aging retina: Relationship to lipofuscin accumulation and macular degeneration. Invest Ophthalmol Vis Sci 30:1691-1699

Eldred GE, Katz ML (1991) The lipid peroxidation theory of lipofuscinogenesis cannot yet be confirmed. Free Radic Biol Med 10:445-447

Eldred GE, Lasky MR (1993) Retinal age pigments generated by self-assembling lysosomotropic detergents. Nature 361(6414):724-726

Feeney L (1978) Lipofuscin and melanin of human retinal pigment epithelium. Invest Ophthalmol Vis Sci 17:583-600

Feeney-Burns L, Eldred GE (1983) The fate of the phagosome: Conversion to 'age pigment'and impact in human retinal pigment epithelium. Trans Ophthalmol Soc UK 103:416-421

Gaillard ER, Atherton SJ, Eldred G, Dillon J (1995) Photophysical studies on human retinal lipofuscin. Photochem Photobiol 61:448-453

Handelman GJ, Dratz EA (1986) The role of antioxidants in the retina and retinal pigment epithelium and the nature

of prooxidant induced damage. Adv Free Rad Biol Med 2:1–89
Holz FG, Pauleikhoff D (1997) Altersabhängige Makuladegeneration. Springer, Berlin
Holz FG, Sheraidah G, Pauleikhoff D, Bird AC (1994) Analysis of lipid deposits extracted from human macular and peripheral Bruch's membrane. Archives of Ophthalmology 112:402-406
Holz FG, Bellmann C, Margaritidis M, Schütt F, Otto TP, Völcker HE (1999a) Patterns of increased in vivo fundus autofluorescence in the junctional zone of geographic atrophy of the retinal pigment epithelium associated with age-related macular degeneration. Graefe Arch Exp Clin Ophthalmol 237:145–152
Holz FG, Schuett F, Kopitz J, Eldred GE, Kruse FE, Völcker HE, Cantz M (1999b) Inhibition of lysosomal degradative functions in RPE cells by a retinoid component of lipofuscin. Invest Ophthalmol Vis Sci 40:737–743
Kahn HA, Moorhead HB (1973) Statistics on blindness in the model reporting areas 1969–1970. United States Department of Health, Education and Welfare (NIH). U.S. Government Printing Office, Washington, D.C., pp 73–427
Katz ML, Eldred DE, Robison WG (1987) Lipofuscin autofluorescence: Evidence for vitamin A involvement in the retina. Mech Ageing Dev 39:81–90
Katz ML, Gao CL, Rice LM (1996) Formation of lipofuscin-like fluorophores by reaction of retinal with photoreceptor outer segments and liposomes. Mech Ageing Dev 92:159–174
Kennedy CJ, Rakoczy PE, Constable IJ (1995) Lipofuscin of the retinal pigment epithelium: A review. Eye 9:763–771
Killingsworth MC (1987) Age-related components of Bruch's membrane in the human eye. Graefes Arch Clin Exp Ophthalmol 225:406–412
Klaver CCW, Wolfs RCW, Assink JJM et al (1998) Genetic risk of age-related maculopathy. Arch Ophthalmol 116:1646–1651
Klein ML, Mauldin WM, Stoumbos VD (1994) Heredity and age-related macular degeneration. Arch Ophthalmol 112:932–937
Klein R (1999) Epidemiology. In: Berger JW, Fine SL, Maguire M (eds) Age-related macular degeneration. Mosby, St Louis, pp 31–56
Meyers SM, Zachary AA (1988) Monozygotic twins with age-related macular degeneration. Arch Ophthalmol 106:651–653
Morimura H, Fishman GA, Grover SA, Fulton AB, Berson EL, Dryja TP (1998) Mutations in the RPE65 gene in patients with autosomal recessive retinitis pigmentosa or Leber congenital amaurosis. Proc Natl Acad Sci U S A 17;95:3088–3093
Pauleikhoff D, Harper CA, Marshall J, Bird AC (1990) Aging changes in Bruch's membrane. A histochemical and morphologic study. Ophthalmology 97:171–178
Penfold PL, Killingworth M, Sarks S (1985) Senile macular degeneration: The involvement of immunocompetent cells. Graefes Arch Clin Ophthalmol 223:69
Piguet B, Wells JA, Palmwang IB et al (1993) Age-related Bruch's membrane change: A clinical study of the relative role of heredity and environment. Br J Ophthalmol 77:400–403
Ramrattan RS (1994) Morphometric analysis of Bruch's membrane, the choriocapillaris, and the choroid in aging. Invest Ophthalmol Vis Sci 35:2857–2864
Rozanowska M, Jarvis-Evans J, Korytowski W, Boulton M, Burke JM, Sarna T (1995) Blue light induced reactivity of retinal age pigment: In vitro generation of oxygen reactive species. J Biol Chem 270:18825–18830
Rückmann Av, Fitzke FW, Bird AC (1997) Fundus autofluorescence in age-related macular disease imaged with a laser scanning ophthalmoscope. Invest Ophthalmol Vis Sci 38:478–486
Samorajski T, Keefe J, Ordy JM (1964) Intracellular localization of lipofuscin age pigment in the nervous system. J Gerontol 19:262–276
Sarks JP, Sarks SH, Killingsworth MC (1994) Evolution of soft drusen in age-related macular degeneration. Eye 8:269–283
Schraermeyer U, Heimann K (1999) Current understanding on the role of retinal pigment epithelium and its pigmentation. Pigment Cell Res 12:219–236
Schütt F, Davies S, Kopitz J, Holz FG, Boulton M (2000) A2-E, a retinoid of lipofuscin, is photo-damaging to human RPE cells. Invest ophthalmol Vis Sci (in press)
Seddon JM, Ajani UA, Mitchell BD (1997) Familial aggregation of age-related macular maculopathy. Am J Ophthalmol 123:199–196
Silvestri G, Johnston PB, Hughes AE (1994) Is genetic predisposition an important risk factor in age-related macular degeneration? Eye 8:564–568
Spitznas M, Hogan MJ (1970) Outer segments of photoreceptors and the retinal pigment epithelium. Interrelationship in the human eye. Arch Ophthalmol 84:810–819
Sunness JS, Rubin GS, Applegate CA et al (1997) Visual function abnormalities and prognosis in eyes with age-related geographic atrophy of the macula and good visual acuity. Ophthalmology;104:1677–1691
Sunness JS, Gonzales-Baron J, Applegate CA et al (1999) Enlargement of atrophy and visual acuity loss in the geographic atrophy form of age-related macular degeneration. Ophthalmology 106:1768–1779
Weingeist TA, Kobrin JL, Watz KE (1982) Histopathology of Best's macular dystrophy. Arch Ophthalmol 100:1108–1114
Weiter JJ, Delori FC, Wing GL, Fitch KA (1986) Retinal pigment epithelial lipofuscin and melanin and choroidal melanin in human eyes. Invest Ophthalmol Vis Sci 27:145–152
Wing GL, Gordon CB, Weiter JJ (1978) The topography and age relationship of lipofuscin concentration in the retinal pigment epithelium. Invest Ophthalmol Vis Sci 17:601
Wormald R (1995) Assessing the prevalence of eye disease in the community. Eye 9:674–6
Young RW (1987) Pathophysiology of age-related macular degeneration. Surv Ophthalmol 31:291–306
Zinn K, Marmor MF (1979) The retinal pigment epithelium. Harvard University Press, Cambridge, Mass

2 Clinical Manifestations and Natural History of Age-Related Macular Degeneration

JAN ZURDEL and GISBERT RICHARD

CONTENTS

2.1 Introduction

This chapter presents an overview of the relevant findings in patients with different stages of age-related macular degeneration (ARMD) from a clinician's point of view, and the natural course of the disease and its dependencies. It follows the guidelines of the classification and grading system of the International ARM Epidemiological Study Group (1995).

2.2 Classification System

The classification and grading system used here is based on morphological abnormalities in the macular area assessed on color fundus transparencies. The entity "ARMD" is subdivided into different stages and forms which share common clinical hallmarks. In this system, visual acuity is not used to define the presence of any form of ARMD. Other definitions and grading systems have used different approaches to define and grade ARMD, but since the system proposed by the International ARM Epidemiological Study Group is widely accepted, this discussion is entirely based on it.

Early ARMD is characterized by the presence of drusen and pigmentary abnormalities. Drusen are yellow-white deposits of various size, configuration, and shape beneath the retinal pigment epithelium (RPE) (Fig. 2.1). Therefore, numerous types of drusen can be distinguished: hard, soft, distinct, indistinct, etc. Some forms are known to be associated with greater risk of progression of ARMD, which will be addressed in detail later.

Pigmentary abnormalities are defined as small areas (<175 μm wide) of focal hypopigmentation and hyperpigmentation. Sometimes they may be seen overlying drusen, which can possibly be explained by their interaction: drusen accumulation leads to hyperplasia of the RPE but later causes its atrophy.

Late ARMD consists of geographic atrophy and exudative ARMD. Geographic atrophy of the retinal pigment epithelium creates a large, well-demarcated area (>175 μm in width) of RPE loss and hypopigmented RPE, which may be the result of regressing soft drusen or follow serous detachment of the RPE (Fig. 2.2).

Exudative ARMD consists of choroidal neovascularization (CNV), pigment epithelial detachment, and disciform scarring. CNV is characterized by the ingrowth of new vessels originating from the choroid through breaks in Bruch's membrane and can further be subdivided into classic and occult CNV, depending on its appearance on fluorescein angiography. Whereas classic CNV displays an area of well-defined hyperfluorescence and dye leakage in the early phase (Fig. 2.3), occult CNV will show blurred, stippled hyperfluorescence with leakage in late phases of fluorescein angiography.

J. ZURDEL, MD
G. RICHARD, MD, Professor
Augenklinik und Poliklinik, University Hospital Eppendorf, Martinistrasse 52, 20246 Hamburg, Germany

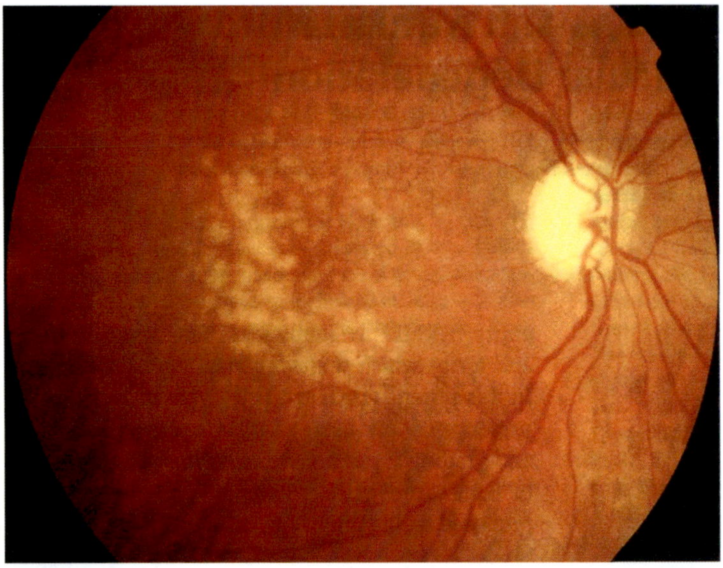

Fig. 2.1. Early ARMD on color fundus photograph: confluent serous drusen

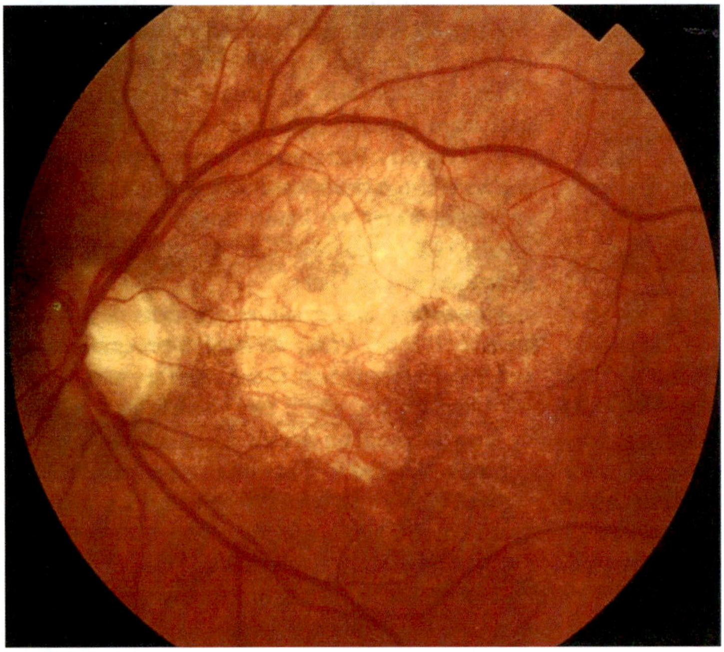

Fig. 2.2. Geographic atrophy of the retinal pigment epithelium: sharply demarcated area of RPE atrophy with large choroidal vessels visible

Serous detachment of the retinal pigment epithelium is a sharply demarcated area of elevated RPE and may be accompanied by detachment of the neurosensory retina. It may occur in association with CNV or independently of it.

A disciform scar is the fibrous end stage of any form of CNV and displays a variety of features, e.g., fibrous tissue replacing the retina and RPE, detachment of the sensory retina, subretinal blood, and lipid exudates (Fig. 2.4).

2.3 Early Age-Related Macular Degeneration

2.3.1 Morphological Changes

Clinical hallmarks of early ARMD include drusen formation and pigmentary abnormalities in the macula. Drusen vary considerably in appearance and are located between the basement membrane of the RPE

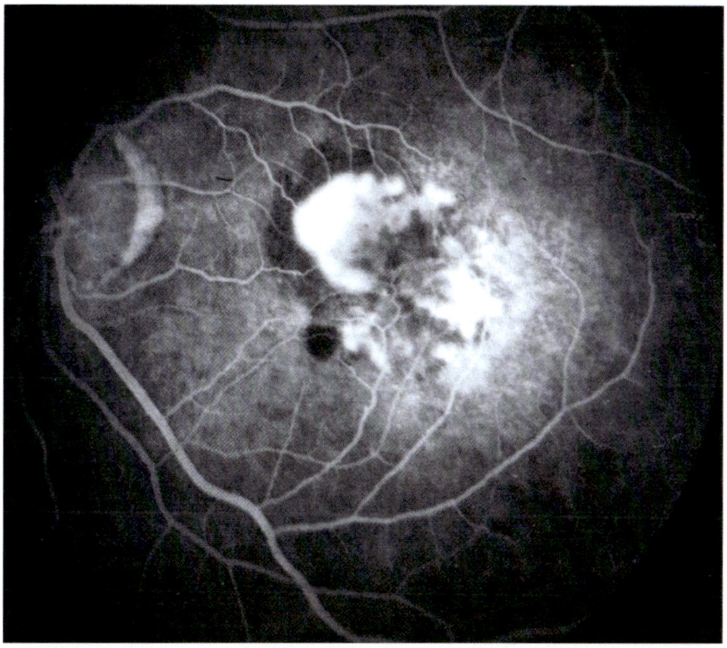

Fig. 2.3. CNV on fluorescein angiography: well-demarcated borders of hyperfluorescence indicative of classic CNV

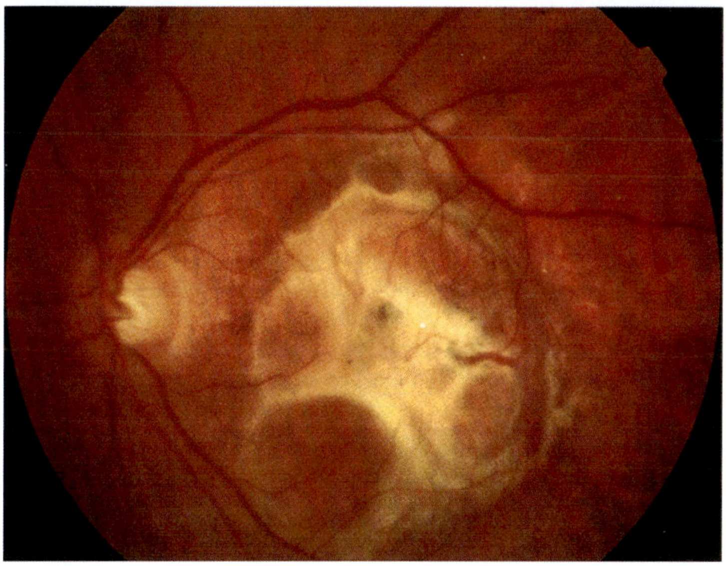

Fig. 2.4. Disciform scar extending over the entire macula

and Bruch's membrane. They are visible on color fundus photographs and on fluorescein angiography. Several subgroups of drusen can be distinguished, depending on size, shape, confluence, and distinctness of borders. Soft drusen (>63 μm) are considered to be a sign of early ARMD, whereas hard drusen alone are not considered as lesions of early ARMD since they can be found in nearly 100% of the elderly population and do not bear an excess risk of progression to the advanced forms of ARMD (Klein et al. 1997).

Pigmentary abnormalities include focal areas of hyperpigmentation and hypopigmentation, both of which are signs of early ARMD and associated with increased risk of progression to late ARMD. Pigmentary alterations are usually to be found in the vicinity of drusen, and prevalence increases with the size of the largest drusen and with age (Bressler et al. 1990).

The incidence of early ARMD was 5.7% overall in the Beaver Dam Eye Study and increased significantly with age.

2.3.2 Functional Changes

Visual acuity in patients is usually good or mildly reduced, e.g., between 20/20 and 20/32. More severe reduction is uncommon and should arouse suspicion of other lesions, namely when patients complain about deterioration of visual acuity or additional symptoms, e.g., metamorphopsia. In these cases, late forms of ARMD or other diseases must be excluded.

Over time, visual loss progresses slowly. Other deficits include reduced contrast sensitivity (KLEINER et al. 1988), impaired dark adaptation and abnormal scotopic sensitivity (STEINMETZ et al. 1993). The extent of functional change is related to the severity of early ARMD. Contradictory reports exist about color vision abnormalities in these patients. Whereas MIDENA et al. (1997) reported no deficits in color vision, EISNER et al. (1987, 1991) found worse scores on the D-15 test and in red/green Rayleigh color matching. Together, these data illustrate that patients with signs of early ARMD have only mild functional impairment.

2.3.3 Progression of Early ARMD

The risk of progression from early to late ARMD has been the subject of a number of investigations. In the population-based Beaver Dam Eye Study, KLEIN et al. (1997) reported an annual risk of less than 0.01% of developing late ARMD if no signs of ARMD or only hard drusen were present at baseline. Among people initially having bilateral early ARMD, 11.7% developed late ARMD over a 5-year period; 7.1% were diagnosed with exudative ARMD and 4.6% with geographic atrophy. Thus, patients with bilateral early ARMD have approximately 100 times the risk of contracting some form of late ARMD compared to patients with hard drusen only or no signs of early ARMD at all. In a study by HOLZ et al. (1994), the annual risk was estimated to be 3%.

Patients with unilateral choroidal neovascularization are at much higher risk of developing exudative ARMD in the fellow eye with early ARMD than patients with bilateral early ARMD. Risk factors known to be associated with the development of CNV in the fellow eye are larger drusen (>63 μm), focal hyperpigmentation, the presence of five or more drusen, and systemic hypertension. Risk depends strongly on the number of risk factors present. Within 5 years, only 7% of patients with none of these risk factors developed CNV, compared to 87% of patients with all four risk factors present (MACULAR PHOTOCOAGULATION STUDY GROUP 1997).

2.4 Geographic Atrophy of the Retinal Pigment Epithelium

Geographic atrophy (GA) of the retinal pigment epithelium is characterized by sharply demarcated areas of RPE loss and subsequent atrophy of the choriocapillaris which is accompanied by retinal thinning and loss of the outer layers of the retina.

Drusen and pigmentary abnormalities are the most common antecedent lesions of GA. In these cases, GA evolves in several stages and good visual acuity is usually preserved until late in the course of the disease. However, patients with relatively good visual acuity have profound visual function abnormalities.

MAGUIRE and VINE (1986) proposed three stages of GA:

- In the initial phase, focal areas of RPE atrophy appear in the parafoveal area and enlarge and coalesce over time. Due to the sparing of the fovea, these eyes retain good visual acuity. The tendency to form an incomplete ring of atrophy around the fovea – sometimes referred to as a horseshoe configuration – has been noted. The RPE in the fovea itself remains intact; foveal involvement at that time is usually limited to numerous drusen.
- In the second phase, visual acuity is lost rapidly as the ring of atrophy spreads into the fovea.
- In the last stage, the macula presents with a confluent area of RPE atrophy and visual acuity is very poor, as patients have to use eccentric areas of intact retina for vision.

The rate of spread of the atrophic area involved has been calculated at 1.8 Macular Photocoagulation Study (MPS) disc areas over a 2-year period (SUNNESS et al. 1996). A tendency to faster expansion was found in patients under 75 years, whereas in patients over 75 years the zones of atrophy expanded more slowly.

Overall, the progression to the end stage of GA may well take a decade, which is an important part of the remaining lifetime of elderly patients. Therefore, the natural course of GA is generally more benign compared to the rapid loss in visual acuity in patients with exudative ARMD.

SCHATZ and McDONALD (1989) reported an annual rate of severe visual loss (defined as vision loss from 20/50 or better to 20/100 or worse) of 8%.

Visual acuity changes in patients with GA describe visual function deficits only incompletely. Due to the late involvement of the foveal center, patients may still be able to read single numbers or letters on visual acuity charts but may have severe problems in reading texts with a small zone of fovea remaining intact. Sunness and coworkers found reduced maximum reading rates of 110 words per minute in patients with baseline visual acuity of 20/50 or better (median VA 20/35). After 2 years, the maximum reading rate had deteriorated to 51 words per minute, whereas patients lost a median of three lines on ETDRS charts, representing a doubling of the minimum angle of resolution. Moreover, in this study, patients with GA experienced significant changes in dark adaptation and contrast sensitivity despite good visual acuity. Both were associated with an increased relative risk of doubling of the visual angle by 2 years (SUNNESS et al. 1997).

Altogether, these data suggest that in the earlier stage of GA, patients have already developed considerable abnormalities in visual function and may experience difficulties despite well-preserved visual acuity. Paracentral scotomata caused by areas of atrophy leave an "island" of foveal vision which affects the ability to read and to recognize faces, as the field of vision is not big enough. It is noteworthy that these patients are not helped by magnification, e.g., with low vision aids, where even fewer features are recognized.

Somewhat conflicting data exist about bilateral involvement in GA due to differing numbers of patients and varying follow-up times in these studies, but conventional clinical wisdom holds that bilateral manifestation of GA is very common.

The risk of developing choroidal neovascularization depends on the status of the fellow eye. Patients with bilateral GA and no evidence of CNV are at low risk of developing CNV. SUNNESS et al. (1998) followed up 152 patients and reported an 11% rate of CNV by 4 years. In contrast, patients with GA and CNV in one eye are at significantly higher risk of developing CNV in the fellow eye with GA at baseline: 34% by 4 years. The border of the atrophy zone is the most common location for CNV to develop, followed by the spared fovea.

In some cases, GA may follow RPE detachment, which has been described as decompensation of the RPE. In these cases, the extent of visual loss is determined primarily by the location of RPE detachment. An extrafoveal location will have less impact than foveal involvement. Visual function deficits are essentially the same as described above.

2.5 Choroidal Neovascularization

Eyes with choroidal neovascularization have varying degrees of reduced visual acuity, depending on location, size, type, and age of the neovascular lesion. Depending on the location of CNV, three subtypes can be distinguished:

- Extrafoveal CNV does not extend closer than 200 µm to the center of the foveal avascular zone (FAZ) with the posterior border.
- In juxtafoveal CNV, the border of the neovascular membrane or associated blood or blocked fluorescence is between 1 µm and 199 µm from the center of the FAZ.
- In subfoveal CNV, the eye has CNV under the geometric center of the FAZ.

A large proportion of the knowledge about the natural history of eyes with CNV comes from patients assigned to no treatment in randomized clinical trials of laser photocoagulation. The MPS group has initiated the largest of these trials. They have provided data based on standardized enrollment requirements, clinical assessment, and fluorescein photographic evaluation for follow-ups of up to 5 years.

2.5.1 Extrafoveal CNV

In 1982, 1983, and 1991, the MPS group's results for treatment of extrafoveal CNV with argon laser photocoagulation compared to no treatment were reported. The MPS group did not differentiate between classic and occult CNV during recruitment of participants into this trial. However, the majority of lesions were likely to have well-demarcated borders and would now be called classic. To be eligible, eyes were required to have visual acuity of 20/100 or better at study entry. After 5 years, mean visual acuity had fallen to 20/200, representing a loss of 7.1 lines on Bailey-Lovie visual acuity charts. A loss of six or more lines was defined as severe. On the Bailey-Lovie chart, a decrease of six lines represents a fourfold increase in the visual angle, e.g., a change from 20/100 to 20/400. The greatest proportion of severe visual loss occurred by around 2 years of follow-up (56%) and stabilized thereafter. By the 5-year examination, 64% of eyes with no treatment experienced severe visual loss, as the neovascular lesion extended through the foveal center. In contrast, eyes assigned to laser treatment experienced a lesser decrease in visual acuity (mean after 5 years: 20/125), and fewer eyes had severe visual loss (46% at 5 years). Therefore, laser photocoagulation is now standard treatment for extrafoveal CNV (Macular Photocoagulation Study Group 1991, 1993).

2.5.2 Juxtafoveal CNV

At the time of recruitment, the MPS group did not distinguish between classic and occult CNV. In the 1990s, all baseline fluorescein angiograms of participants enrolled in the Krypton Photocoagulation Study were reviewed and regraded retrospectively to differentiate the angiographic features of classic and occult CNV: 52% (237 eyes) had classic CNV only, 35% (158 eyes) had classic and occult CNV, and 13% (61 eyes) had occult CNV only. At the initial examination, visual acuity was required to be 20/400 or better.

After 5 years, the average visual acuity was 20/250 among participants assigned to no treatment, down from 20/50 for occult CNV and 20/62 for both the classic only and the combined forms of CNV. Due to the wide range of initial visual acuity, the change from baseline visual acuity rather than average visual acuity at the final examination illustrates the natural course of the condition. Sixty-one percent of the participants who received no treatment and 52% in the treatment group experienced severe visual loss of six or more lines. Again, severe visual loss was more likely to occur early during follow-up, and the proportion stabilized at around 24 months. Comparing the course over time for classic CNV, classic and occult CNV, and occult CNV, patients with occult CNV tended to lose visual acuity over a more prolonged period than other subgroups. Patients with classic CNV were most likely to suffer a rapid decline in visual acuity, whereas those with occult CNV lost vision more slowly, with a considerable proportion (40%) remaining almost stable during the first year of follow-up. However, after 5 years this difference was no longer seen and all subgroups had suffered the same visual loss. Essentially, this means that the natural course of eyes with occult CNV is more variable and patients preserve better vision for a limited period. Interestingly, in eyes with juxtafoveal CNV, the benefit of laser treatment depended largely on hypertensive status, and patients with systemic hypertension fared no better with laser treatment than without, whereas a benefit for normotensive patients was shown (Macular Photocoagulation Study Group 1994).

2.5.3 Subfoveal CNV

In the Subfoveal New CNV trial, all participants recruited were required to have some classic CNV component. New lesions were <3.5 times larger than the MPS disc areas and baseline visual acuity had to be 20/320 or better.

At 4-year examination, mean visual acuity in patients assigned to no treatment had decreased to 20/500, down from 20/160 at the initial examination. Small and medium-sized lesions with better levels of visual acuity at baseline were more likely to have severe vision loss. On average, visual acuity decreased by 5.0 lines, with 45% of participants experiencing severe visual loss. Plainly, these findings mean that nearly one half of observed eyes were unable to read by 3 or 4 years (Macular Photocoagulation Study Group 1993).

At first glance, the loss of five lines appears less severe than in patients with juxtafoveal and extrafoveal CNV. However, attention must be paid to the initial requirements at baseline, where visual acuity had to be considerably better in extrafoveal and juxtafoveal lesions. Therefore, the prospect of losing an additional five lines from a low starting point in subfoveal lesions must be assessed as being significant and has considerable impact. For instance, visual acuity in patients with juxtafoveal occult CNV was about 20/100 after 3 years, compared to 20/500 in patients with subfoveal CNV after 4 years. Although none of those can be labeled good vision, this difference affects the chances of preserving many abilities in everyday life as well as the ability to use low-vision aids.

Over time, CNV is transformed into fibrous tissue of varying size and appearance to form a disciform scar. Visual acuity in affected eyes is usually very poor and the decrease in visual function has reached its final stage.

2.6 Serous Detachment of the Retinal Pigment Epithelium

According to the classification and grading system of the International ARM Epidemiological Study Group, serous detachment of the retinal pigment epithelium is a separate form of exudative ARMD. Serous detachment of the RPE must be distinguished from fibrovascular pigment epithelial detachment, a form of occult CNV defined by its appearance on fluorescein angiography.

The natural course of the condition depends strongly on whether CNV is present or not. In about 49% of these eyes, CNV develops within 3 years (Poliner et al. 1986) or may be present from baseline. Fluorescein angiographic features associated with the development of CNV and adverse visual outcome were: older patient age, notching on one side of the pigment epithelial detachment (PED), irregular shape and filling of the PED, late filling, increased size, and additional sensory retinal detachment (Poliner et al. 1986; Elman et al. 1986). In some of these cases, indocyanine green angiography may be helpful to visualize CNV as a hotspot of focal hyperfluorescence. Indocyanine green angiography employs a different dye than fluorescein angiography and, due to the different maximum absorption and emission wavelengths, shows a better penetration of ocular pigment (RPE) and medium opacity and is better able to demonstrate choroidal circulation and sub-RPE pathologies (Richard 1998).

If no CNV is present, the prognosis for maintenance of visual acuity is favorable; little deterioration occurs over timeand visual acuity usually remains within three lines of the status at the time of presentation. Severe visual loss is unlikely to occur and affects less than 10% of these patients. In patients with no evidence of CNV, pigment epithelial detachment persists over years and may then resolve to leave an area of GA of the RPE, which has been described as decompensation of the RPE.

The development of CNV dramatically worsens the natural course of the condition. Between 57% (Elman et al. 1986) and 78% (Poliner et al. 1986) of eyes deteriorate to a visual acuity of 20/200 or worse. Eyes with CNV at presentation fare even worse. In the study by Poliner et al., 88% of these patients had dropped to visual acuity of 20/200 or worse after a mean follow-up of 2.3 years. Singerman and Stockfish (1989) reported visual acuity of less than 20/200 in 65% of these patients at 1 year. This outcome is comparable to the poor prognosis of visual function in patients with subfoveal CNV. Both groups tend to form a disciform scar over time.

References

Bressler SB, Maguire MG, Bressler NM, Fine SL, Macular Photocoagulation Study Group (1990) Relationship of drusen and abnormalities of the retinal pigment epithelium to the prognosis of neovascular macular degeneration. Arch Ophthalmol 108:1442–1447

Eisner A et al (1987) Sensitivities in older eyes with good acuity: Eyes whose fellow eye has exudative AMD. Invest Ophthalmol Vis Sci 28:1832–1837

Eisner A et al (1991) Relation between fundus appearance and function: Eyes whose fellow eye has exudative age-related macular degeneration. Invest Ophthalmol Vis Sci 32:8–20

Elman MJ et al (1986) The natural history of serous retinal pigment epithelium detachment in patients with age-related macular degeneration. Ophthalmology 93:224–230

Holz FG et al (1994) Bilateral macular drusen in age-related macular degeneration: Prognosis and risk factors. Ophthalmology 101:1522–1528

Klein R, Klein BEK, Jensen SC, Meuer SM (1997) The 5-year incidence and progression of age-related maculopathy. The Beaver Dam Eye Study. Ophthalmology 104:7–21

Kleiner RC et al (1988) Contrast sensitivity in age-related macular degeneration. Arch Ophthalmol 106:55–57

Macular Photocoagulation Study Group (1991) Argon laser photocoagulation for neovascular maculopathy after 5 years: Results from randomized clinical trials. Arch Ophthalmol 109:1109–1114

Macular Photocoagulation Study Group (1993a) Laser photocoagulation of subfoveal neovascular lesions of age-related macular degeneration: Updated findings from two clinical trials. Arch Ophthalmol 11:1200–1209

Macular Photocoagulation Study Group (1993b) Five-year follow-up of fellow eyes of patients with age-related macular degeneration and unilateral extrafoveal choroidal neovascularization. Arch Ophthalmol 111:1189–1199

Macular Photocoagulation Study Group (1994) Laserphotocoagulation for juxtafoveal choroidal neovascularization: Five-year results from randomized clinical trials. Arch Ophthalmol 112:500–509

Macular Photocoagulation Study Group (1997) Risk factors for choroidal neovascularization in the second eye of patients with juxtafoveal or subfoveal neovascularization secondary to age-related macular degeneration. Arch Ophthalmol 115:741–747

Maguire P, Vine AK (1986) Geographic atrophy of the retinal pigment epithelium. Am J Ophthalmol 102:621–625

Midena E et al (1997) Macular function impairment in eyes with early age-related macular degeneration. Invest Ophthalmol Vis Sci 38: 469–477

Poliner LS et al (1986) Natural history of retinal pigment epithelial detachments in age-related macular degeneration. Ophthalmology 93:543–551

Richard G (1998) Fluorescein and ICG angiography, 2nd edn. Thieme, Stuttgart

Schatz H, McDonald HR (1989) Atrophic macular degeneration: Rate of spread of geographic atrophy and visual loss. Ophthalmology 96:1541–1551

Singerman LJ, Stockfish JH (1989) Natural history of subfoveal pigment epithelial detachments associated with subfoveal or unidentifiable choroidal neovascularization complicating age-related macular degeneration. Graefes Arch Clin Exp Ophthalmol 227:501–507

Sunness JS et al (1996) The enlargement of geographic atrophy over time in age-related macular degeneration. Invest Ophthalmol Vis Sci 37:S21

Sunness JS et al (1997) Visual function abnormalities and prognosis in eyes with age-related geographic atrophy of the macula and good visual acuity. Ophthalmology 104:1677–1691

Sunness JS et al (1998) The development of choroidal neovascularization in eyes with the geographic atrophy form of age-related macular degeneration. Ophthalmology 106:910–919

The International ARM Epidemiological Study Group (1995) An international classification and grading system for age-related maculopathy and age-related macular degeneration. Surv Ophthalmol 39(5):367–374

3 Diagnostic Workup

ANDREA HASSENSTEIN and GISBERT RICHARD

CONTENTS

3.1 Fluorescein Angiography

Fluorescein angiography (FAG) of the fundus is a main step in investigating the circulation of the retina and choroid and especially for visualizing macular pathology. When excited, molecules with short wavelengths emit light of longer wavelengths; this phenomenon is called fluorescence. Fluorescein angiography was described first by Novotny and Alvis, medical students from Indianapolis, USA.

The light is not reflected but is changed in its quality. Physically, the incoming light elevates electrons to a higher level and the resulting energy is transmitted as light of a longer wavelength. The maximum of fluorescein absorption is at 490 nm, in the blue part of the spectrum. The light issued has maximum wavelength at 530 nm, in the green part of the spectrum. Seventy to 85% of the fluorescein is attached to serum proteins, mainly albumin, in the bloodstream. The remainder is called „free fluorescein." The zonulae occludentes of the retinal endothelium form the inner blood-retina barrier, which is not permeable to fluorescein. Leakage of fluorescein from retinal vessels is pathologic.

A. HASSENSTEIN, MD
G. RICHARD, MD, Professor
Department of Ophthalmology, University of Hamburg, Martinistrasse 52, 20246 Hamburg, Germany

The choroidal vessels are not permeable to fluorescein, but the choriocapillaris has multiple fenestrations and is permeable to free fluorescein, which penetrates the intercellular part of the retinal pigment epithelium (RPE). The tight junctions of the RPE are not permeable to free fluorescein and are called the „outer blood-retina barrier". Leakage of fluorescein through the RPE is also pathologic.

The fluorescein reaches the eye via the ophthalmic artery and follows the short posterior ciliary arteries to the choroid and the central retinal artery to the retinal circulation. The retinal circulation follows the choroidal circulation 1 s later.

The choroidal filling is either segmental or patchy, or diffuse. Choroidal fluorescence depends on the pigmentation of the fundus. Because of the quick filling of the choriocapillaris, differentiation of choroidal filling is not possible except in pathologic hypoperfusion of the choroid, such as choroidal infarction (Elschnig's bodies). Late fluorescence of the optic nerve head is normal.

The dark foveal presentation is due to the lack of vessels within the foveal avascular arcade and to the high concentration of xanthophyll in the neuroretina (HASSENSTEIN and RICHARD 1998; HOLZ and PAULEIKHOFF 1997; KANSKI and SPITZNAS 1987; RICHARD 1998).

3.1.1 Technique

A fundus camera with serial photographs and a high-energy flash, including a locking filter, is used. The camera is focussed on the central 30° to 50°. The first picture is taken in red-free light. Essential for angiograms of good quality are dilated pupils and clear media. After injection of the fluorescein (5% concentration, 5 ml) pictures are taken in quick succession. The early phase is important for diagnosis and photographs are taken every second during this time. After 5–10 min, late photographs are taken. Today, photographs are transferred to a computer so that digital processing for better contrast is possible and the photographs are immediately available.

Usually, fluorescein causes only minor side effects, sometimes nausea or a yellowish tint in the skin or urine. Allergic reactions such as bronchospasm or shock are rare.

The four phases of fluorescein vascular filling are:
1. Prearterial phase: filling of the choroid, no fluorescein in the retinal circulation
2. Arterial phase: 1 second later, from beginning to complete filling of retinal arteries
3. Arteriovenous phase: complete filling of retinal arteries and laminar flow in retinal veins
4. Venous phase: complete filling of retinal veins and clearance from the retinal arteries

3.1.2 Fluorescein Angiography in Age-Related Macular Degeneration

There are various stages of age-related macular degeneration (AMD). The first presentation might be drusen, which are either hard and sharply demarcated or soft and confluent. Soft drusen have a higher risk for the development of exudative disease (Fig. 3.1) (Berger et al. 1999; Holz and Pauleikhoff 1997)

The drusen show a focal depigmentation of the RPE and, therefore, a window-like defect in the underlying choroidal fluorescence. At the posterior pole, you may see a lawn of hyperfluorescent drusen which stain in the late phase. In patients with geographic atrophy, a sharply demarcated hyperfluorescent central lesion is visible, sometimes with thick choroidal vessels. This is the nonexudative form of AMD with a better visual prognosis.

In some patients, detachment of the RPE occurs, which is sometimes due to an underlying fibrovascular membrane. The fluorescein angiography shows hyperfluorescent circular leakage and pooling of fluorescein within the detachment and a sharp demarcation in the late phase. There is no progressive leakage in the late phase, in contrast to choroidal neovascularization (CNV).

The classic choroidal neovascular membrane shows, in the early phase, the hyperfluorescent neovascular vessels as a lacy pattern which then presents in the late phase typically as a diffuse leakage because of the lack of tight junctions. In classic neovascular membranes, the newly formed vessels fluoresce brightly during the early filling phase, when the boundaries of the membrane are clearly visible.

By definition, classic CNV has well-demarcated boundaries, allowing for accurate determination of the location and size of these lesions. Occult CNV is characterized by diffuse late leakage of undetermined source. In some cases, we find simultaneous detachment of the RPE (Figs. 3.2, 3.3).

3.2 Indocyanine Green Angiography

For better overall visualization of the choroidal circulation, indocyanine green (ICG) angiography was developed. Indocyanine is an organic substance with maximum of absorption at 805 nm and fluorescence at 835 nm, near infrared. It is even more attached to proteins (98%) than is fluorescein (60%–80%). The dye cannot penetrate the choroidal vessels because of the strong attachment to high molecular albumin. Today, it is possible to visualize the choroidal vessels without the choriocapillaris, which is important mainly in cases of CNV and chorioretinal anastomosis before laser treatment (Figs. 3.4, 3.5).

Indications for ICG are CNV, choroidal tumors, and detachment of the RPE or sensory retina. A disadvantage of ICG is the low contrast of the photographs.

As with fluorescein angiography, a modified fundus camera is used that allows maximum infrared transmission.

In classic CNV, the ICG shows a pattern of hyperfluorescence similar to that with FAG. In occult CNV, the ICG presents various lesions such as hot spots (29%), plaque lesions (61%), and combinations of both (8%). Hot spots are smaller than 1 disc area, well demarcated by ICG, and represent an active proliferation, typically found outside the foveolar avascular arcade. A plaque CNV is more than 1 disc area in size, ill-defined, and represents inactive occult CNV, commonly subfoveal.

At this time, it is not possible to guide laser treatment by ICG, but future improvements in technique will lead to more information about choroidal neovascularization (Richard 1998).

3.3 Optical Coherence Tomography

Optical coherence tomography (OCT) is a new, noninvasive technology providing us with pictures of retinal structures with a high optical resolution of up to 10 μm. It is the first method which enables the demonstration of different retinal layers and of the vitreoretinal interface. OCT is a technique for the quantitative assessment of pathological findings of retinal structures.

The OCT is analogous to conventional ultrasound, except that optical rather than acoustic properties of tissues are measured. The imaging depends on the contrast in optical reflectivity between different tissue microstructures. Light beams of a defined wavelength (850 nm, near infrared) are used. The technique is based on an optical measurement technique known as low-coherence interferometry. The OCT device measures the time delays of optical echoes by comparing the reflected light beam with a reference beam.

One hundred A-scans within 1 s produce a B-picture. The resulting picture is two-dimensional with an axial optical resolution of 10 μm and a transverse resolution of 20–50 μm, depending on the scan length. The scans can be performed in a circular or linear manner.

The images are displayed in a false color representation, meaning that the highest back reflections are red and white colors whereas the lowest backscattering shows up as blue or black. The colors represent different optical properties and not necessarily different tissue morphology. The nerve fiber layer exhibits medium to high reflectivity, followed by the sensory retina divided into the inner and outer plexiform layers. Subsequently the RPE, including the choriocapillaris, is visualized as a strong red line with high reflectivity. The dark green to bluish-black layer is the choroid. Limitations to OCT are opacified media and the inability to fixate in cases of severe visual loss or peripheral fundus pathology (Berger et al. 1999; Hassenstein and Richard 2000) (Figs. 3.6–3.9).

References

Berger JW, Fine SL, Maguire MG (1999) Age-related macular degeneration. Mosby, St. Louis, pp 219–247

Hassenstein A, Richard G (1998) Geschichte und Entwicklung der Fluoreszenzangiographie. Ophthalmochirurgie 10:75-84

Hassenstein A, Richard G (2000) Die optische Kohärenztomographie in der Diagnostik der Makulaerkrankungen. Der Augenspiegel 3:16–23

Holz FG, Pauleikhoff D (1997) Altersabhängige Maculadegeneration. Springer, Berlin Heidelberg New York, pp 40–46

Kanski JJ, Spitznas M (1987) Lehrbuch der klinischen Ophthalmologie. Thieme, Stuttgart

Richard G (1998) Fluorescein and ICG angiography, textbook and atlas. Thieme, Stuttgart, pp 142–153

a

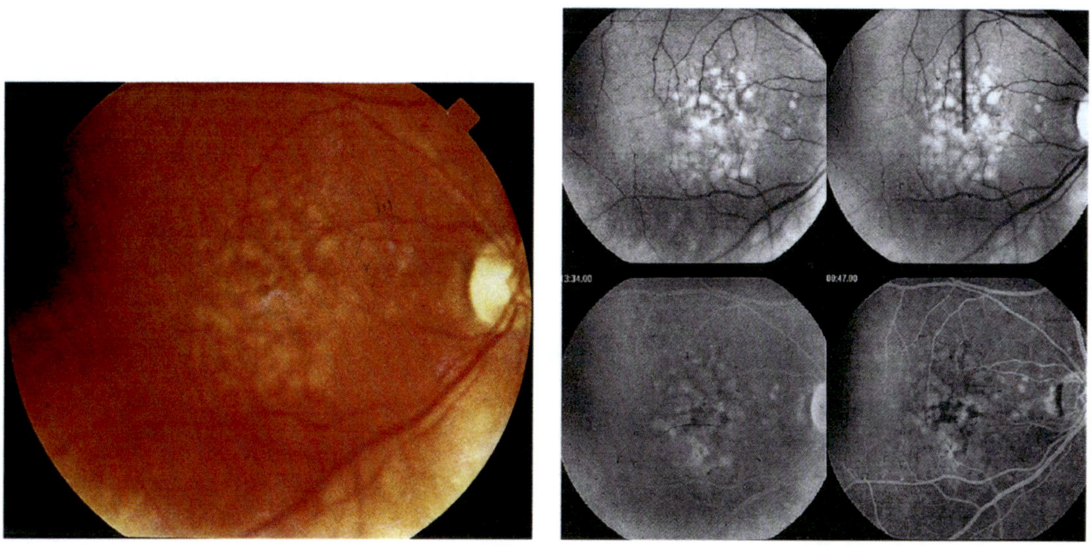

b

Fig. 3.1. a Soft drusen on funduscopy. Biomicroscopy of the fundus of a patient with soft drusen in the right eye who has a high risk of developing exudative ARMD. Visual acuity is 20/200. The retina shows confluent yellowish spots in the macula. **b** Soft drusen on FAG: hyperfluorescent, ill-defined confluent lesions including focal hyperpigmentation of the macula

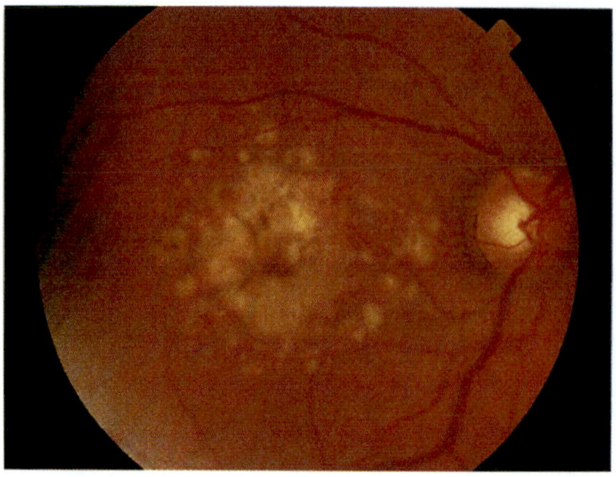

a

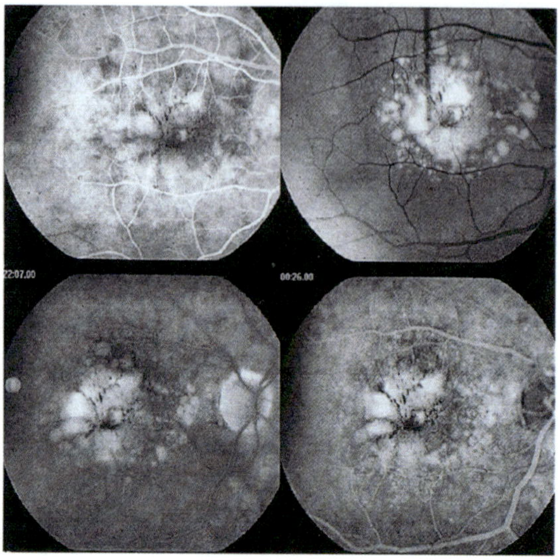

b

Fig. 3.2. **a** Occult CNV on funduscopy. Biomicroscopy of a patient with visual acuity of 20/40 in the left eye with occult CNV and subretinal hemorrhage. **b** Occult CNV on FAG: a central, ill-defined hyperfluorescence and surrounding hypofluorescent hemorrhage. In the late phase, the fluorescein dye leaks out of the choroidal neovascular membrane

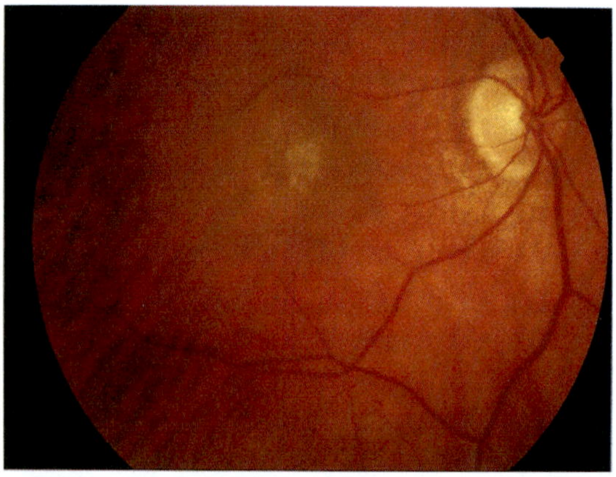

a

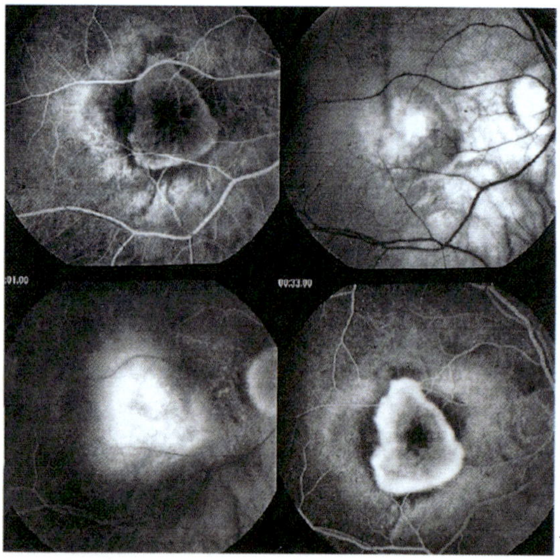

b

Fig. 3.3. **a** Classic CNV on funduscopy. This patient has a prominent gray-brown lesion of the macula at funduscopy, with visual acuity of 10/200 in the right eye. **b** Classic CNV on FAG: a huge, subretinal, hyperfluorescent neovascular membrane of the macula with surrounding hypofluorescence and leakage in the late phase. In contrast to occult CNV, the border of this CNV is well-defined

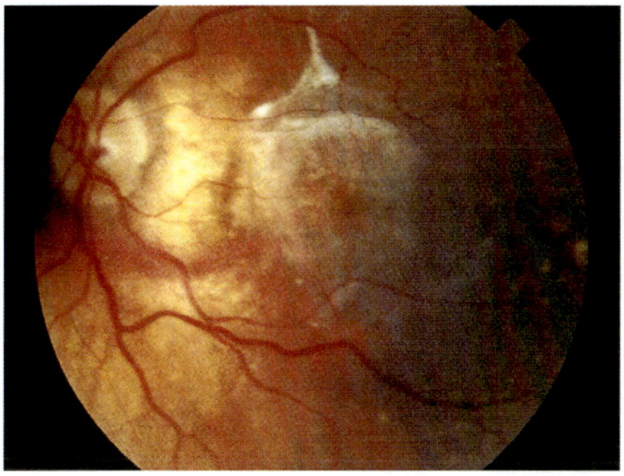
a

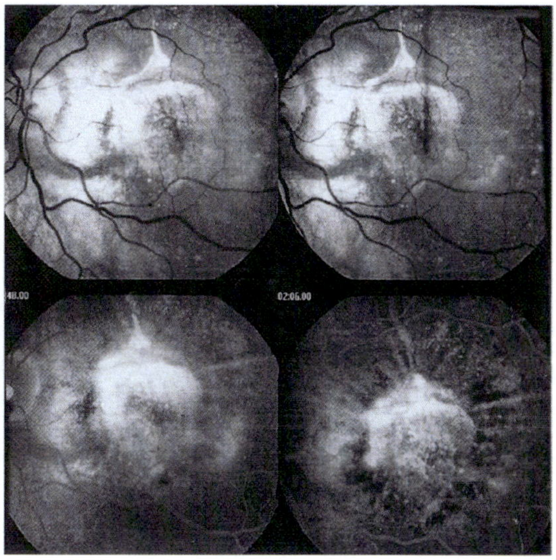
b

Fig. 3.4. a Subretinal scar, funduscopy. This patient suffers subretinal scarring following CNV and the visual acuity in the left eye deteriorated to detecting hand movements. The macula shows a gray subretinal membrane which wrinkles the retina. **b** Subretinal scar on FAG. The imaging reveals hyperfluorescent staining of the fibrovascular membrane. The membrane causes a circular wrinkling of the retina

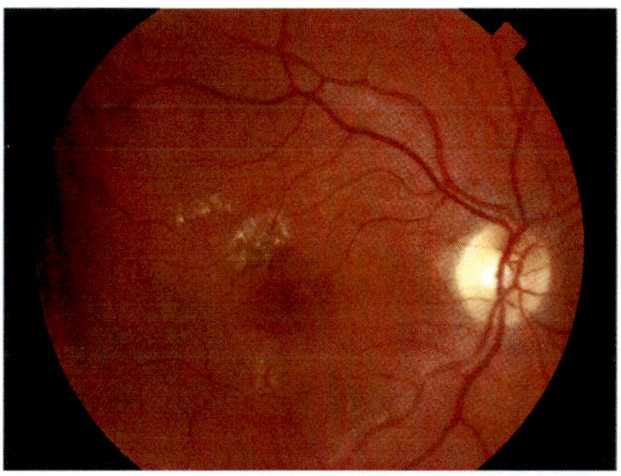
a

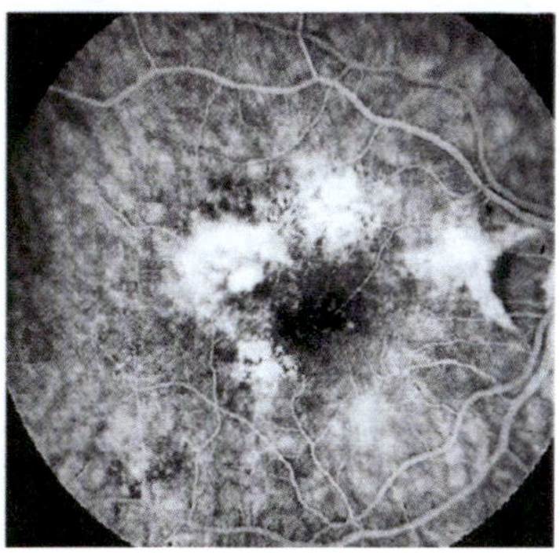
b

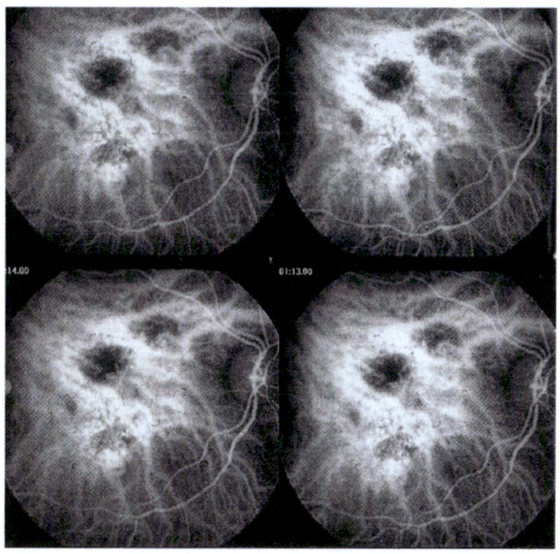
c

Fig. 3.5. a Funduscopy of a CNV scar after laser treatment. Biomicroscopy shows a gray laser scar temporally and superiorly to the macula without edema. **b** Angiography of CNV scar after laser treatment shows hyperfluorescent leakage temporal to the macula and hyperfluorescent staining of the laser scar. **c** CNV scar after laser treatment. ICG angiography reveals the large choroidal vessels and hypofluorescent CNV scar. Below the laser scar, hyperfluorescent staining is visible which might represent new occult CNV

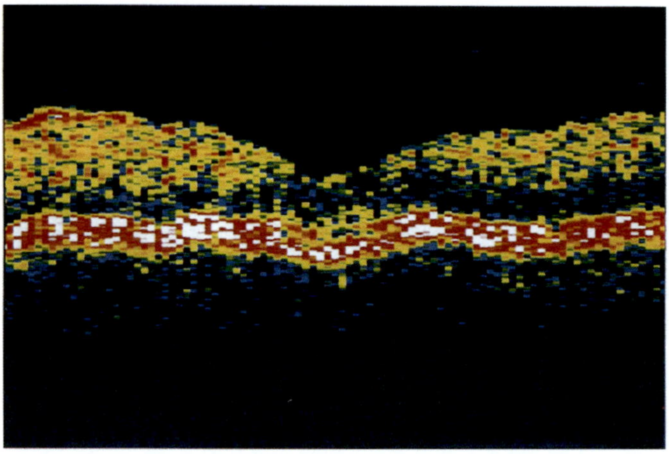

Fig. 3.6. Normal OCT. The horizontal red line represents the highly reflective pigment epithelium and the overlying yellow layer the sensory retina. The foveolar depression is visible. The outer retinal layers are less reflective, as are the underlying choroid and choriocapillaris

a

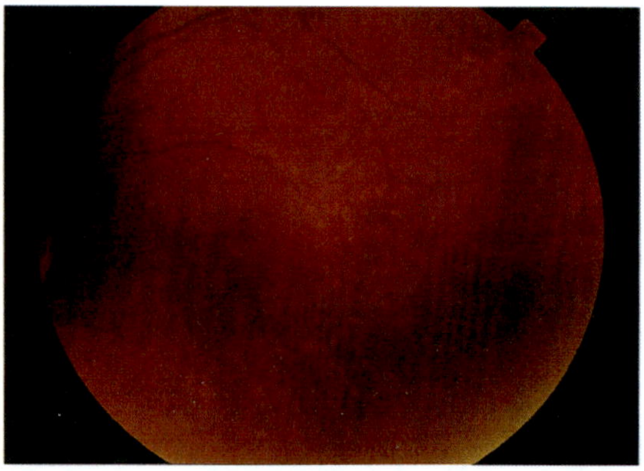

b

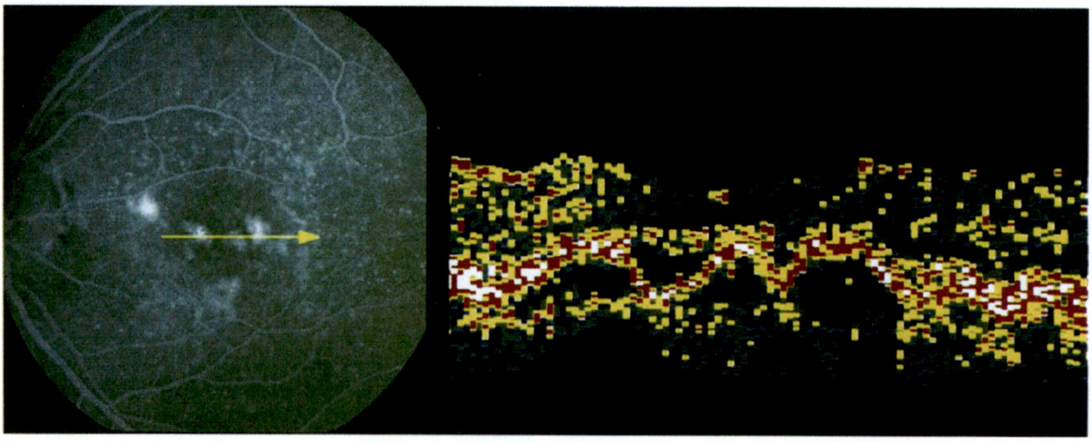

Fig. 3.7. a Soft drusen on funduscopy. Biomicroscopy of soft drusen show yellow-white lesions which are ill-defined. **b** Soft drusen, OCT. As soft drusen are almost nonreflective, they present here as small focal detachments of the RPE. In OCT, the soft drusen represent the wavy detachment of the RPE. Between the wavelines, the sensory retinal is stretched and detached

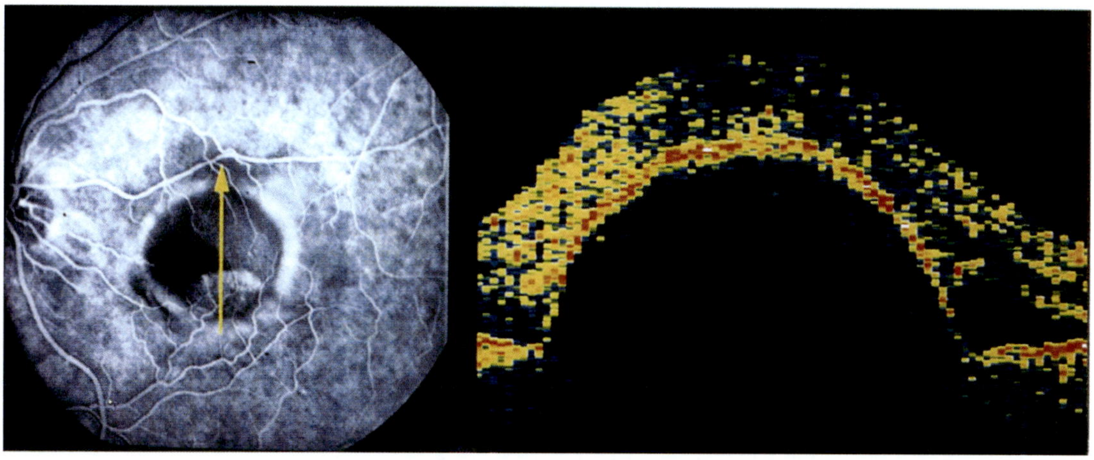

Fig. 3.8. Detachment of the RPE on FAG and OCT. The fluorescein angiography (*left*) shows a serous detachment of the RPE and hyperfluorescent pooling of the fluorescein dye at the detached border. There is no hyperfluorescent CNV visible. OCT presents very clearly the detachment of the RPE and the optically empty space beneath the RPE layer, as in serous detachments

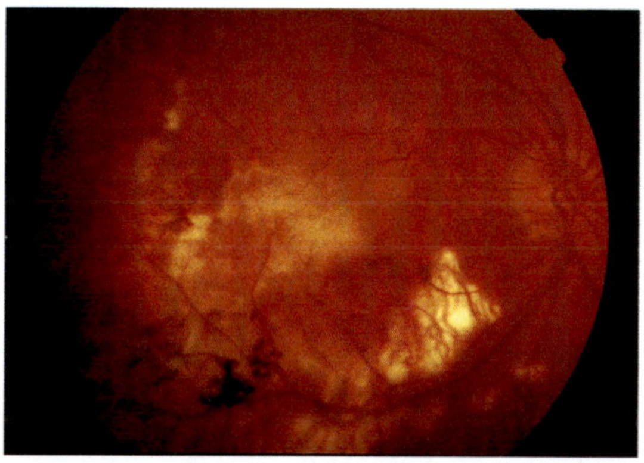

a

Fig. 3.9. **a** Fibrovascular scar in CNV: funduscopy. This patient shows a large central CNV and surrounding atrophy of the RPE and choriocapillaris. A prominent gray-brown lesion in the macula is visible. **b** Fibrovascular scar in CNV: OCT. The highly reflective RPE layer is thickened like a spindle, which is typical for membranes. Furthermore, there is detachment of the sensory retina and cystic formation in the neurosensory retina. The fovea does not show any depression; rather, there is cystic elevation of the retina

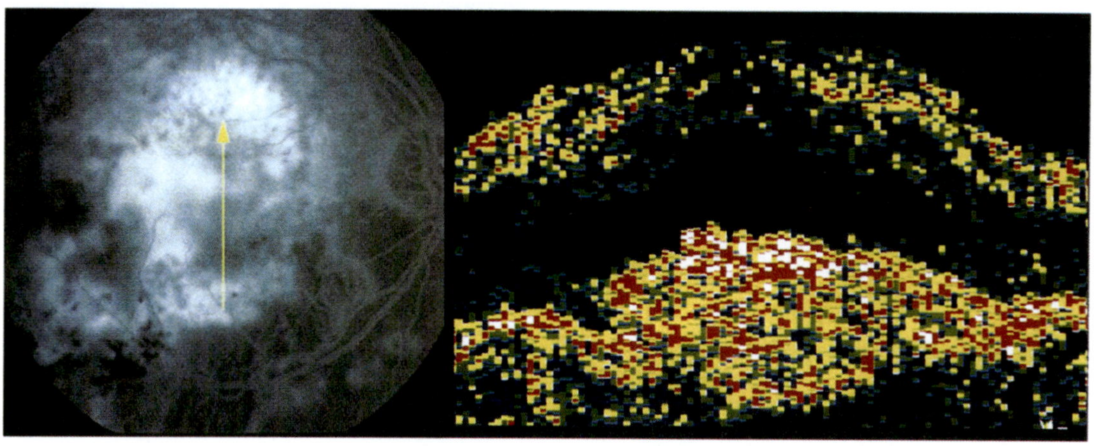

b

4 Planimetry of Age-Related Macular Degeneration

R. Schwartz

CONTENTS

4.1 Introduction

Planimetry is a suitable tool for follow-up of choroidal neovascularizations (CNV). By means of manual, computer-assisted, or automated image processing, areas of interest such as hemorrhages, drusen, CNV, detachment of pigment epithelium, or atrophy are delineated. We describe an easy method of obtaining semiquantitative data from fluorescence angiographic findings in classic CNV.

4.2 History

In the past, the sizes of retinal areas under investigation have been compared to the diameter of the optic disc. This procedure, which is based on a nonstandardized calculation, does not satisfy the requirements for exact quantitation. For standardized analysis and follow-up of areas of interest, a method of exact quantitation must be implemented, thereby allowing reference reading centers (Bird et al. 1995) to assess the success of clinical therapeutical trials. Many previous studies of the treatment of age-related macular degeneration (ARMD) (Klein et al. 1997) have only followed up subjective parameters such as visual acuity, visual fields, contrast sensitivity, and metamorphopsias; however, the size and activity of CNV and hemorrhages have been neglected.

4.3 Planimetry

4.3.1 Imaging Methods

Storage and transmission of digital fundus images allow for exact image analysis, image comparison, and detection of changes and have resulted in an important diagnostic tool (Akita, Kuga 1992; Berger 1998; Goldbaum et al 1990). Photographs are transformed from analog to digital formats by a scanner digitizer. The loss of information during subsequent digitization usually does not influence the planimetric analysis of fundus features, although the resolution of film-based analog images is clearly superior. For the follow-up of classic CNV in ARMD after treatment with external beam radiotherapy, we propose a simple planimetric method to achieve highly accurate images for comparison of drusen, hemorrhages, CNV, pigment epithelial detachment, or retinal pigment epithelium (RPE) atrophy (Goldbaum et al. 1993; Kirkpatrick et al. 1995; Peli, Lahav 1986; Morgan et al. 1994). Despite the availability of automated image processing, we prefer manual methods. In this way, the examiner can define the areas of interest in angiographic images. To control the accuracy of our method, two different angiography readers analyzed the same sequential angiographic frames. We used a Topcon TRC 50X camera for our study. A demarcation line was drawn around areas of interest with a computer mouse. Subsequently, two prominent anatomic markers, e.g., the bifurcation of retinal vessels, were determined by the mouse (Hart, Goldbaum 1994). To increase accuracy, these characteristic markers were localized as far from the areas of interest as possible. The square

R. Schwartz, MD
Augenklinik und Poliklinik, University Hospital Eppendorf, Martinistrasse 52, 20246 Hamburg, Germany

of the distance between the two marking points was compared to the area of interest. The number of pixels of both areas was calculated using our computer software. From the follow-up, we compared the ratio between the area of interest and reference area. To achieve semiquantitative data for the areas of interest in square millimeters, one needs data about the camera, patient refraction, and biometrics. In comparing dimensions of the areas of interest, our planimetric method does not depend on the angle of the image frame. Images created by different cameras or from different angles are comparable if both images include the same markers for calculating the reference area.

Planimetry may be combined with other methods (Phillips et al. 1991; Nagin et al. 1995; von Ruckmann et al. 1997) to calculate the activity and amount of hyperfluorescent leakage.

4.3.2 Planimetric Calculation of Classic CNV

Our first example shows fluorescein angiogram images of the same classic CNV. Figure 4.1 shows a frame of 20°, Fig. 4.2 a frame of 35°, and Fig. 4.3 a frame of 50°. As characteristic markers, we determined the same bifurcations of retinal vessels. In Fig. 4.1, the square of the distance between the two marked points was 177,874 pixels and the area of interest contained 8129 pixels. The ratio of area of interest to reference area was 0.045. In Fig. 4.2, the square of the distance between the two marked points was 79,380 pixels and the area of interest contained 3665 pixels. The ratio of area of interest to reference area was 0.046. In Fig. 4.3, the square of the distance between the two marked points was 45,316 pixels and the area of interest contained 1889 pixels. The ratio of area of interest to reference area was 0.041.

This example demonstrates the high reliability of our method. The difference between the ratios of images 1 and 2 is 2.2%, and that between images 1 and 3 is 8.9%. As expected, the accuracy of the ratio calculation decreases with a decrease in the size of the reference area.

In our second example, one sees fluorescein angiogram images of a classic CNV before and 6 months after treatment with external beam radiotherapy. Figure 4.4 shows two reference points and the demarcation line around the CNV before external beam radiotherapy. Figure 4.5 shows the same reference points and the demarcation line around the CNV 6 months after radiotherapy. In Fig. 4.4, the square of the distance between the two reference points is 234,397 pixels and the area of interest contains 19,522 pixels. The ratio of area of interest to reference area was 0.083. In Fig. 5, the square of the distance between the two reference points is 226,120 pixels and the area of interest contains 31,937 pixels. The ratio of area of interest to reference area is 0.141.

The difference between the ratios of the two areas of interest is about 70%, which indicates an increase in the CNV despite external beam radiotherapy.

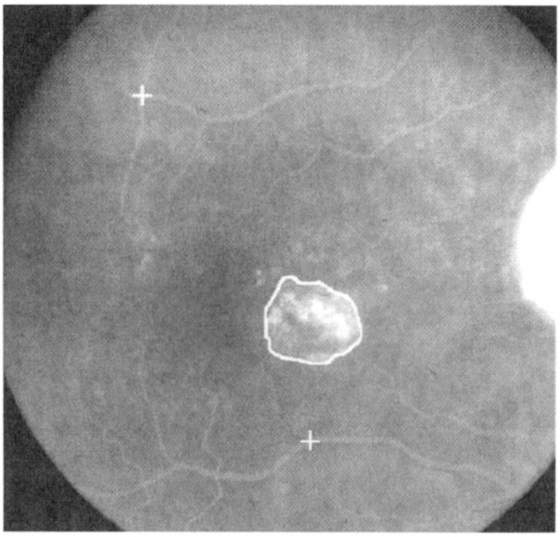

Fig. 4.1. Fluorescein angiogram image with demarcation line around a classic choroidal neovascularization and two reference points in a 20° frame

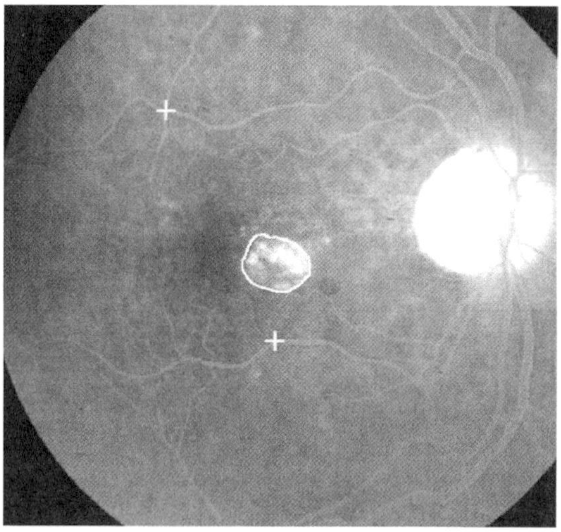

Fig. 4.2. The same classic choroidal neovascularization as in Fig. 4.1 in a 35° frame

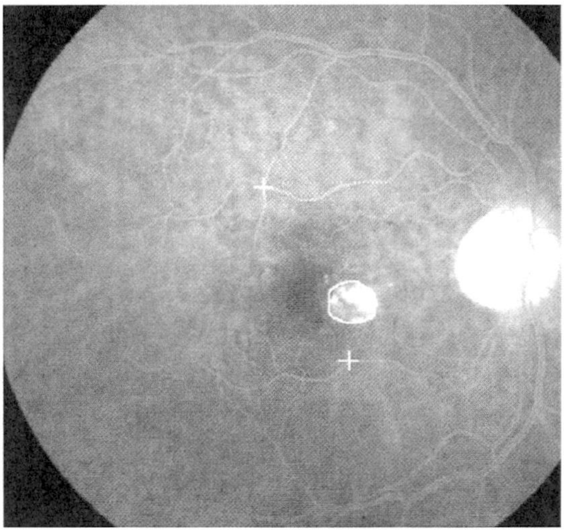

Fig. 4.3. The same classic choroidal neovascularization as in Fig. 4.1 in a 50° frame

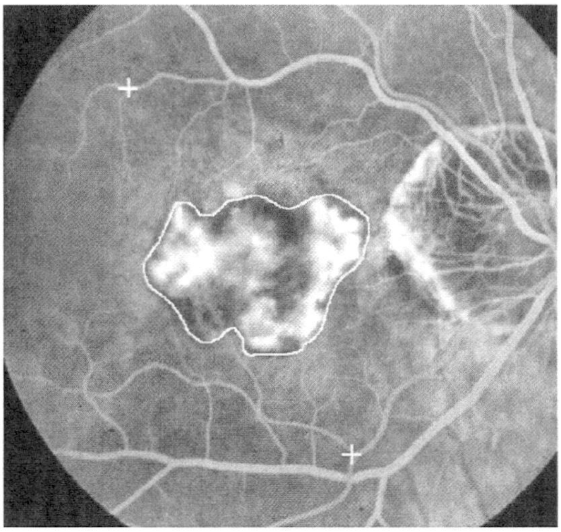

Fig. 4.5. Fluorescein angiogram image with demarcation line around the same choroidal neovascularization as in Fig. 4.4, 6 months after external beam radiotherapy

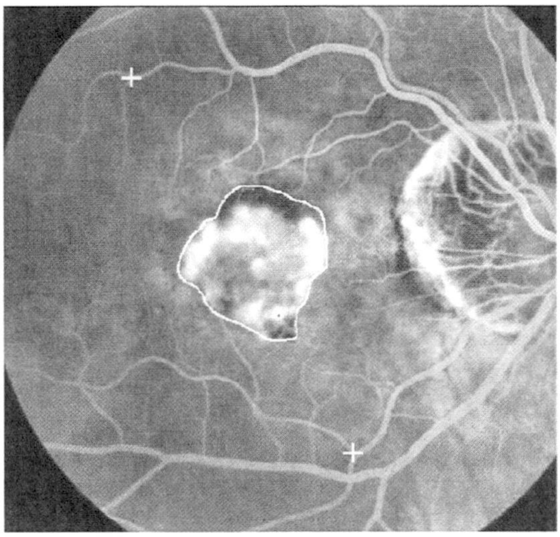

Fig. 4.4. Fluorescein angiogram image with demarcation line around a classic choroidal neovascularization and two reference points before radiotherapy

4.4 Conclusion

Planimetry is an accurate and simple method for the follow-up of many and various areas of interest on digital images. Comparing the ratio of the number of pixels of the area of interest to a reference area, one is able to calculate the extent of change.

References

Akita K, Kuga H (1992) A computer method of understanding ocular fundus images. Pattern Recognition 15:431–433

Berger JW (1998) Quantitative, spatiotemporal image analysis of fundus features in age-related macular degeneration. Proc SPIE 3246:48–53

Bird AC et al (1995) An international classification and grading system for age-related maculopathy and age-related macular degeneration: The International ARM Epidemiological Study Group. Surv Ophthalmol 39:367–374

Goldbaum MH et al (1990) Digital image processing for ocular fundus images. Ophthalmol Clin North Am 3:447–466

Goldbaum MH et al (1993) Automated registration of digital ocular fundus images for comparison of lesions. Proc SPIE 1877:94–99

Hart WE, Goldbaum MH (1994) Registering retinal images using automatically selected control point pairs. In: IEEE Proceedings of International Conference of Computer Vision, pp 576–580

Kirkpatrick JN et al (1995) Quantitative image analysis of macular drusen from fundus photographs and scanning laser ophthalmoscope images. Eye 9:48–55

Klein R et al (1997) The five-year incidence and progression of age-related maculopathy: The Beaver Dam Eye Study. Ophthalmology 104:7–21

Morgan WH et al (1994) Automated extraction and quantification of macular drusen from fundal photographs. Aust N Z J Ophthalmol 22:7–12

Nagin P et al (1985) Measurement of fluorescein angiograms of the optic disc and retina using computerized image analysis. Ophthalmology 92:547–552

Peli E, Lahav M (1986) Drusen measurement from fundus photographs using computer image analysis. Ophthalmology 93:1575–1580

Phillips RP et al (1991) Detection and quantification of hyperfluorescent leakage by computer analysis of fundus fluorescein angiograms. Graefe's Arch Clin Exp Ophthalmol 229:329–335

Von Ruckmann A et al (1997) Fundus autofluorescence in age-related macular disease imaged with a laser scanning ophthalmoscope. Invest Ophthalmol Vis Sci 38:478–486

Surgery of
Age-Related Macular Degeneration (ARMD)

5 Surgery – an Overview

Jan Zurdel and Katrin Engelmann

CONTENTS

5.1 Introduction

Since the late 1980s, surgical techniques have become available for submacular surgery in choroidal neovascularization (CNV) and associated subretinal hemorrhages secondary to age-related macular degeneration (ARMD). Results of surgical removal of CNV are encouraging, given the poor prognosis for visual acuity in the natural course of the disease, and stabilization of vision seems to be the most likely outcome. However, although removal of CNV can be accomplished, the strong tendency toward recurrence is a pending threat for patients who have undergone surgery. Moreover, the operation itself causes damage to the tissue in the vicinity of the choroidal neovascular membrane and thus limits the benefits.

Removal of subretinal hemorrhages can be achieved by using tissue plasminogen activator and expansible gas, possibly in combination with vitrectomy but, again, long-term results depend on the underlying cause of the bleeding.

A general therapeutic regimen does not exist and the decision for treatment should be individually designed according to the patient's specific circumstances.

J. Zurdel, MD
K. Engelmann, MD, Professor
Department of Ophthalmology, University of Hamburg, Martinistrasse 52, 20246 Hamburg, Germany

5.2 Surgical Removal of Choroidal Neovascular Membranes

Among the first patients to undergo subretinal surgery to remove CNV in ARMD were four reported in 1988 by De Juan and Machemer. At that time, due to retinal detachment and proliferative vitreoretinopathy, visual outcome was very poor, with none of the patients having visual acuity (VA) better than 5/200. Thereafter, some encouraging reports with favorable visual outcomes were reported (Slusher 1989), reigniting hopes that this approach might be beneficial in these patients who were otherwise threatened by severe visual loss.

Until now, indications for surgical removal of choroidal neovascular membranes (CNVM) have not been defined unambiguously, since data consist of small case series and no large randomized clinical trials are available. However, reliable data on the natural history of patients come from large control groups of the Macular Photocoagulation Study (MPS). Therefore, data from surgically treated patients may well be compared to these control groups.

5.2.1 Surgical Technique

A standard three-port vitrectomy is performed and the posterior hyaloid is elevated. Then, a small retinotomy is needed in the vicinity of the neovascular lesion, usually temporally to the macula, and balanced salt solution or viscoelastic is injected into the subretinal space to separate the retina from the underlying tissue, including the CNVM. The CNVM is mobilized and removed using a subretinal forceps. Endolaser coagulation or endocryocoagulation may be performed at the site of the retinotomy. Finally, fluid is exchanged for air or expansible gas, and the patient is positioned face-down for several days to allow tamponade of the macula by the gas bubble.

5.2.2 Results

Several studies indicate that it is possible to stabilize visual acuity (VA) in the majority of patients, whereas considerable improvement or severe worsening of VA are less frequent (MERRILL et al. 1999; THOMAS et al. 1994). The mean changes of VA in these studies have been about zero. Nonetheless, attention must be paid to the duration of follow-up and the inclusion criteria. With longer follow-up, more patients experience recurrences and related visual loss. The overall rate of recurrence is estimated to be 30%, somewhat lower than after laser photocoagulation; in the MPS trials, the rates of recurrence were slightly above 50%, depending on the location of CNV.

In ARMD, neovascular membranes usually grow underneath and above the RPE, a pattern causing significant damage to the RPE and choriocapillaris during removal of the CNVM. Surgery may, therefore, cause severe trauma to underlying tissues necessary for survival of photoreceptors and thus limit the benefits of the procedure, as demonstrated in a 1-year follow-up after surgery in a case series (CASTELLARIN et al. 1998). Therefore, preoperative selection of patients appears to be important with respect to visual outcome.

However, other evidence suggests that surgical removal of CNVM did not benefit patients. TSUJIKAWA et al. (1999) demonstrated that excision of CNVM did not improve central retinal sensitivity, and patients had poor visual outcome in most cases. However, in some cases sensitivity could be preserved and visual outcome was relatively good following surgical CNV removal. So far, it is not well understood why, in some patients, the surgically damaged area remains functionally well preserved postoperatively (LOEWENSTEIN et al. 1998). SCHEIDER et al. (1999) reported a prospective study including 54 eyes which were subcategorized into three subtypes according to the MPS: well-defined (classic) CNV, ill-defined (occult) CNV, and submacular hemorrhage. They demonstrated that subfoveal surgery might preserve remaining retinal function in eyes with well-defined CNV but that eyes with occult CNV or hemorrhages did not benefit from surgery. In contrast to this prospective study, retrospective analyses revealed no correlation between visual outcome and type of CNV, presence of hemorrhage, or duration of visual symptoms (BENSON et al. 1998).

Interestingly, results of surgery seem to be better with different CNV etiology, e.g., results were remarkably good in CNV associated with presumed ocular histoplasmosis syndrome (THOMAS and KAPLAN 1991)

All in all, removal of CNVM in ARMD seems to be a viable method of halting visual loss which otherwise threatens the majority of patients. Stabilization of VA, which most of the studies suggest is the average outcome, is a considerably better prospect for these patients compared to the natural history of the disease (see chapter 2). Meanwhile, other surgical techniques, namely macular translocation, have evolved and their results will have to be compared to conventional removal of CNVM.

5.2.3 Complications

Excision of CNV may lead to RPE loss followed by atrophy of neighboring tissue. Some clinical studies indicate benefit only for removal of membranes lying above the RPE. After CNVM excision, 75% of patients showed new areas of decreased choriocapillaris perfusion (NASIR et al. 1997).

Development of cataract is a known postoperative complication after vitrectomy for other indications, e.g., removal of epiretinal membranes or macular hole surgery. The rate of complications increased with the size of CNV and the extent of manipulation. In conclusion, results now do not warrant a general recommendation for CNVM surgery (STRMEN and HASA 1996) and an individual approach and assessment of possible benefits and risks appear to be necessary (ECKARDT 1996).

5.3 Surgery in Subretinal Hemorrhage

Subretinal hemorrhage may be a complication of CNV. Small amounts of blood are frequently seen associated with these lesions, but extensive subretinal bleeding is relatively rare. Surgical removal of subretinal hemorrhages and membranes in ARMD eyes is feasible from a technical point of view. However, an advantage over the natural course has not yet been established. Nevertheless, a reduction of central scotoma size can be achieved by surgical intervention (PETERSEN et al. 1998). Other studies demonstrated that only intravitreal injection of tissue plasminogen activator (TPA; 25–100 μg) followed by an additional injection of expansible gas (0.3–0.4 ml perfluoropropane or sulfur hexafluoride) without surgery led to an improvement of vision (FRAMME et al. 2000; HASSAN et al. 1999).

Surgery may be helpful in cases where blood clots are present beneath the retina (SAIKA et al. 1998). In the long term, the benefit of surgery vs. the complication rate depends largely on the treatability and recurrence of the underlying CNVM, e.g., on the possibility to remove the CNVM or apply laser photocoagulation postoperatively. In many patients, no definite treatment for the underlying cause of the subretinal bleeding is applicable and therefore it must be suspected that the postoperative course resembles the natural history of CNV and that the benefits from surgery may be temporary. KAMEI et al. (1996) concluded that the use of TPA may improve the outcome of surgery by reducing the surgically induced retinal damage. However, a general therapeutic regimen in case of such severe ARMD-related subretinal hemorrhages cannot be given yet.

References

Benson MT et al (1998) Surgical excision of subfoveal neovascular membranes. Eye 12:768–774

Castellarin AA et al (1998) Progressive presumed choriocapillaris atrophy after surgery for age-related macular degeneration. Retina 18(2):143–149

De Juan E, Machemer R (1988) Vitreous surgery for hemorrhagic and fibrous complications of age-related macular degeneration. Am J Ophthalmol 105:25–29

Eckardt C (1996) Surgical removal of submacular neovascularization membranes. Ophthalmologe 93(6):688–693

Framme et al (2000) Clinical results of intravitreal administration of tissue-type plasminogen activator (tPA) and gas for removal of subretinal hemorrhage in senile macular degeneration. Klin Monatsbl Augenheilkd 216(1):33–39

Hassan AS et al (1999) Management of submacular hemorrhage with intravitreous tissue plasminogen activator injection and pneumatic displacement. Ophthalmology 106(10):1900–1906

Kamei M et al (1996) Surgical removal of submacular hemorrhage using tissue plasminogen activator and perfluorocarbon liquid. Am J Ophthalml 121(3):267–275

Loewenstein A et al (1998) Scanning laser ophthalmoscope fundus perimetry after surgery for choroidal neovascularization. Am J Ophthalmol 125(5):657–665

Merrill et al (1999) Surgical removal of choroidal neovascularization in age-related macular degeneration. Ophthalmology 106:782–789

Nasir MA, Sugino I, Zarbin MA (1997) Decreased choriocapillaris perfusion following surgical excision of choroidal neovascular membranes in age-related macular degeneration. Br J Ophthalmol 81(6):481–489

Petersen J et al (1998) Visual fields after removal of subretinal hemorrhages and neovascular membranes in age-related macular degeneration. Graefe's Arch Clin Exp Ophthalmol 236(4):241–247

Saika S et al (1998) Subretinal administration of tissue-type plasminogen activator to speed the drainage of subretinal hemorrhage. Graefe's Arch Clin Exp Ophthalmol 236(3):196–201

Scheider A et al (1999) Surgical extraction of subfoveal choroidal new vessels and submacular hemorrhage in age-related macular degeneration: Results of a prospective study. Graefe's Arch Clin Exp Ophthalmol 237(1):10–15

Slusher MM (1989) Evacuation of submacular hemorrhage: technique and timing. In: Vitreoretinal surgery and technology, vol 1. Slack, Thorofare, New Jersey, USA

Strmen P, Hasa J (1996) Surgical removal of large subretinal neovascular membranes: Results and complications. Int Ophthalmol 20(4):165–169

Thomas MA, Kaplan HJ (1991) Surgical removal of subfoveal neovascularization in the presumed ocular histoplasmosis syndrome. Am J Ophthalmol 111:1–7

Thomas MA et al (1994) Visual results after surgical removal of choroidal neovascular membranes. Ophthalmology 101:1384–1396

Tsujikawa M et al (1999) Change in retinal sensitivity due to excision of choroidal neovascularization and its influence on visual acuity outcome. Retina 19(2):135–140

6 Limited Macular Translocation in Age-Related Macular Degeneration

KAH-GUAN AU EONG, DANTE J. PIERAMICI, GILDO Y. FUJII, and EUGENE DE JUAN JR.

CONTENTS

6.1 Introduction

Age-related macular degeneration (ARMD) is the leading cause of blindness and a major public health problem in many developed countries, particularly in Europe and North America (HAWKINS et al. 1999; KRUMPASZKY et al. 1999; KLEIN et al. 1992; LEIBOWITZ et al. 1980). neovascular complications of ARMD account for 80%–90% of cases of blindness from this disease, while atrophic changes are responsible for the remainder. Despite intensive research efforts worldwide to combat the disease, no treatment is currently available for the non-neovascular variety, while only limited therapy can be offered to patients with the neovascular form.

The Macular Photocoagulation Study (MPS) documented that laser photocoagulation of extrafoveal and juxtafoveal choroidal neovascularization (CNV) secondary to ARMD reduces the risk of severe visual loss (MACULAR PHOTOCOAGULATION STUDY GROUP 1991a, 1994a). It also proved that laser photocoagulation of the entire area of age-related subfoveal CNV is beneficial with regard to long-term visual acuity when compared to no treatment (MACULAR PHOTOCOAGULATION STUDY GROUP 1991b, c, 1993). However, because laser photocoagulation damages the overlying neurosensory retina, treatment of sub-

K.-G. AU EONG, MBBS, Mmed (Ophth), FRCS (Edin), FRCS (Glasg), DRCOphth, FAMS
Clinical Fellow in Diseases and Surgery of the Vitreous and Retina, Vitreoretinal Service, Wilmer Ophthalmological Institute, Johns Hopkins University School of Medicine, Johns Hopkins Hospital, Maumenee 719, 600 North Wolfe Street, Baltimore, MD 21287-9277, USA
Consultant Ophthalmologist, Department of Ophthalmology, Tan Tock Seng Hospital, 11 Jalan Tan Tock Seng, Singapore 308433, Singapore
Adjunct Associate Scientist, Singapore Eye Research Institute, 500 Dover Road, Singapore Polytechnic Workshop 2 (W212), Singapore 139651, Singapore

D.J. PIERAMICI, MD
Assistant Professor of Ophthalmology, Wilmer Ophthalmological Institute, Johns Hopkins University School of Medicine, Johns Hopkins Hospital, Maumenee 719, 600 North Wolfe Street, Baltimore, MD 21287-9277, USA
G.Y. FUJII, MD
Research Fellow in Diseases and Surgery of the Vitreous and Retina, Wilmer Ophthalmological Institute, Johns Hopkins University School of Medicine, Johns Hopkins Hospital, Maumenee 719, 600 North Wolfe Street, Baltimore, MD 21287-9277, USA
E. DE JUAN Jr., MD
Joseph E. Green Professor of Ophthalmology, Wilmer Ophthalmological Institute, Johns Hopkins University School of Medicine, Johns Hopkins Hospital, Maumenee 719, 600 North Wolfe Street, Baltimore, MD 21287-9277, USA

foveal CNV was associated with an immediate average reduction of three Bailey-Lovie lines in visual acuity. In addition, the benefits of treatment over the natural history of the condition only became apparent after 6 months, and retention or recovery of good vision rarely occurred in treated patients. None of the 77 eyes in the subfoveal new CNV study had visual acuity of 20/80 or better, while 88% had visual acuity of 20/200 or worse at the 48-month examination following laser ablation of the subfoveal lesion (MACULAR PHOTOCOAGULATION STUDY GROUP 1993). Recurrence or persistence of the CNV was also common following treatment, with close to half of the treated eyes having persistent or recurrent CNV within 3 years (MACULAR PHOTOCOAGULATION STUDY GROUP 1994b). For these reasons, it is not surprising that a recent survey in the United Kingdom and the Republic of Ireland by BEATTY et al. (1999) disclosed that only 13.6% of 339 consultant ophthalmologists whose practice includes laser photocoagulation of age-related CNV treat subfoveal CNV with laser ablation.

Most cases of age-related CNV do not meet the MPS criteria for laser photocoagulation because the lesion is subfoveal and too large, has poorly demarcated boundaries, or has only occult and no classic CNV (MACULAR PHOTOCOAGULATION STUDY GROUP 1994c). Therefore, many investigators are seeking new treatment modalities that can be used in a larger group of patients than conventional laser photocoagulation and can improve the visual outcome of this disease. Alternative therapies such as interferon alpha-2a (CHAN et al. 1994; Pharmacological Therapy For MACULAR DEGENERATION STUDY GROUP 1997; POLINER et al. 1993; THOMAS and IBANEZ 1993a), radiation (CHAR et al. 1999; SPAIDE et al. 1998), subretinal endolaser photocoagulation (THOMAS and IBANEZ 1993b), and submacular surgery (BERGER and KAPLAN 1992; BLINDER et al. 1991; DE JUAN and MACHEMER 1988; LAMBERT et al. 1992; THOMAS et al. 1992, 1994) have been found to offer little or no benefit. Photodynamic therapy has recently been shown to provide some modest short-term benefits but does not benefit all patients with subfoveal CNV and multiple retreatments are usually necessary (MILLER et al. 1999; SCHMIDT-ERFURTH et al. 1999; Treatment of Age-Related Macular Degeneration with PHOTODYNAMIC THERAPY STUDY GROUP 1999).

Macular translocation surgery recently emerged as a novel strategy for the management of subfoveal CNV. It is also known by several other names, including retinal relocation (LINDSEY et al. 1983), retinal translocation (DE JUAN et al. 1998; IMAI et al. 1998), macular relocation (IMAI and DE JUAN 1996; MACHEMER and STEINHORST 1993a, b), macular rotation (ECKARDT et al. 1999), and foveal translocation (CEKIC et al. 1999; FUJIKADO et al. 1998a, b; NINOMIYA et al. 1996; OHJI et al. 1998).

The different techniques currently used for macular translocation surgery may be classified into two broad groups based on the size of the retinotomy/retinotomies created: (1) macular translocation with non-self-sealing retinotomy and (2) macular translocation with self-sealing or no retinotomy (Fig. 6.1). Procedures with non-self-sealing retinotomy require retinopexy and silicone oil internal tamponade, while those with self-sealing or no retinotomy do not.

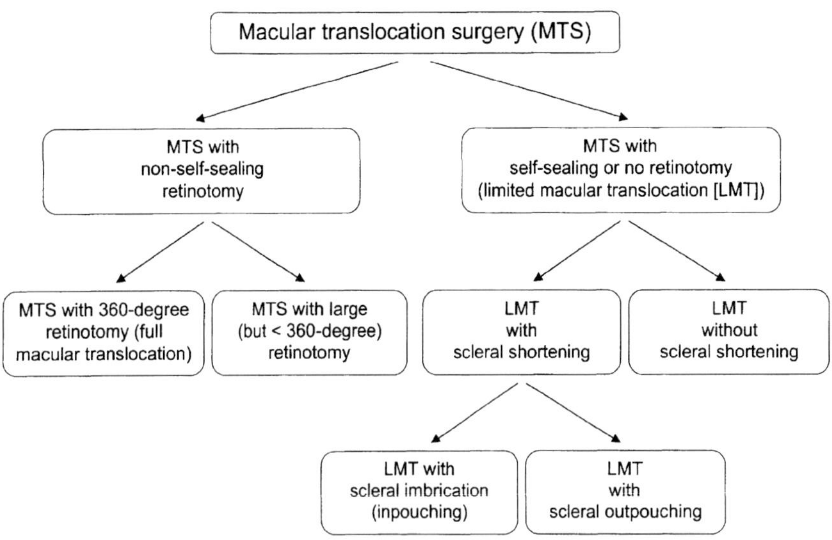

Fig. 6.1. Classification of macular translocation surgery

Macular translocation with non-self-sealing retinotomy may be further subdivided into (a) macular translocation with 360° peripheral circumferential retinotomy (also known as full macular translocation: MACHEMER and STEINHORST 1993a, b; SEABER and MACHEMER 1997; TOTH and MACHEMER, 1999) and (b) macular translocation with large (but less than 360°) circumferential retinotomy (CEKIC et al. 1999; FUJIKADO et al. 1998a, b; NINOMIYA et al. 1996; OHJI et al. 1998). Macular translocation with self-sealing or no retinotomy is also known as limited macular translocation and may be further subdivided into types with and without scleral shortening (DE JUAN and VANDER 1999). Scleral shortening may be effected by either scleral imbrication (scleral inpouching) (DE JUAN et al. 1998; HARLAN et al. 1999; IMAI and DE JUAN 1996; IMAI et al. 1998) or scleral outpouching (KAMEI et al. 2000; MEYER et al. 2000). This chapter reviews the current state of knowledge and technique of inferior limited macular translocation with scleral imbrication for the management of age-related subfoveal CNV.

6.2 Rationale of Macular Translocation Surgery

The surgical goal of macular translocation surgery is to displace the neurosensory retina of the fovea in an eye with recent-onset subfoveal CNV to a new location with a presumably healthier bed of the retinal pigment epithelium (RPE)–Bruch's membrane–choriocapillaris complex devoid of CNV. The rationale is that this displacement may allow the fovea to recover or maintain its visual function over relatively more normal subretinal tissues. In addition, relocating the fovea to an area outside the CNV allows conventional laser ablation of the CNV without destroying the fovea, thereby preserving central vision while arresting the progression of the CNV. When combined with submacular surgery, macular translocation surgery also allows the fovea to be relocated to an area outside the RPE defect associated with the CNV removal.

The density and pigmentation of RPE cells and the pattern of choroidal circulation are not uniform throughout the ocular fundus. It has been shown that the macular area has the greatest density of RPE melanin pigmentation (T'so and FRIEDMAN 1967) and a lobular choroidal angioarchitecture that allows for extremely fast circulation (YONEYA and T'so 1987). Therefore, although the concept of macular translocation surgery is attractive, how well the extrafoveal or extramacular RPE and choriocapillaris can support good foveal function is relatively unknown. TOLLER and HAINSWORTH (1998) reported an 18-year-old man who retained good visual acuity despite foveal displacement to an area of extramacular RPE and choroid following an open-globe injury, thus demonstrating that extramacular RPE and choroid can indeed support some foveal function.

6.3 History of Macular Translocation Surgery

Lindsey et al. first reported their experiments with retinal relocation to study the anatomic dependency of the foveal retina on foveal RPE and choroid in 1983. The idea of using retinal relocation as a treatment for subfoveal CNV secondary to ARMD was conceived by TIEDEMAN et al. (1985). They reported that it was feasible to rotate the macula approximately 45° around the optic disc in animal eyes. The proposed treatment was not pursued for some time until MACHEMER and STEINHORST (1993b) finally demonstrated its feasibility in humans.

Their technique involves lensectomy, complete vitrectomy, planned retinal detachment by trans-scleral infusion of fluid under the retina, 360° peripheral circumferential retinotomy, rotation of the retina around the optic disc, and retinal reattachment with silicone oil tamponade. A number of modifications have since been made to this technique by several investigators, but many still require large (NINOMIYA et al. 1996) or 360° peripheral circumferential retinotomy (WOLF et al. 1999; ECKARDT et al. 1999; TOTH and MACHEMER 1999) for effective macular translocation. In an attempt to reduce the incidence and severity of the proliferative vitreoretinopathy (PVR) that has been reported to occur with macular translocation surgery with large or 360° peripheral circumferential retinotomy, IMAI and DE JUAN developed a new technique of macular translocation without the need for any retinotomy in 1996. They were able to achieve predictable macular relocation of greater than 500 μm in rabbit eyes with their technique of planned retinal detachment by trans-scleral subretinal hydrodissection, anterior-posterior scleral shortening near the equator, and retinal reattachment. The risk of developing PVR was thought to be lower with this technique than with earlier techniques because no retinal break was created. Since the initial description in 1996, de Juan and associates have made several modifications to their technique (de Juan et al. 1998; de Juan and Vander 1999; Harlan et al. 1999a; Imai et al. 1998; Pieramici et al. in press).

6.4 Indications of Limited Macular Translocation

The spectrum of conditions in which limited macular translocation is clinically useful has not been fully ascertained. Currently, the most common indication for limited macular translocation is subfoveal CNV. The CNV may be secondary to a number of etiologies, but given the high prevalence of ARMD and its poor visual prognosis without treatment, ARMD is the most common disease that has been treated with this procedure. Besides displacing the fovea away from the underlying CNV in eyes with new or recurrent CNV, we have also used limited macular translocation to displace the fovea away from RPE defects created by submacular surgery in a few eyes.

6.5 Preoperative Considerations of Limited Macular Translocation

Since not all cases of ARMD are suited to limited macular translocation, careful and detailed preoperative assessment is crucial to select the appropriate surgical candidates. Proper selection ensures that patients have an acceptable risk:benefit ratio and a reasonable chance of good anatomic and functional outcome following surgery.

The precise relationship of the CNV to the geometric center of the foveal avascular zone is determined from a recent good quality fluorescein angiogram, preferably obtained within 1 week of the surgery. Besides paying attention to the characteristics of the lesion in the macula, care should also be taken to exclude concurrent pathology such as retinal breaks elsewhere in the retina that may affect the surgery.

Our experience has shown that several pathophysiologic and anatomic factors are important in determining the postoperative functional and anatomic outcome following limited macular translocation, and these should be considered during the preoperative evaluation of the patient.

6.5.1 Pathophysiologic Considerations

The mechanisms responsible for visual loss during the different stages of neovascular ARMD may be broadly divided into "reversible" and "irreversible" components.

6.5.1.1 *"Reversible" Components of Visual Loss*

"Reversible" components of visual loss in ARMD include (1) impaired photoreceptor function secondary to abnormal RPE function (retinal metabolism) and impaired nutrient/waste exchange across the RPE and Bruch's membrane, (2) relative retinal ischemia/hypoxia secondary to an abnormal RPE–Bruch's membrane–choriocapillaris complex, (3) retinal edema and subretinal fluid, and (4) retinal and subretinal hemorrhages. These mechanisms operate early in the course of the disease process. Because their effects are not immediately devastating, affected eyes often retain foveal fixation. Metamorphopsia and central blurring are common symptoms. Theoretically, if one or more of these factors are reduced or reversed by reestablishment of a relatively more normal subretinal space following effective macular translocation and subsequent ablation of the CNV, visual recovery may occur. The best candidates for this procedure are therefore those with recent-onset metamorphopsia or disturbances in central vision due to new or recurrent CNV, before the onset of more permanent mechanisms that damage the fovea irreversibly.

6.5.1.2 *"Irreversible" Components of Visual Loss*

Fibrovascular scarring occurs in untreated long-standing neovascular ARMD and results in permanent photoreceptor cell loss. The size and thickness of the resultant disciform scar have been found to relate directly to loss of photoreceptors (Green and Enger 1993). The visual loss is often severe and may result in loss of foveal fixation, but metamorphopsia becomes less prominent. Because the foveal photoreceptor loss is "irreversible," affected eyes are unlikely to achieve good functional recovery even after effective macular translocation.

A number of clinical tests may be used to assess foveal function prior to surgery. Visual acuity is a good guide and has been shown to be associated with better postoperative visual outcome (Pieramici et al. in press). Other guides include scanning laser ophthalmoscope (SLO) microperimetry and focal electroretinography. SLO microperimetry, By identifying eyes that are able to maintain foveal fixation, appears to be an excellent test for functional foveal photoreceptors (LOEWENSTEIN et al. 1998).

6.5.2 Anatomic Considerations

When the surgical goal of macular translocation has been achieved, the operation may be called *effective*. We define effective macular translocation as (1) successful postoperative relocation of the fovea to an area outside the border of the CNV, i.e., a previously subfoveal CNV becomes either juxtafoveal (1–199 μm from the foveal center) or extrafoveal (+200 μm from the foveal center) following surgery or (2) successful postoperative relocation of the fovea to an area outside the border of the RPE defect associated with CNV removal during the surgery. For the surgery to be effective, the postoperative foveal displacement must *exceed* the minimum desired translocation (see below) for a particular patient. Although not fully predictable before surgery, some idea of the postoperative foveal displacement that is likely to be achieved can be gained by knowing the *median* postoperative foveal displacement of a series of cases performed by the surgeon.

6.5.2.1 Minimum Desired Translocation

The minimum desired translocation for inferior macular translocation is the distance between the foveal center and a point on the inferior border of the lesion, these two points being equidistant from the temporal edge of the optic disc (Fig. 6.2). This distance is related to the size, shape, and eccentricity of the subfoveal lesion (CNV or RPE defect) (Figs. 6.3, 6.4). Since the papillomacular bundle enters the disc from the temporal side, the temporal edge of the optic disc rather than the center of the disc is the pivot point for the papillomacular bundle when the fovea is relocated during macular translocation surgery. The postoperative foveal displacement must *exceed* this

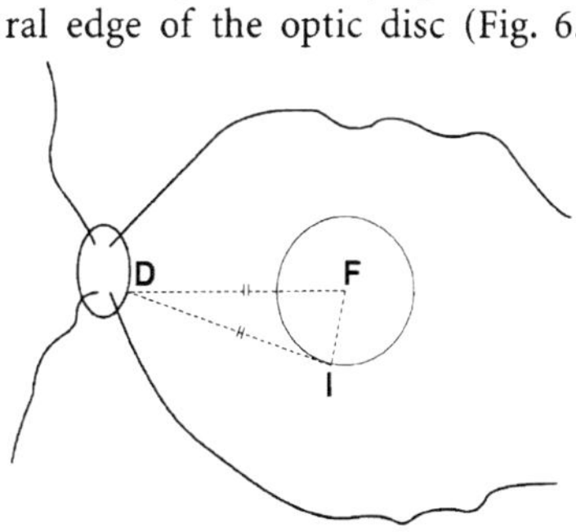

Fig. 6.2. Schematic diagram showing fundus of the left eye. *F* is the foveal center, *D* is a point on the temporal edge of the optic disc, and *I* is a point on the inferior border of the subfoveal lesion (*circle*) such that DF=DI. The distance *FI* is the minimum desired translocation for an inferior translocation

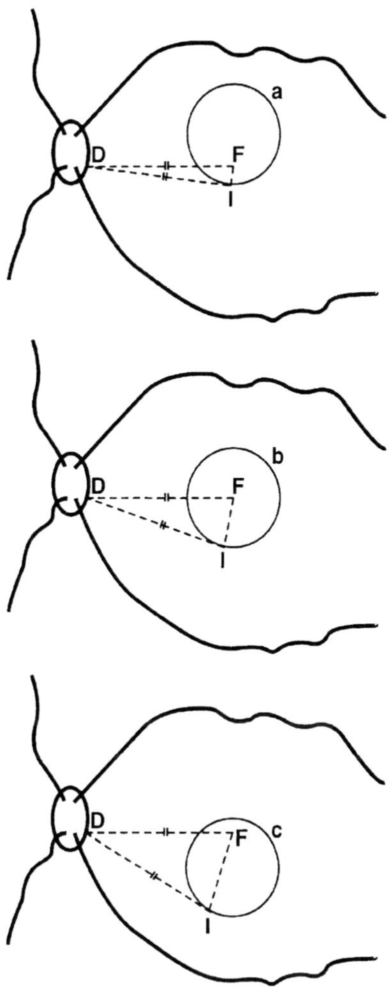

Fig. 6.3. Schematic diagram showing the fundi of three eyes with subfoveal lesions (*circles a, b*, and *c*) of equal size but different eccentricity relative to the foveal center (*F*). Lesion a (*top*) is centered eccentrically upwards relative to F, lesion b (*middle*) is centered on F, and lesion c (*bottom*) is centered eccentrically downwards relative to F. *D* is a point on the temporal edge of the optic disc and *I* is a point on the inferior border of the subfoveal lesions such that DF=DI. The minimum desired translocation (*FI*) for inferior translocation is smallest for lesion a and greatest for lesion c. Lesion a is therefore more likely to achieve effective macular translocation compared to lesions b and c following inferior macular translocation

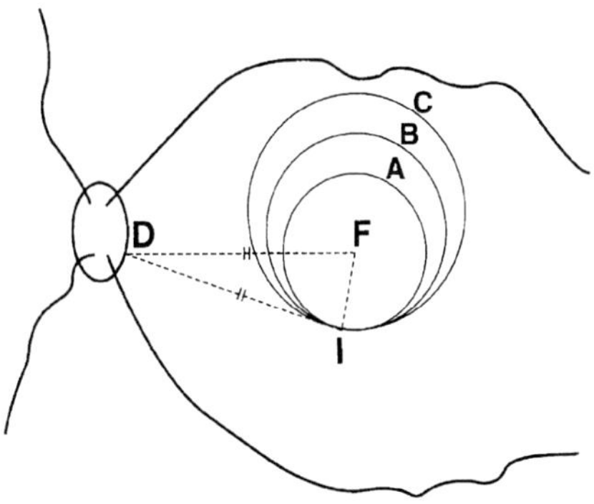

Fig. 6.4. Schematic diagram showing ocular fundus with three possible subfoveal lesions (*circles A*, *B*, and *C*) of different sizes and eccentricities. *F* is the foveal center, *D* is a point on the temporal edge of the optic disc, and *I* is a point on the inferior border of the subfoveal lesions such that DF=DI. The minimum desired translocations (*FI*) for inferior translocation for lesions A, B, and C are identical. These lesions therefore have the same likelihood of achieving effective macular translocation following inferior macular translocation

distance for the macular translocation to be effective.

6.5.2.2 Median Postoperative Foveal Displacement

A surgeon who is aware of the *median* postoperative foveal displacement he has achieved in his previous cases will have some idea of the likelihood of effective macular translocation for a particular *minimum* desired translocation. The median postoperative foveal displacement can be derived by analyzing data collected retrospectively or prospectively in a series of consecutive cases operated by the surgeon.

We estimate the postoperative foveal displacement from the preoperative and postoperative fluorescein angiograms without resorting to sophisticated imaging equipment. First we measure the distance between a predetermined "retinal" landmark such as a retinal vascular bifurcation situated superior to the macular lesion and a fixed "choroidal" landmark such as the inferior edge of the CNV or a laser scar on the preoperative fluorescein angiogram. We then use the same landmarks to obtain a similar measurement on the postoperative angiogram. The absolute difference between these two measurements is an estimate of the amount of foveal displacement (Fig. 6.5). The size and characteristics of the CNV on the postoperative angiogram tend not to change significantly if the time between the preoperative and postoperative angiograms is short.

If the median postoperative foveal displacement achieved by a surgeon in previous cases is *equal* to the minimum desired translocation in a particular case, barring any complication, the eye theoretically has about a 50% chance of achieving effective macular translocation following the surgery. It should be noted that because the size and shape of the RPE defect accompanying CNV removal may differ significantly from those of the CNV, the minimum desired translocation might change following CNV removal. In addition, the median postoperative foveal displacement for a particular surgeon is not static and may change with experience or technical modifications in macular translocation surgery.

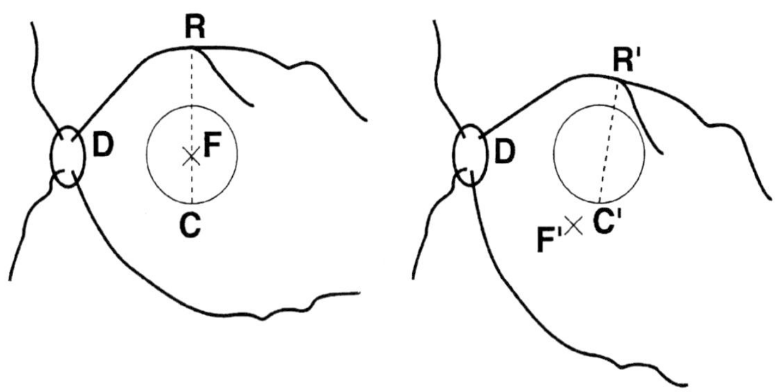

Fig. 6.5. Schematic diagram showing the fundus of an eye before (*left*) and after (*right*) inferior macular translocation. *R* is a point on a retinal vascular bifurcation ("retinal" landmark) situated superior to the subfoveal lesion (*circle*). *C* is a point on the inferior border of the subfoveal lesion ("choroidal" landmark) such that the line *RC* is close to and roughly parallel to the "path" of the foveal displacement. *F* and *F'* are the foveal centers before and after macular translocation respectively. *R'* and *C'* are the same retinal and choroidal landmarks respectively following macular translocation. The absolute difference between the distances RC and R'C' estimates the postoperative foveal displacement achieved

6.6 Surgical Principles and Operative Technique of Limited Macular Translocation

Since the initial descriptions of the technique of limited macular translocation (DE JUAN et al. 1998; IMAI and DE JUAN 1996; Imai et al. 1998), modifications and refinements have evolved as our experience with the surgery increased (DE JUAN and VANDER 1999; HARLAN et al. 1999a; PIERAMICI et al. in press). Although limited macular translocation may be either inferior or superior relative to the underlying RPE and choroid, our experience shows that inferior translocation achieves a greater median postoperative foveal displacement than superior translocation for the same amount of scleral imbrication used. With the usual upright postoperative head positioning, the weight of the subretinal fluid in a partially air-filled eye pulls the retina downwards. This probably contributes to the greater downward displacement of the fovea during inferior translocation and reduces the upward displacement of the fovea during superior translocation. For this reason, we currently perform inferior limited macular translocation for the vast majority of eyes undergoing macular translocation surgery and rarely perform superior limited macular translocation, except for the very occasional case in which the CNV is markedly eccentrically centered inferiorly relative to the fovea. The subsequent discussion in this chapter will be confined to inferior limited macular translocation.

Our current technique for inferior limited macular translocation is as follows: a limbal conjunctival peritomy is made to expose about three quadrants of the sclera for scleral imbrication and for the three sclerostomies for standard pars plana vitrectomy. The limbal peritomy is made from the 7 o'clock position clockwise to the 4 o'clock position for surgery in the right eye and from the 8 o'clock position clockwise to the 5 o'clock position in the left eye. The superior and lateral recti are isolated on 2-0 silk sutures to help with movement of the globe and surgical exposure. Five nonabsorbable imbricating (mattress) 5-0 dexon or 4-0 silk sutures are placed on the sclera prior to pars plana vitrectomy. The imbricating sutures straddle the equator of the globe and are first placed partial-thickness through the sclera circumferentially 3 mm posterior to the insertions of the recti, and then 6 mm posterior to the anterior scleral bite. Three imbricating sutures are placed in this fashion between the superior and lateral recti, one is placed medial to the superior rectus, and the final one is placed inferior to the lateral rectus (Fig. 6.6). The imbricating sutures are initially left untightened until the planned subtotal retinal detachment has been achieved.

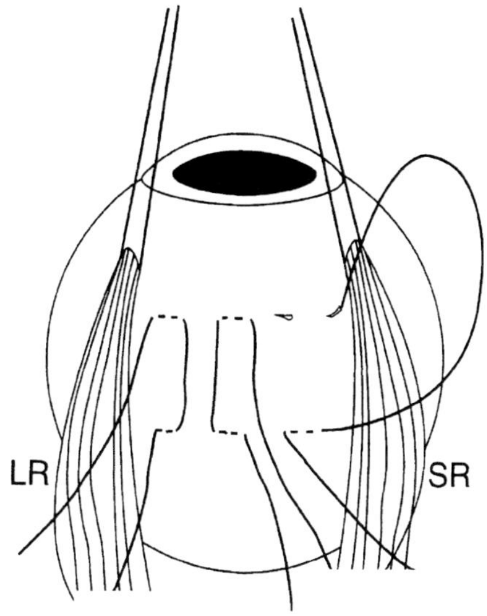

Fig. 6.6. Nonabsorbable imbricating sutures are placed straddling the equator of the globe prior to pars plana vitrectomy. The anterior scleral bites are placed 3 mm posterior to the recti insertion and the posterior scleral bites are placed 6 mm posterior to the anterior bites. Three imbricating sutures are placed between the superior rectus (*SR*) and lateral rectus (*LR*). The fourth imbricating suture is placed medial to the superior rectus and the final one is placed inferior to the lateral rectus (not shown)

Conventional three-port pars plana vitrectomy is then performed with a wide-angle viewing system, taking special care to peel the posterior hyaloid face off the posterior pole if a posterior vitreous detachment is not already present in the eye. Temporal to an imaginary vertical line bisecting the optic disc the retina is detached by injecting balanced salt solution under the retina through several tiny retinotomies with a 41 gauge retinal hydrodissection cannula (MADLAB, Bausch and Lomb Surgical, St. Louis, Mo., USA) (Figs. 6.7, 6.8). We usually place one retinotomy near the superotemporal vascular arcade to detach the superior retina up to or near the ora serrata, taking special care to detach the peripheral retina beyond the zone of intended scleral imbrication (Fig. 6.9). A second retinotomy is placed near the inferotemporal vascular arcade to detach the inferior retina, and one or more retinotomies are placed a few disc diameters temporal to the fovea to detach the temporal retina (Fig. 6.10). The total number of retinotomies required to achieve the desired planned subtotal retinal detachment ranges from three to

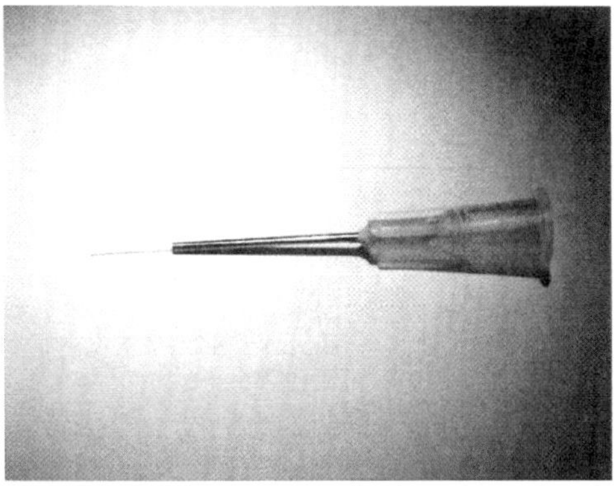

Fig. 6.7. Forty-one gauge retinal hydrodissection cannula (MADLAB retinal hydrodissection cannula, Bausch and Lomb Surgical, St, Louis, MO, USA)

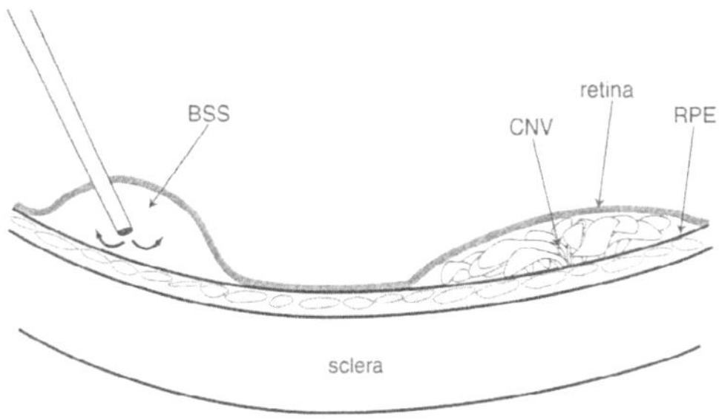

Fig. 6.8. The retina is detached by injecting balanced salt solution (*BSS*) between the neurosensory retina and the retinal pigment epithelium (*RPE*) with a 41-gauge retinal hydrodissection cannula through a tiny retinotomy. *CNV* choroidal neovascularization

eight, with an average of about four. The retinal "bullae" created by subretinal hydrodissection in this fashion tend to expand outward toward the retinal periphery instead of toward the fovea, presumably because the macula has greater adherence to the underlying RPE than the peripheral retina. The macula is therefore rarely fully detached by subretinal hydrodissection alone. To detach the macula fully, a complete fluid-air exchange is performed and the subretinal fluid is allowed to gravitate posteriorly and dissect the macula from the underlying RPE (Fig. 6.11). The separate retinal "bullae" will often coalesce and become a large retinal detachment after the fluid-air exchange, although it may take 4–5 min before this is achieved. To minimize posterior capsular opacification in phakic patients during fluid-air exchange, we use an air humidifying chamber (MoistAir, RetinaLabs.com, Atlanta, Ga., USA) (Fig. 6.12) (Harlan et al. 1999b). The humidified air may also potentially reduce excessive nerve fiber layer dehydration during this stage of the procedure.

To achieve effective macular translocation, it is important to detach the macula completely up to the temporal margin of the optic disc (Fig. 6.13). Failure to do so is likely to jeopardize the anatomic outcome of the operation. In this regard, prior laser photocoagulation to a previously juxtafoveal or extrafoveal CNV with resultant abnormal chorioretinal adhesions can increase the difficulty of detaching the macula

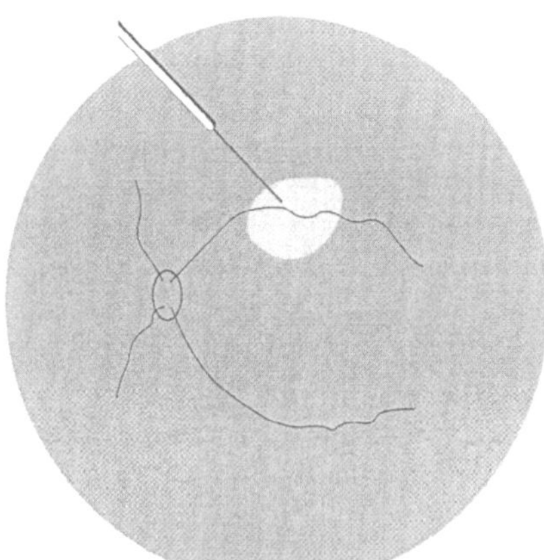

Fig. 6.9. The first retinotomy for subretinal hydrodissection is placed near the superotemporal vascular arcade to detach the superior retina

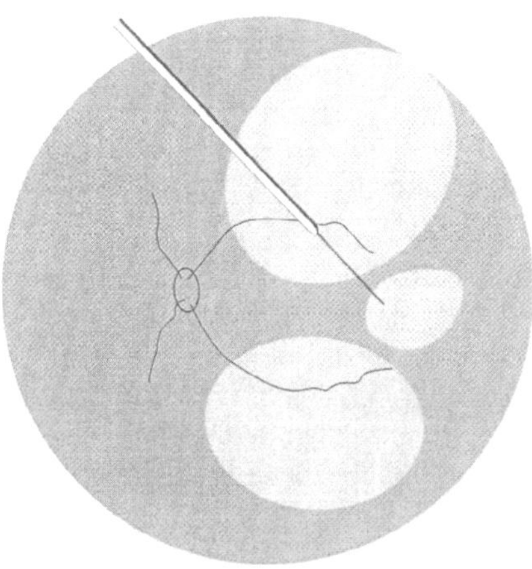

Fig. 6.10. The third retinotomy for subretinal hydrodissection is placed a few disc diameters temporally to the fovea to detach the temporal retina. The inferior retina had been detached earlier with a retinotomy near the inferotemporal vascular arcade. Note that the retinal detachment from the first retinotomy extends anteriorly beyond the zone of intended scleral imbrication

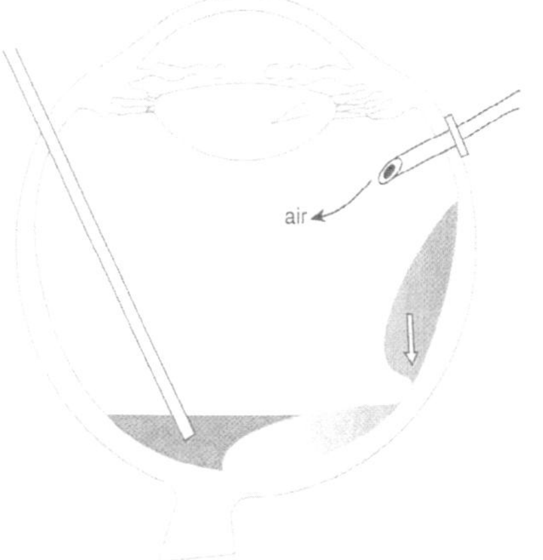

Fig. 6.11. A complete fluid-air exchange allows the subretinal fluid to gravitate posteriorly (*arrow*) and dissect the macula from the underlying retinal pigment epithelium

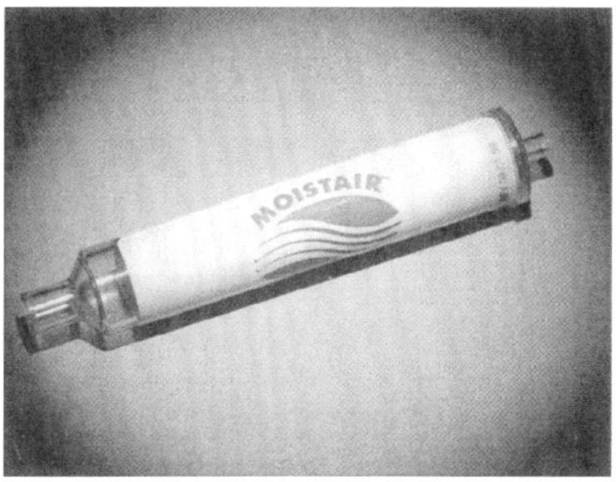

Fig. 6.12. Air humidifier (MoistAir humidifying chamber, RetinaLabs.com, Atlanta, GA, USA)

during surgery. This should be considered preoperatively, although it is not an absolute contraindication to surgery. Chorioretinal adhesion from recent (several weeks) laser photocoagulation is usually not strong and the weight of the subretinal fluid during fluid-air exchange will often be sufficient to dissect the macula off the underlying RPE. In cases with strong chorioretinal adhesions in the macula, gentle traction of the retina as well as the scar with a retinal manipulator (Bausch and Lomb Surgical, St Louis, Mo., USA) (Figs. 6.14, 6.15) or subretinal blunt dissection using a blunt pick between the retina and RPE through a tiny eccentric retinotomy will usually detach the macula completely (Fig. 6.16) (Lewis et al. 1999).

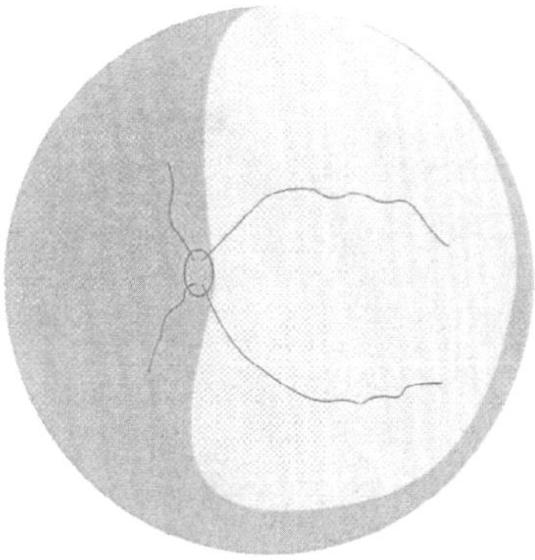

Fig. 6.13. A large retinal detachment temporal to an imaginary vertical line bisecting the optic disc is obtained following coalescence of the multiple smaller localized retinal detachments. It is important to ensure that the macula is completely detached and that the retinal detachment extends anteriorly beyond the zone of intended scleral imbrication

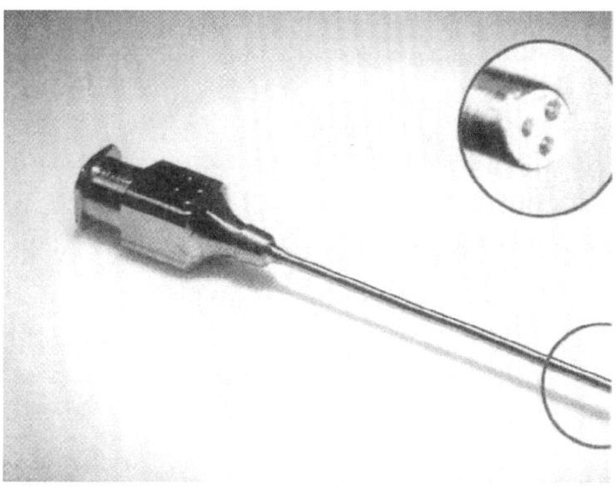

Fig. 6.14. Retinal manipulator (Bausch and Lomb Surgical, St. Louis, MO, USA). The tip of the instrument is enlarged to show the three small openings of the retinal manipulator

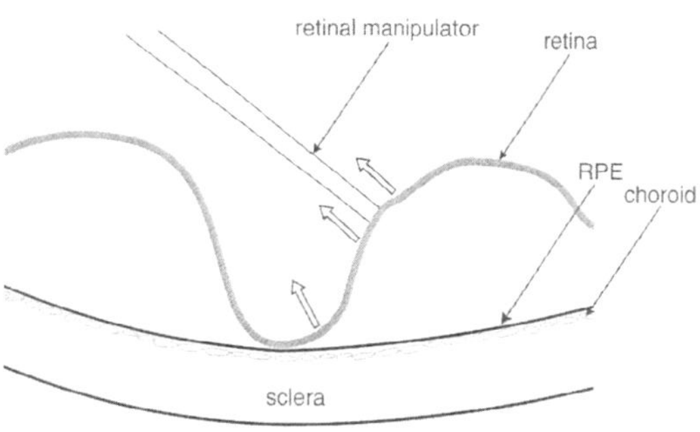

Fig. 6.15. Gentle traction on the retina (*white arrows*) with a retinal manipulator helps to break abnormal chorioretinal adhesions and fully detach the macula from the retinal pigment epithelium (*RPE*)

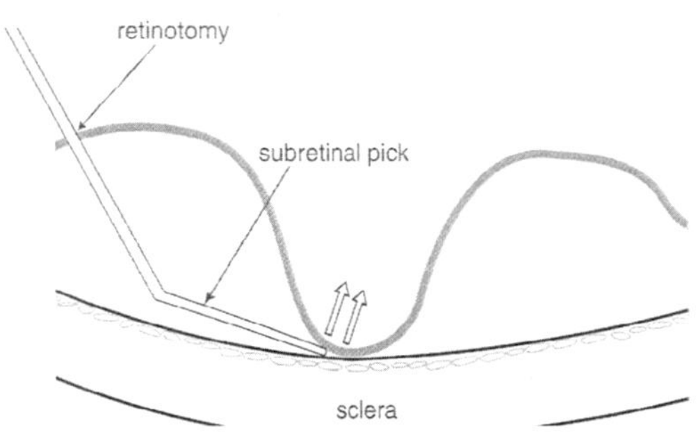

Fig. 6.16. Subretinal blunt dissection (*white arrows*) with a pick through a small eccentric retinotomy may be necessary to break abnormal chorioretinal adhesions in the macula

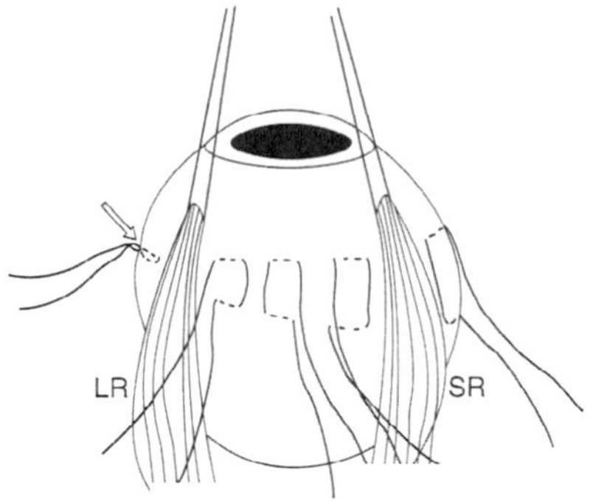

Fig. 6.17. Tightening the imbricating sutures (*arrow*) causes the sclera to be imbricated under the detached retina and creates redundancy of the retina relative to the eyewall (sclera, choroid, and retinal pigment epithelium). *LR* lateral rectus, *SR* superior rectus

When detaching the retina, care should be taken to avoid inadvertently detaching the superior retina nasal to the imaginary vertical line bisecting the optic disc, as this is associated with a higher incidence of postoperative macular or foveal fold.

After detaching the macula completely, the intravitreal air is replaced with fluid and the eye is left soft momentarily to allow the imbricating sutures to be tightened (Fig. 6.17). Tightening the imbricating sutures causes imbrication of the sclera beneath the detached retina, producing a redundancy of the retina that allows the fovea to be displaced relative to the choroid. This stage of the procedure is probably the most hazardous, as prolonged hypotony may be complicated by suprachoroidal and subretinal hemorrhages, especially if subretinal dissection has been performed. In addition, retinal incarceration is possible at this stage, especially at the superotemporal sclerostomy.

Following scleral imbrication, fluid-air exchange is repeated and the vitreous cavity is filled with air to about 75%–90% of capacity (Fig. 6.18). The subretinal fluid is not drained. Because the retinotomies created during subretinal hydrodissection or subretinal manipulation are self-sealing, no retinopexy is necessary.

After the final fluid-air exchange, the sclerostomies and conjunctival incisions are closed with absorbable sutures, and a combination corticosteroid-antibiotic subconjunctival injection is given to the eye. The eye is then patched and the patient turned onto the side of the operative eye for about 4–5 min to allow the subretinal fluid to gravitate temporally to detach the temporal peripheral retina. From this position (without turning the patient onto his back), the patient is sat upright and instructed to keep his head upright overnight. Besides allowing the temporal peripheral retina to be completely detached, this maneuver also causes all the subretinal fluid to accumulate in the inferior retina, reducing the risk of a macular or foveal fold postoperatively (Fig. 6.19). If the superonasal retina has been inadvertently detached during surgery, sitting the patient upright from the supine position may cause some subretinal fluid to be trapped under the superonasal retina, causing a retinal "bulla" or retinal fold to overhang from the superonasal retina. This "bulla" or fold will often cause a retinal fold to stretch from the superior margin of the optic disc into the macula. When such a macular or foveal fold persists postoperatively, severe visual impairment is often present and remedial surgery may be necessary to remove the fold.

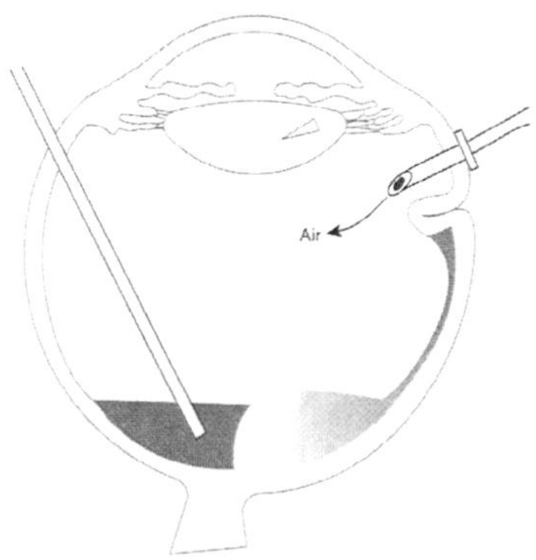

Fig. 6.18. Following scleral imbrication, a final subtotal fluid-air exchange is performed without draining the subretinal fluid

When the patient's head is upright, the weight of the subretinal fluid pulls the retina downward in the air-filled eye (Fig. 6.20). The superior retina is the first to become reattached, and this is quickly followed by the macula and the rest of the retina over the next several days.

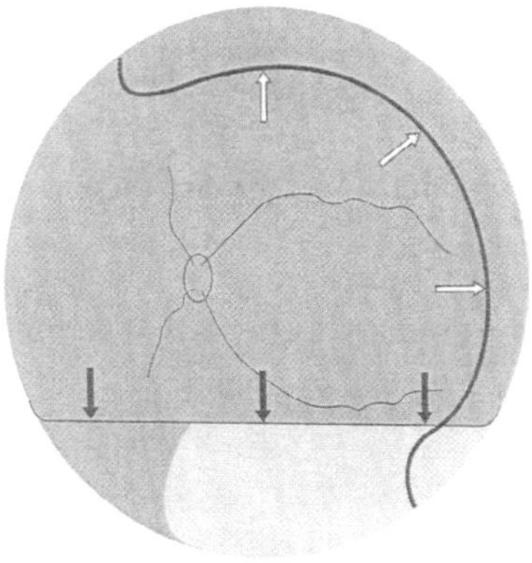

Fig. 6.19. The immediate postoperative head-positioning maneuver (see text) causes all the subretinal fluid to accumulate under the inferior retina. The inferior retina is detached. Note the scleral imbrication (*white arrows*) and the fluid-air interface in the vitreous cavity (*black arrows*)

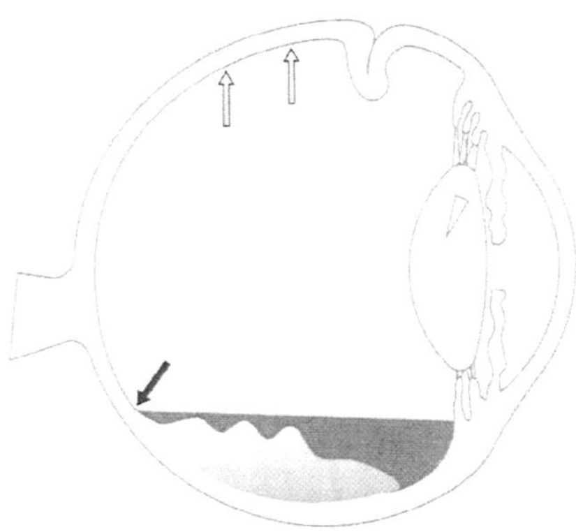

Fig. 6.20. With the head in an upright position following surgery, the buoyancy of the air bubble supports the superior retina (*white arrows*) while the weight of the subretinal fluid stretches the retina downwards (*black arrow*), displacing the fovea downwards relative to the underlying eyewall (sclera, choroid, and retinal pigment epithelium)

We perform anterior-posterior shortening of the eye wall with scleral imbrication for the vast majority of cases. However, it is interesting to note that this is not always necessary, and effective macular translocation may still be achieved without scleral imbrication for subfoveal lesions with very small minimum desired translocations (DE JUAN and VANDER 1999).

Although it is possible to combine inferior limited macular translocation with removal of the CNV during the surgery (LEWIS et al. 1999), we prefer to treat the CNV postoperatively with laser photocoagulation. The retinotomy for CNV removal often enlarges inadvertently as the CNV is extracted, and postoperative face-down positioning to tamponade the enlarged retinotomy may reduce the amount of inferior foveal displacement. In addition, the avulsed choroidal feeder vessels may bleed when the eye is left soft momentarily during tightening of the imbricating sutures. The unpredictability of the size of the RPE defect that may occur can reduce the likelihood of achieving effective macular translocation.

6.7 Postoperative Management of Limited Macular Translocation

6.7.1 Postoperative Head Positioning

Following surgery, patients are routinely instructed to keep their heads upright overnight until the first postoperative day. Some have found anorthopedic cervical collar helpful for the upright head positioning. After the first postoperative day, patients can lie on their sides, preferably with the cheek opposite the operative eye resting on the pillow to allow the air bubble to tamponade the macula. Patients are discouraged from lying supine before the air bubble is completely absorbed, which usually takes 4–7 days.

6.7.2 Postoperative Review, Fluorescein Angiography, and Laser Photocoagulation

Patients are reviewed on the first postoperative day for early complications of surgery such as raised intraocular pressure, infection, rhegmatogenous retinal detachment, and intraocular hemorrhage. The visual acuity at this point is often in the range of counting fingers to hand motion because the air bubble fills about half of the vitreous cavity and the macula may still be detached. Usually the inferior retina is shallowly detached. Complete reattachment of the retina is often achieved by the third postoperative day. A fold of redundant retina is sometimes present in the inferior periphery following retinal reattachment.

Our routine postoperative fluorescein angiogram is obtained on the third to sixth postoperative day. It is not necessary to wait for the entire air bubble to be absorbed before fluorescein angiography is performed. On the other hand, a large air bubble may obscure the superior portion of a large CNV, preventing laser ablation to the entire lesion. In this situation, additional laser treatment to the obscured portion of the CNV may be necessary later when the air bubble becomes smaller. CNV that have become juxtafoveal or extrafoveal are ablated with laser photocoagulation following the guidelines outlined in the MPS (Macular Photocoagulation Study Group 1990). Following laser treatment, the patient is reviewed about 3–4 weeks later with repeat fluorescein angiography to detect persist or recurrent CNV.

6.7.3 Management of Persistent or Recurrent Subfoveal Choroidal Neovascularization

When the CNV remains under the foveal center postoperatively due to insufficient macular translocation or when CNV recurs under the displaced foveal center following surgery and laser treatment, further management options include observation, laser ablation, submacular surgery, and photodynamic therapy. In many of these cases, the area of destruction of the perifoveal tissues by laser photocoagulation may be less than if macular translocation had not been performed before the laser treatment. Photodynamic therapy appears to be a reasonable option, although we do not currently know if prior limited macular translocation alters the response of the eye to this treatment modality. Repeat macular translocation is not recommended, because of the high risk of retinal detachment and PVR. Extrafoveal or juxtafoveal recurrences are treated with laser photocoagulation.

6.7.4 Postoperative Sensory Adaptation

Some patients, especially those with good vision bilaterally, may experience postoperative diplopia and/or cyclotropia following limited macular translocation. Because the amount of foveal displacement is smaller in this procedure than in macular translocation with 360° peripheral circumferential retinotomy, the incidence of this complication is lower and the symptoms less severe following limited macular translocation. In addition, the symptoms tend to disappear spontaneously within a few months (Lewis et al. 1999). Prisms may be used to relieve diplopia in those few patients with persistent symptoms, but corrective muscle surgery as described by Eckardt et al. (1999) is not necessary.

6.8 Outcomes of Limited Macular Translocation

The potential for significant visual improvement is the greatest advantage of macular translocation surgery over other current experimental or established treatment for ARMD (Figs. 6.21–6.23). Although some authors have found limited macular translocation unpredictable (Lewis et al. 1999), others have had more encouraging results (de Juan et al. 1998; Pieramici et al. in press).

Pieramici et al. (in press) reported the outcomes of inferior limited macular translocation for new or recurrent CNV secondary to ARMD by a single surgeon in 102 consecutive eyes of 101 patients aged 41–89 years (median 76 years) (Pieramici et al. in press). The postoperative foveal displacement achieved ranged from 200 μm to 2800 μm, with a median of 1200 μm. Effective macular translocation was achieved in 62% of eyes. Thirty-one percent of the eyes achieved a visual acuity greater than 20/100 at 3 months postoperatively while 49% achieved this vision at 6 months postoperatively. At 3 and 6 months postoperatively, 37% and 48% of the eyes respectively experienced two or more Snellen lines of visual improvement and, at 6 months postoperatively, 16% experienced six or more lines of improvement.

Pieramici et al. (in press) found that factors associated with better visual acuity at 3 and 6 months postoperatively were good preoperative visual acuity, achievement of the desired amount of translocation, a greater amount of postoperative foveal displacement, and recurrent CNV at baseline. Poor preoperative visual acuity and the development of complications either during or after surgery were associated with worse visual acuity at 3 and 6 months postoperatively (Lewis et al. 1999; Pieramici et al. in press). The subfoveal disease in patients with recurrent CNV at baseline may be of shorter duration and less severe than in those with new CNV, since this group of patients with previous laser photocoagulation for juxtafoveal or extrafoveal lesions were more likely to be aware of the need for early treatment and were on close follow-up by their ophthalmologists.

Lewis et al. (1999) reported the outcome of a smaller series of ten eyes of ten patients with subfoveal CNV secondary to ARMD treated by one surgeon. The postoperative foveal displacement in this prospective series ranged from 114 μm to 1919 μm, with a median of 1286 μm. The best-corrected visual acuity, as measured with the Early Treatment Diabetic Retinopathy Study chart, improved in four

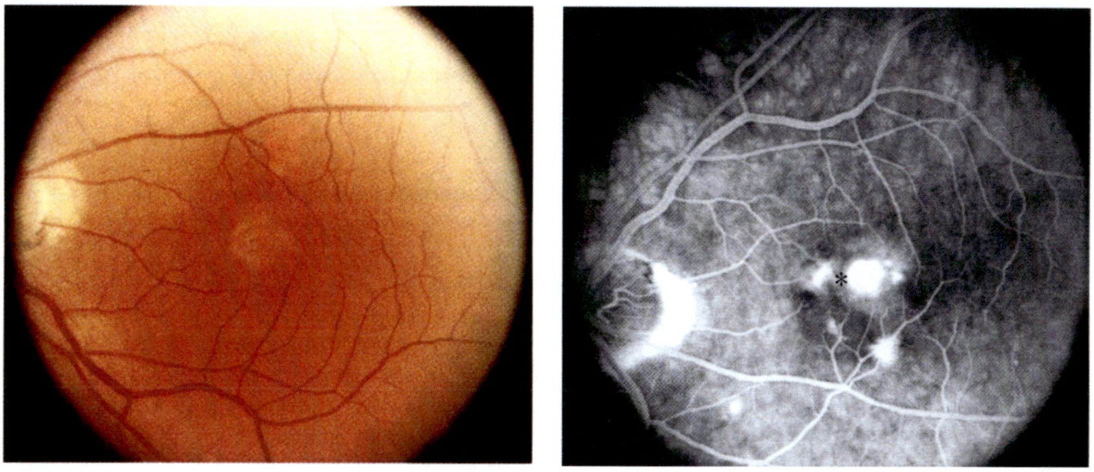

Fig. 6.21. Fundus photograph (*left*) and fluorescein angiogram (*right*) of a 57-year-old man at presentation demonstrate a choroidal neovascular membrane secondary to age-related macular degeneration under the geometric center of the foveal avascular zone (*asterisk*) in the left eye. Visual acuity is 20/80

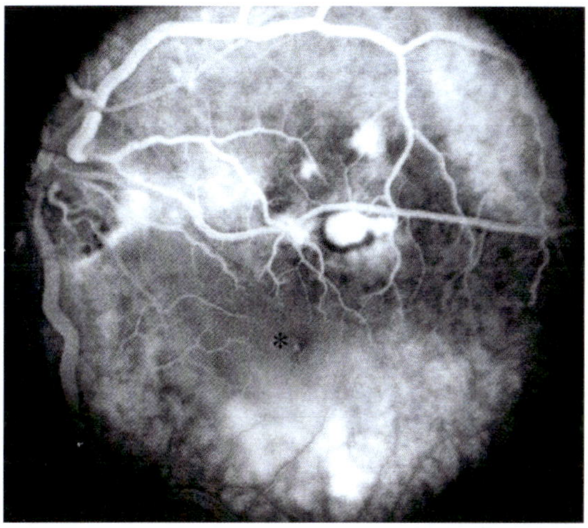

Fig. 6.22. Fluorescein angiogram of the same eye as in Fig. 6.21, 3 days following inferior limited macular translocation demonstrates effective macular translocation with displacement of the geometric center of the foveal avascular zone (*asterisk*) to an area inferior to the choroidal neovascular membrane

Fig. 6.23. Fundus photograph (*left*) and fluorescein angiogram (*right*) of the same eye as in Fig. 6.21, 7 months after inferior limited macular translocation show successful laser ablation of the choroidal neovascular membrane with no evidence of recurrence. The geometric center of the foveal avascular zone (*asterisk*) is preserved. Visual acuity is 20/60

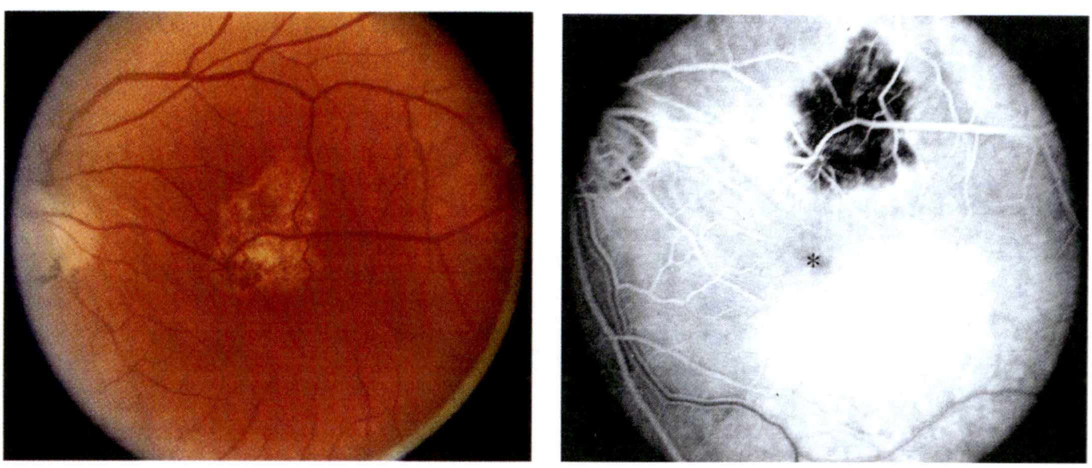

eyes (median, 10.5 letters) and decreased in six eyes (median, 14.5 letters). The median change in visual acuity was a decrease of 5 letters for the entire series. Six months postoperatively, visual acuity was 20/80 in two eyes, 20/126 in one eye, 20/160 in four eyes, and 20/200, 20/250, and 20/640 in one eye each. Although a direct comparison cannot be made between these results and those of the MPS, it is worthwhile noting that the mean visual acuity of 83 untreated eyes in the subfoveal new CNV study was 20/500 at the 48-month follow-up examination, with 89.2% of these eyes having visual acuity of 20/200 or worse (Macular Photocoagulation Study Group 1993).

6.9 Complications of Limited Macular Translocation

A number of intraoperative and postoperative complications are associated with limited macular translocation (Table 6.1). Some of these, such as unplanned retinal breaks and scleral perforation, are common to vitreoretinal procedures involving pars plana vitrectomy and placement of partial-thickness scleral sutures, while a few, such as new CNV formation at the retinotomy site for subretinal hydrodissection and postoperative transient formed visual hallucinations, are more confined to limited macular translocation.

Table 6.1. Complications associated with limited macular translocation

Timing of complication	Complication
Intraoperative	Scleral perforation Unplanned retinal break Suprachoroidal hemorrhage Subretinal hemorrhage Vitreous hemorrhage Macular hole Unplanned translocation of retinal pigment epithelium
Postoperative	Rhegmatogenous retinal detachment Proliferative vitreoretinopathy Endophthalmitis Cataract Vitreous hemorrhage Macular or foveal fold New CNV at site of retinotom Acute angle-closure glaucoma Transient formed visual hallucinations

The intraoperative and postoperative complications documented in the series reported by Pieramici et al. (in press) are summarized in Table 6.2.

6.9.1 Intraoperative Complications

Inadvertent scleral perforation during suture placement for scleral imbrication may be complicated by suprachoroidal hemorrhage, vitreous hemorrhage, and retinal break. Unintended retinal break may also be caused by the vitreous cutter, vitreous traction near the sclerostomies, retinal incarceration at the sclerostomies, and retinal manipulation during planned retinal detachment (Lewis et al. 1999). Retinal break(s) should be treated with laser retinopexy or cryoretinopexy, either intraoperatively or during the early postoperative period. In addition, a longer-acting gas such as sulfur hexafluoride should be used for internal tamponade. Failure to treat an unplanned non-self-sealing retinal break may result in postoperative rhegmatogenous retinal detachment. Of 102 consecutive cases in the series reported by Pieramici et al. (in press), unintended retinal breaks occurred in ten eyes. Long-acting gas may also be necessary for eyes complicated by macular hole formation (Figs. 6.24, 6.25).

The retinal hydrodissection cannula used for subretinal hydrodissection and the subretinal pick used for blunt subretinal dissection during planned detachment of the retina can inadvertently traumatize the vascular choroid and cause subretinal hemorrhage. A patch of RPE abnormally adherent to the overlying neurosensory retina may be avulsed when the retina detaches, resulting in unplanned translocation of the RPE (Harlan et al. 1999a).

The short period when the eye is deliberately kept soft to allow the imbricating sutures to be tightened is considered by some surgeons to be the most hazardous part of the operation. This is because the eye is at risk of severe intraocular hemorrhage, including suprachoroidal and subretinal hemorrhages during this state of hypotony. In addition, retinal incarceration at the sclerostomies may occur, and it is possible that negative pressure within the eye during this maneuver may aspirate fluids or air from outside the eye into the vitreous cavity and increase the risk of postoperative endophthalmitis.

Table 6.2. Intra- and postoperative complications associated with inferior limited macular translocation in Pieramici and associates' series (n=102)

Types of complication	Intraoperative (n eyes)	Postoperative (n eyes)	Total (n eyes)
Macular hole	9	0	9
Scleral perforation	2	0	2
Choroidal hemorrhage	1	0	1
Subretinal hemorrhage	1	0	1
Unintended retinal break	6	4	10
Vitreous hemorrhage	2	2	4
Unplanned retinal detachment	0	9	9
Macular fold	0	3	3
New CNV at site of retinotomy	0	2	2

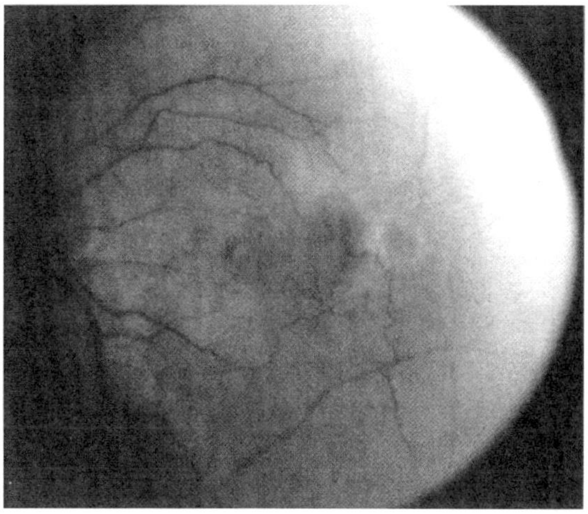

Fig. 6.24. Red-free photograph of a left eye at presentation demonstrates a subfoveal choroidal neovascular membrane. Visual acuity is 20/150

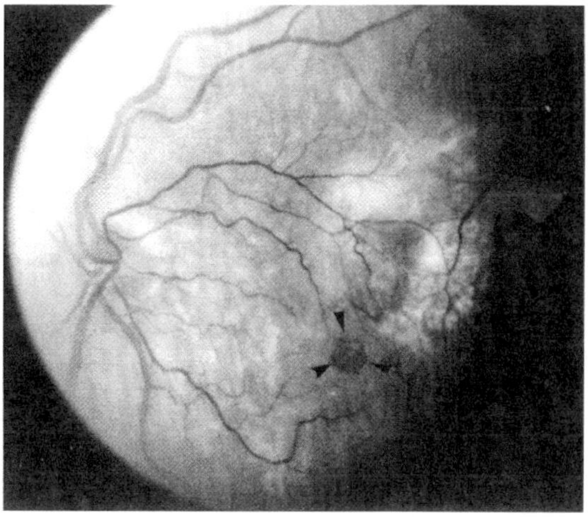

Fig. 6.25. Red-free photograph of the same eye as in Fig. 6.24, 3 months after inferior limited macular translocation and laser photocoagulation to the choroidal neovascular membrane shows a macular hole (*arrowheads*) that had formed during the surgery. Visual acuity is 20/125

6.9.2 Postoperative Complications

The most common serious postoperative complication of limited macular translocation is rhegmatogenous retinal detachment. Selected cases with breaks in the superior retinal periphery may be treated by pneumoretinopexy. When associated with PVR, repeat pars plana vitrectomy and membrane peeling is often necessary. Postoperative endophthalmitis, although rare, is another potentially sight-threatening complication.

The incidence of cataract formation appears to be similar to that following other vitrectomy procedures. Cataract in the immediate postoperative period can impair visualization of the ocular fundus and interfere with the subsequent management of the CNV. Early cataract extraction may be indicated in such cases. Other complications such as vitreous hemorrhage can also interfere with visualization of the fundus and management of the CNV.

Macular or foveal fold (Figs 6.26–6.28) can be associated with poor vision and was reported in three out of ten eyes by Lewis et al. (1999). Focal damage to Bruch's membrane by the retinal hydrodissection cannula may cause new CNV formation at the retinotomy site. We have seen a case of acute angle-closure glaucoma following limited macular translocation that may have been related to the scleral shortening. We have also seen two patients who developed formed visual hallucinations within 24 h after the procedure while the retina was detached in the immediate postoperative period. The hallucinations ceased completely following retinal reattachment 3–7 days postoperatively.

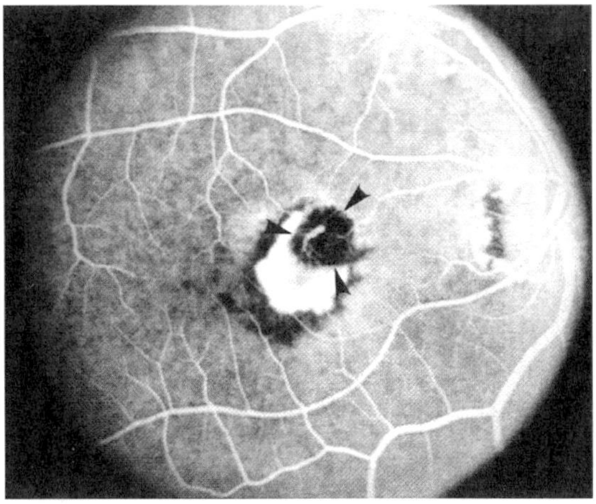

Fig. 6.26. Fluorescein angiogram of a right eye demonstrates a recurrent subfoveal age-related choroidal neovascular membrane adjacent to a scar (*arrowheads*) from previous laser photocoagulation. Visual acuity is 20/150

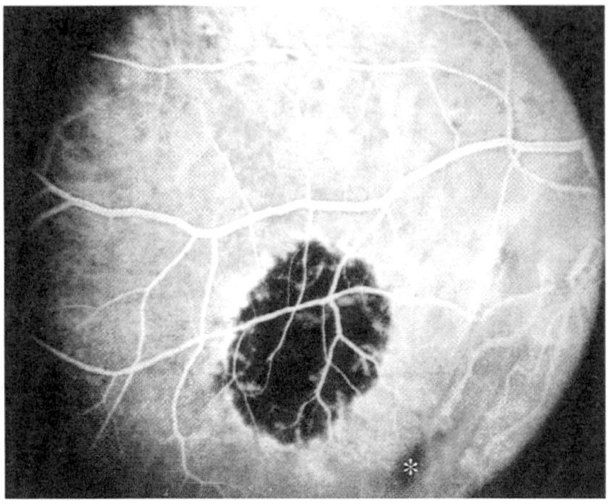

Fig. 6.28. Fluorescein angiogram of the same eye as in Fig. 6.26, 3 months after inferior limited macular translocation shows successful laser ablation of the choroidal neovascular membrane with no evidence of recurrence. The geometric center of the foveal avascular zone (*asterisk*) is preserved. The macular fold just spares the foveal center (*asterisk*). Visual acuity is 20/32

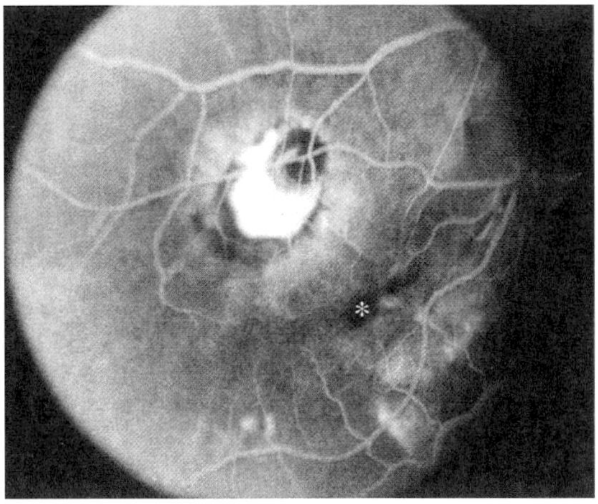

Fig. 6.27. Fluorescein angiogram of the same eye as in Fig. 6.26, 3 days following inferior limited macular translocation demonstrates effective macular translocation with displacement of the geometric center of the foveal avascular zone (*asterisk*) inferonasally to the choroidal neovascular membrane. Submacular dissection of the chorioretinal adhesion with a pick was necessary to achieve complete macular detachment during surgery. Note the small macular fold near the foveal center (*asterisk*)

6.10 Conclusion

Limited macular translocation is a promising new option for the management of recent-onset subfoveal CNV secondary to ARMD. It is currently the only treatment with the potential to restore excellent vision in these individuals. It is in early stages of development, and continued modifications and refinements are likely to make it safer and more predictable. Besides treatment of subfoveal CNV from a variety of etiologies, its use may be extended to other foveal diseases in the future. A few surgeons including Machemer (1998) have expressed hope that macular translocation surgery may one day also be applied as prophylaxis in diseases such as relentlessly progressive non-neovascular ARMD or other inherited subfoveal diseases such as Best disease, Stargardt disease and central areolar chorioretinal dystrophy. We hope that the precise role of limited macular translocation in ophthalmology can be established in the near future with further experience and more controlled evaluation of this procedure.

Acknowledgements. The authors wish to thank Morvarid Behmanesh, MA, from the Johns Hopkins Microsurgery Advanced Design Laboratory (http://www.madlab.jhu.edu), the Wilmer Ophthalmological Institute, and the Johns Hopkins University School of Medicine, Baltimore, Maryland, for the illustrations. K.-G. Au Eong was supported by a National Medical Research Council–Singapore Totalisator Board Medical Research Fellowship.

Figures 6.2–6.20 and Tables 6.1 and 6.2 are reprinted with permission from: Au Eong KG, Pieramici DJ, Fujii GY, de Juan Jr E (2001) Limited macular translocation. In: Lim JI (ed) Age-related macular degeneration. Marcel Dekker Inc., New York (in press)

References

Beatty S, Au Eong KG, McLeod D, Bishop PN (1999) Photocoagulation of subfoveal choroidal neovascular membranes in age-related macular degeneration: The impact of the macular photocoagulation study in the United Kingdom and Republic of Ireland. Br J Ophthalmol 83(10):1103–1104

Berger AS, Kaplan HJ (1992) Clinical experience with the surgical removal of subfoveal neovascular membranes. Ophthalmology 99(6):969–976

Blinder KJ, Peyman GA, Paris CL, Gremillion CM (1991) Submacular scar excision in age-related macular degeneration. Int Ophthalmol 15(4):215–222

Cekic O, Ohji M, Hayashi A, Fujikado T, Tano Y (1999) Foveal translocation surgery in age-related macular degeneration. Lancet 354(9175):340–340

Chan CK, Kempin SJ, Noble SK, Palmer GA (1994) The treatment of choroidal neovascular membranes by alpha interferon. Ophthalmology 101(2):289–300

Char DH, Irvine AI, Posner MD, Quivey J, Phillips TL, Kroll S (1999) Randomized trial of radiation for age-related macular degeneration. Am J Ophthalmol 127(5):574–578

de Juan E, Machemer R (1988) Vitreous surgery for hemorrhagic and fibrous complications of age-related macular degeneration. Am J Ophthalmol 105(1):25–29

de Juan E, Vander JF (1999) Effective macular translocation without scleral imbrication. Am J Ophthalmol 128(3):380–382

de Juan E, Loewenstein A, Bressler NM, Alexander J (1998) Translocation of the retina for management of subfoveal choroidal neovascularization. II. A preliminary report in humans. Am J Ophthalmol 125(5):635–646

Eckardt C, Eckardt U, Conrad H-G (1999) Macular rotation with and without counter-rotation of the globe in patients with age-related macular degeneration. Graefe's Arch Clin Exp Ophthalmol 237(4):313–325

Fujikado T, Ohji M, Hayashi A, Kusaka S, Tano Y (1998a) Anatomic and functional recovery of the fovea after foveal translocation surgery without large retinotomy and simultaneous excision of a neovascular membrane. Am J Ophthalmol 126(6):839–842

Fujikado T, Ohji M, Saito Y, Hayashi A, Tano Y (1998b) Visual function after foveal translocation with scleral shortening in patients with myopic neovascular maculopathy. Am J Ophthalmol 125(5):647–656

Green WR, Enger C (1993) Age-related macular degeneration histopathologic studies. The 1992 Lorenz E. Zimmerman lecture. Ophthalmology 100(10):1519–1535

Harlan JB, de Juan E, Bressler NM (1999a) Retinal translocation with unplanned translocation of the retinal pigment epithelium. The Wilmer Retina Update 5(1):3–8

Harlan JB, Lee ET, Jensen PS, de Juan E (1999b) Effect of humidity on posterior lens opacification during fluid-air exchange. Arch Ophthalmol 117(6):802–804

Hawkins BS, Bird AC, Klein R, West SK (1999) Epidemiology of age-related macular degeneration. Mol Vis 3(5):26

Imai K, de Juan E (1996) Experimental surgical macular relocation by scleral shortening. ARVO abstracts. Invest Ophthalmol Vis Sci 37 [Suppl]:S116

Imai K, Loewenstein A, de Juan E (1998) Translocation of the retina for management of subfoveal choroidal neovascularization I: Experimental studies in the rabbit eye. Am J Ophthalmol 125(5):627–634

Kamei M, Roth DB, Lewis H (2000) Macular translocation using scleral clips to create an outpouching radial fold of the sclera, choroid, and retinal pigment epithelium. ARVO Abstracts. Invest Ophthalmol Vis Sci 41 [Suppl]:S540

Klein R, Klein BEK, Linton LKP (1992) Prevalence of age-related maculopathy. The Beaver Dam Eye Study. Ophthalmology 99(6):933–943

Krumpaszky HG, Ludtke R, Mickler A, Klauss V, Selbmann HK (1999) Blindness incidence in Germany: A population-based study from Wuerttemberg-Hohenzollern. Ophthalmologica 213(3):176–182

Lambert HM, Capone AJ, Aaberg TM, Sternberg PJ, Mandell BA, Lopez PF (1992) Surgical excision of subfoveal neovascular membranes in age-related macular degeneration. Am J Ophthalmol 113(3):257–262

Leibowitz HM, Krueger DE, Maunder LR, Milton RC, Kini MM, Kahn HA, Nickerson RJ, Pool J, Colton TL, Ganley JP, Loewenstein JI, Dawber TR (1980) The Framingham Eye Study Monograph: An ophthalmological and epidemiological study of cataract, glaucoma, diabetic retinopathy, macular degeneration, and visual acuity in a general population of 2631 adults. 1973–1975. Surv Ophthalmol 24 [Suppl]:335–610

Lewis H, Kaiser PK, Lewis S, Estafanous M (1999) Macular translocation for subfoveal choroidal neovascularization in age-related macular degeneration: A prospective study. Am J Ophthalmol 128(2):135–146

Lindsey P, Finkelstein D, D'Anna S (1983) Experimental retinal relocation. ARVO asbtracts. Invest Ophthalmol Vis Sci 24 [Suppl]:242–242

Loewenstein A, Sunness JS, Bressler NM, Marsh MJ, de Juan E (1998) Scanning laser ophthalmoscope fundus perimetry after surgery for choroidal neovascularization. Am J Ophthalmol 125(5):657–665

Machemer R (1998) Macular translocation (editorial). Am J Ophthalmol 125(5):698–700

Machemer R, Steinhorst UH (1993a) Retinal separation, retinotomy, and macular relocation: I. Experimental studies in the rabbit eye. Graefe's Arch Clin Exp Ophthalmol 231(11):629–634

Machemer R, Steinhorst UH (1993b) Retinal separation, retinotomy, and macular relocation: II. A surgical approach for age-related macular degeneration? Graefe's Arch Clin Exp Ophthalmol 231(11):635–641

Macular Photocoagulation Study Group (1990) Krypton laser photocoagulation for neovascular lesions of age-related macular degeneration: results of a randomized clinical trial. Arch Ophthalmol 108(6):816–824

Macular Photocoagulation Study Group (1991a) Argon laser photocoagulation for neovascular maculopathy: Five-year results from randomized clinical trials [published correction appears in Arch Ophthalmol 110:761]. Arch Ophthalmol 109(8):1109–1114

Macular Photocoagulation Study Group (1991b) Laser photocoagulation of subfoveal neovascular lesions in age-related macular degeneration: Results of a randomized clinical trial. Arch Ophthalmol 109(9):1220–1231

Macular Photocoagulation Study Group (1991c) Laser photocoagulation of subfoveal recurrent neovascular lesions in age-related macular degeneration: Results of a randomized clinical trial. Arch Ophthalmol 109(9):1232–1241

Macular Photocoagulation Study Group (1993) Laser photocoagulation of subfoveal neovascular lesions of age-related macular degeneration: updated findings from two clinical trials. Arch Ophthalmol 111(9):1200–1209

Macular Photocoagulation Study Group (1994a) Laser photocoagulation for juxtafoveal choroidal neovascularization: Five-year results from randomized clinical trials. Arch Ophthalmol 112(4):500–509

Macular Photocoagulation Study Group (1994b) Persistent and recurrent neovascularization after laser photocoagulation for subfoveal choroidal neovascularization of age-related macular degeneration. Arch Ophthalmol 112(4):489–499

Macular Photocoagulation Study Group (1994c) Visual outcome after laser photocoagulation for subfoveal choroidal neovascularization secondary to age-related macular degeneration: The influence of initial lesion size and initial visual acuity. Arch Ophthalmol 112(4):480–488

Meyer CH, Benner JD, Winter KP, Caldwell JV, Heinis RM, Toth CA (2000) Distance of movement with three different macular translocation techniques in humans (scleral outpouching, scleral imbrication, 360 retinotomy). ARVO abstracts. Invest Ophthalmol Vis Sci 41 [Suppl]:S540

Miller JW, Schmidt-Erfurth U, Sickenberg M., Pournaras CJ, Laqua H, Barbazetto I, Zografos L, Piguet B, Donati G, Lane A-M, Birngruber R, van den Berg H, Strong A, Manjuris U, Gray T, Fsadni M, Bressler NM, Gragoudas ES (1999) Photodynamic therapy with verteporfin for choroidal neovascularization caused by age-related macular degeneration: Results of a single treatment in a phase 1 and 2 study. Arch Ophthalmol 117(9):1161–1173

Ninomiya Y, Lewis JM, Hasegawa T, Tano Y (1996) Retinotomy and foveal translocation for surgical management of subfoveal choroidal neovascular membranes. Am J Ophthalmol 122(5):613–621

Ohji M, Fujikado T, Saito Y, Hosohata J, Hayashi A, Tano Y (1998) Foveal translocation: A comparison of two techniques. Seminars in Ophthalmol 13(1):52–61

Pharmacological Therapy for Macular Degeneration Study Group (1997) Interferon alfa-2a is ineffective for patients with choroidal neovascularization secondary to age-related macular degeneration: Results of a prospective randomized placebo-controlled clinical trial. Arch Ophthalmol 115(7):865–872

Pieramici DJ, de Juan E, Fujii GY, Reynolds MA, Melia M, Humayun MS, Schachat AP, Hartranft CD (2000) Limited inferior macular translocation for the treatment of subfoveal choroidal neovascularization secondary to age-related macular degeneration. Am J Ophthalmol (in press)

Poliner LS, Tornambe PE, Michelson PE, Heitzmann JG (1993) Interferon alpha-2a for subfoveal neovascularization in age-related macular degeneration. Ophthalmology 100(9):1417–1424

Schmidt-Erfurth U, Miller JW, Sickenberg M, Laqua H, Barbazetto I, Gragoudas ES, Zografos L, Piguet B, Pournaras CJ, Donati G, Lane A-M, Birngruber R, van den Berg H, Strong HA, Manjuris U, Gray T, Fsadni M, Bressler NM (1999) Photodynamic therapy with verteporfin for choroidal neovascularization caused by age-related macular degeneration: Results of retreatments in a phase 1 and 2 study. Arch Ophthalmol 117(9):1177–1187

Seaber JH, Machemer R (1997) Adaptation to monocular torsion after macular translocation. Graefe's Arch Clin Exp Ophthalmol 235(2):76–81

Spaide RF, Guyer DR, McCormick B, Yannuzzi LA, Burke K, Mendelsohn M, Haas A, Slakter JS, Sorenson JA, Fisher YL, Abramson D (1998) External beam radiation therapy for choroidal neovascularization. Ophthalmology 105(1):24–30

T'so MOM, Friedman E (1967) The retinal pigment epithelium, I: Comparative histology. Arch Ophthalmol 78(5):641–649

Thomas MA, Ibanez HE (1993a) Interferon alfa-2a in the treatment of subfoveal choroidal neovascularization. Am J Ophthalmol 115(5):563–568

Thomas MA, Ibanez HE (1993b) Subretinal endophotocoagulation in the treatment of choroidal neovascularization. Am J Ophthalmol 116(9):279–285

Thomas MA, Grand MG, Williams DF, Lee CM, Pesin SR, Lowe MA (1992) Surgical management of subfoveal choroidal neovascularization. Ophthalmology 99(6):952–968

Thomas MA, Dickinson JD, Melberg NS, Ibanez HE, Dhaliwal RS (1994) Visual results after surgical removal of subfoveal choroidal neovascular membranes. Ophthalmology 101(8):1384–1396

Tiedeman J, de Juan E, Machemer R, Hatchell DL, Hatchell MC (1985) Surgical relocation of the macula. ARVO abstracts. Invest Ophthalmol Vis Sci 26 [Suppl]:59

Toller KK, Hainsworth DP (1998) Traumatic foveal relocation with good visual acuity. Arch Ophthalmol 116(11):1536–1537

Toth CA, Machemer R (1999) Macular translocation. In: Berger JW, Fine SL, Maguire MG (eds) Age-related macular degeneration. Mosby, Philadelphia, pp 353–362

Treatment of Age-Related Macular Degeneration with Photodynamic Therapy (TAP) Study Group (1999) Photodynamic therapy of subfoveal choroidal neovascularization in age-related macular degeneration with verteporfin: One-year results of two randomized clinical trials – TAP Report 1. Arch Ophthalmol 117(10):1329–1345

Wolf S, Lappas A, Weinberger AWA, Kirchhof B (1999) Macular translocation for surgical management of subfoveal choroidal neovascularizations in patients with AMD: First results. Graefe's Arch Clin Exp Ophthalmol 237(1):51–57

Yoneya S, T'so MOM (1987) Angioarchitecture of the human choroid. Arch Ophthalmol 105(5):681–687

7 Development of Microelectronic Visual Implants

HEINRICH GERDING, S. TANERI, C. E. UHLIG, and K. KRAUSE

CONTENTS

7.1 Development of Retinal Prostheses

The aim of restoring visual orientation by a retinal prosthetic device implanted either epiretinally or subretinally depends on the availability of useful contacts with neurons that provide a functional afferent connection to the central visual system despite the underlying blinding disease. Diseases that may potentially benefit from the application of retinal implants are hereditary pigmentary degenerations like retinitis pigmentosa or acquired macular diseases such as age-related macular degeneration. Recent quantitative studies on the preservation of retinal cells in donor eyes of legally blind patients with late-stage retinitis pigmentosa have demonstrated that a relevant number of retinal neurons is morphologically preserved despite the underlying disease. STONE et al. (1992) found a 50–75% rate of retained retinal ganglion cells in the macula of patients with retinitis pigmentosa despite a marked reduction in the number of photoreceptors. In a subgroup analysis of patients with far advanced retinitis pigmentosa, about 30% of retained ganglion cells and 78–88% of surviving bipolar neurons were found in the macula area (SANTOS et al. 1997). Although the percentage of preserved ganglion cells in these eyes was lower in the extramacular retina, their number may still be sufficient to restore useful artificial vision (HUMAYUN et al. 1999b). Several studies performed on animal models with chemically induced photoreceptor degeneration and in patients with progressed retinitis pigmentosa have clearly demonstrated that the surviving ganglion cells in retinal areas not providing light perception are preserved histologically and can be stimulated electrically so that evoked cortical responses or localized perception described as regional dots of light could be elicited (HUMAYUN 1994, 1995, 1996, 1999a).

7.2 Development of Subretinal Implants

The idea and conceptual design of a subretinal implant that might serve for the restoration of basic orientation was established by Chow and coworkers in the early 1990s (CHOW 1991a, 1991b, 1993; CHOW and CHOW 1995, 1997). Essentially, the idea was to stimulate surviving neurons in degenerated retinas by electrical currents derived from microphotodiodes integrated within an implant that were driven by incident light. The incoming light served two functions: firstly as the carrier of image information that must be transferred to the light-insensitive degenerated retina

H. GERDING, MD
Professor, Klinik und Poliklinik für Augenheilkunde, Universität Münster, Domagkstrasse 15, 48129 Münster, Germany
S. TANERI, MD
Klinik und Poliklinik für Augenheilkunde, Universität Münster, Domagkstrasse 15, 48129 Münster, Germany
C.E. UHLIG, MD
Klinik und Poliklinik für Augenheilkunde, Universität Münster, Domagkstrasse 15, 48129 Münster, Germany
K. KRAUSE, PhD
Professor, Klinik und Poliklinik für Augenheilkunde, Universität Münster, Domagkstrasse 15, 48129 Münster, Germany

and secondly as the energy source for the microphotodiodes, which must produce adequate electrical energy to stimulate the contacted retina. Presently two groups, Chow et al. (CHOW and CHOW 1995, 1997) and a German SUB-RET group (ZRENNER et al. 1997, 1999), are focusing on this approach. Several attempts have been made to prove the feasibility of such a system using different kinds of retinal stimulation techniques. CHOW and CHOW (1997) have demonstrated that cortical potentials resembling light-evoked responses can be evoked with large subretinal single electrodes (area of 0.36 mm^2) driven by external photodiodes in rabbits. The necessary charge density for a reproducible evoked cortical response was relatively low, in the order of 100 nC/cm^2. Neither electrodes nor photodiodes used in these experiments were of the order of magnitude suitable for a permanently implantable device. In vitro sandwich techniques were used to evaluate parameters necessary for successful stimulation of degenerated RCS (Royal College of Surgeons rat) retinae with electrodes placed on or near the subretinal surface (ZRENNER et al. 1997, 1999). Current threshold in these experiments was less than 10 μA (1 ms) when electrodes were in direct contact with the retina. In vivo tests with subretinally implanted microcontact foils developed for an epiretinal system confirmed the above-mentioned experiments of CHOW and CHOW(1997) using much smaller stimulating electrodes (SCHWAHN et al. 2000) and multifocal cortical field potential recordings. The first data on retinal stimulation elicited by subretinal microphotodiodes are available from several in vitro experiments (ZRENNER et al. 1997, 1999) showing that light intensities of 10,000–100,000 lux, a level that is 100 times the intensity of a normal indoor daylight environment, are necessary to supply enough energy for ensuring suprathreshold retinal stimulation. So far, no in vivo data are available on light-elicited neuronal stimulation effects evoked by subretinally implanted microphotodiodes. An inherent problem of subretinal implants is the creation of a complete barrier eliminating the essential diffusion process between choroid/RPE on one side and the elevated retina on the other. This results in degeneration of the overlying, previously healthy retina in animals with merangiotic retinal vascularization after subretinal placement of implants with a diameter of 3 mm (ZRENNER et al. 1997). Even in case of a holangiotic retina and decreased implant size (0.48 mm^2–0.8 mm^2), degeneration of the overlying retina cannot be completely excluded (ZRENNER et al. 1999). There are several other problems that have to be evaluated and sorted out on the way to creating a subretinal implant that might be an option for clinical testing:

1. Reactions of the subretinal compartment to implanted materials (degradation of the blood-retina barrier).
2. The long-term effect of permanently imbalanced charge delivery by the implant.
3. Identifying which neurons or constituents of the complex overlying retinal structure are stimulated by a subretinal device and whether these stimulations lead to a useful subjective perception in humans.
4. Whether the quality of perception mediated by these implants takes the necessary constant "gestalt" or produces variations with stimulus intensity.
5. Whether it will be necessary to modulate the light-stimulus transfer (in case of permanent signal injection that is below or far above threshold levels or of meaningless or even disturbing information provided by single electrodes).
6. How traumatizing a putative explantation of the implant would be.

7.3 Development of Epiretinal Implants

At present, three cooperative groups are doing basic and developmental research to create retinal prosthetic systems for an epiretinal approach to the partially degenerated retina (ECKMILLER 1997; HUMAYUN et al. 1994, 1995, 1996, 1999a, b; WYATT and RIZZO 1966; RIZZO and WYATT 1997, 1999). All aim to achieve a wireless transfer of image information processed externally to an epiretinal implant for selective stimulation of underlying retinal ganglion cells. Wireless transfer of information and the energy necessary to run the intraocular implant can be achieved either electromagnetically or by optical transfer. Two of the groups aim to use an electromagnetic (HUMAYUN et al. 1994, 1995, 1996, 1999a, b) or optical transfer (RIZZO and WYATT 1996, 1997), and one group is doing developmental work on both (ECKMILLER 1997).

7.3.1 Basic Considerations for the Construction of Epiretinal Implants

The retinal ganglion cell layer is composed of neurons that are heterogeneous in several aspects: size, dendritic stratification, grade of afferent convergence, type of bipolar afferent connections, size and functional organization of the receptive field (RF; on/off), overlapping of dendritic fields, color specificity, and other aspects. So far, there is no definite number of different classes of ganglion cells available; presently, the existence of some 18 cell types is under discussion (KOLB et al. 1992). Regarding the enormous multidimensional possibilities for anatomical and physiological variance of retinal ganglion cells, although classifiable, they appear unique in some aspects – partly a consequence of complex feedback mechanisms during neurogenesis of the visual system. The variability of ganglion cells infers interindividual differences in humans that can be expressed by the ratio of cone and ganglion cell numbers that may vary between 2.9 and 7.5 (CURCIO and ALLEN 1990).

The information process of retinal ganglion cells is essentially an abstract spatiotemporal transformation of an image projected to the retina. The algorithms used for the transformation of visual information into neuronal spike activity depend on the type of ganglion cells and their afferent connections, the nature of the image presented (size, shape, direction, contrast, color, movement, etc.), the current adaptive state of the retina, and, even more complex, the dynamic perception of collateral information processed in parallel or overlapping afferent structures. One of the challenges of the epiretinal approach is to evolve encoding procedures that may substitute the afferent information process of the retina and provide an adequate transformation of a (changing) image into patterns of stimulation that resemble the complex retinal information process and provide stimulus patterns that can be used by the central nervous system. The transformation of visual information into ganglion cell spike activity can be described as an RF filter mechanism (ECKMILLER 1997). RF filters receive the afferent information of a number of photoreceptor-like elements taken from an external camera system. The filtering process has to implement the spatial antagonistic center/surround character of all ganglion cell RFs, even overlapping ones. Besides the spatial aspects, RF filters have to modulate the incoming image information so that typical temporal patterns of ganglion cell output will be achieved. This includes variables such as the basal impulse rate, the rise in impulse rate, maximal impulse rate, temporal aspects of impulse decay, stimulus off response, and others. All these spatial and temporal aspects of RF filters have to be adjustable and moreover, be part of a learning process that can be offered to the carriers of implants.

Comparing putative positions for visual system electronic devices, the retina offers the advantage of a two-dimensional topography with almost identical coordinates of the image projected and the position of cells transducing image information into afferent neuronal spike activity. Although, for the main proportion of the retina, this identity may be accepted as a general rule, it may not be forgotten that in the macula this assumption must be corrected and taken into consideration for the construction of epiretinal implants (RIZZO and WYATT 1999). The fact that the center of the fovea (500 μm) is devoid of any ganglion cells is the basis for a lateral shift of afferent connections originating from the most central photoreceptors towards the ganglion cell layer (SCHEIN 1988). Since the direction of shift is obviously radial, we can propose that neighbouring photoreceptors near the center project to well distantly localized ganglion cells.

When placing epiretinal implants onto the inner surface of the retina, the first neuronal structure to be contacted is the nerve fiber layer of ganglion cell axons. This raises concern that the stimulating electrodes, targeting and processing information for the underlying ganglion cells, might elicit undesired excitation of these axons possibly originating from cells located far away, so that a mismatch of intended localization would result. If stimuli well beyond the axonal threshold were applied, the small size and dense pakking of axons could excite a whole group of distant cells and probably lead to blurred or diffuse, poorly demarcated visual sensations. Recent data derived from axon modeling studies seem to indicate that, simply by varying the spatial orientation of stimuli, the effect can be biased from the overlying axons to the more distant ganglion cells (GRUMET 1994; RIZZO and WYATT 1999). Results of human trials with epiretinal stimulating electrodes indicate so far a dominance of localized but not very discriminant sensations probably originating in the underlying ganglion cells. Disturbing blurring sensations caused by excitation of the axonal layer thus seem to be avoidable (HUMAYUN et al. 1996, 1999a; RIZZO et al. 2000).

7.3.2 Technical Construction of the EPI-RET Retina Implant System

The main components of the EPI-RET retina implant system are schematically depicted in Fig. 7.1. The system consists of several components located outside the eye: (1) camera, (2) retina encoder (RE),

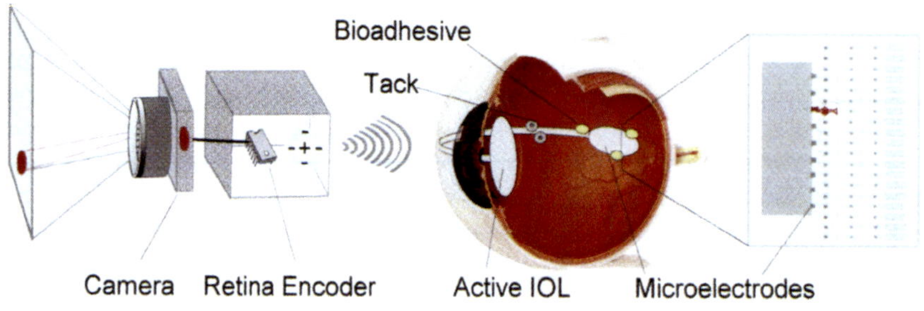

Fig. 7.1. Main components of the EPI-RET retina implant system

and (3) signal and energy transducer. The intraocular implant, or retina stimulator (RS), includes the following components: (4) signal and energy receiver, (5) energy unit, (6) signal demodulator and distributor, and (7) epiretinal microcontacts that will be connected to the main unit of the RS by a flat and flexible microcable. Components 4–6 will be integrated in an anterior IOL-like structure.

The external camera, newly designed and technically optimized for the needs of the EPI-RET system, uses a photosensor array with about 10,000–100,000 pixels at the input site. The camera unit supplies the signal input of the retina encoder (RE). Both the camera and the RE will, in the final version, be integrated into the eyeglass frame together with the signal and energy transducer so that the patient using the system will not have to carry any noticeable or bulky technical equipment. As mentioned above, the RE replaces the natural processing of information normally performed by the afferent retinal layers; in other words, it replaces the RF properties of the retina. It does so by using 100–1000 tunable RF filters representing implementations of approximated typical RF properties of primate retinal ganglion cells. Each RF filter will receive a signal input of 100–1000 photosensor elements from the camera and send one output sequence to the signal and energy transmitter (SE). A very important feature of the RE and essential function of the whole system is the tuning of RF filters. This allows changes in the parameters of the spatiotemporal RF filter functions at any time after implantation. In this way, the RF filter parameters can be matched so that a subjective visual perception elicited by the RS, as reported by the implant carrier, can be optimized with the aim of approaching the optimal visual sensations needed for rehabilitation. Tuning the systems requires a testing and dialog procedure with the implant carrier. In order to optimize precision and reduce the necessary training time, this procedure will be performed as an unsupervised learning process, integrating an adaptive dialog module with an implemented neuronal network learning strategy. Figure 7.2 shows a diagram of the dialog-based procedure used for the tuning of RF filter functions as intended for implant-carrying patients.

7.3.3 Implantation and Mechanical Fixation of Epiretinal Implants

Implantation and mechanical fixation of epiretinal retina implant devices represent a completely new challenge to vitreoretinal and anterior segment surgery. For the first time, a functional implant has to be placed on the retina atraumatically such that it maintains a highly constant intraocular position. Furthermore, the implant itself should not induce major secondary proliferations that would adversely affect precision in position and function of the implant. Concerning the demand for surgical innovation, the process of implantation itself seemed, at the beginning of the project, to be the least problem. The decision to change the design of implants so that they consist not only of a compact one-piece device but

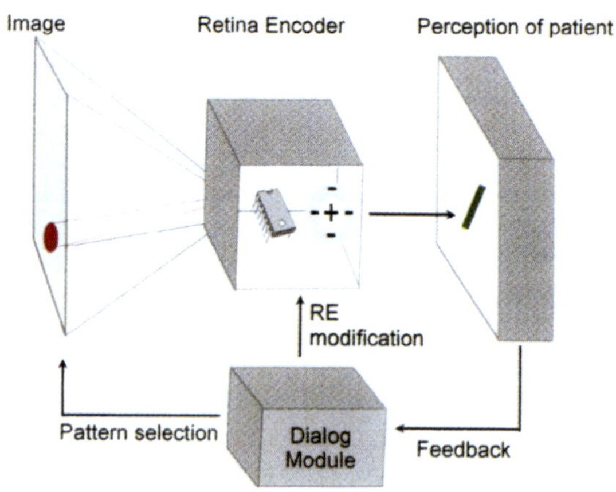

Fig. 7.2. Schematic drawing of the training procedure for patients with an epiretinal implant

of an anterior-segment artificial lens (including the receiving coil and connected circuits) and the posterior segment microcontact foil, connected via a flat and flexible microcable, requires a complex and extensive surgical procedure. The first long-term results of experimental implantations using electrically inactive implants in rabbits proved the possibility of safe and stable positioning of these complex structures without major adverse tissue reactions or other ocular complications (Gerding et al. 1999, 2000b; Vobig et al. 2000). The surgical procedures published so far have in common that they used the lens capsule to stabilize the anterior lens structure of the implant inserted through a wide corneoscleral incision. As the second step of the procedure, the microcontact foil was placed on the retina after creation of a posterior capsulotomy. An even more delicate surgical task is the achievement of mechanical fixation of the implant structures in the posterior segment. Two principally different techniques are now under investigation: (1) intrascleral tack structures and (2) epiretinal bioadhesives. The technique of intraoperative fixation by the application of tacks was introduced by Ando and Kondo (1983, 1986) for the treatment of difficult cases with retinal detachment. Their first reports led to several lines of development focusing on the design of new devices manufactured from different materials. This technique was not adopted widely because other surgical techniques for the achievement of retinal reattachment were established, i.e., the use of liquid perfluorocarbon. For epiretinal fixation of retina implants in the posterior segment of the eye, the use of retinal tacks provides several advantages: a stable anchoring in the sclera and a collar around the epiretinal shaft that can be used for the mechanical stabilization of implants. Conventional tack structures have been experimentally tested and successfully used for the long-term implantation of electrically inactive implants (Gerding et al. 1998; Majji et al. 1999; Taneri et al. 1999; Walter et al. 1999). A disadvantage of currently available conventional retinal tacks is the relatively traumatic and potentially harmful mechanical insertion which may lead to retinal trauma, hemorrhage, partial atrophy of the retina, or the creation of secondary retinal folds. In order to reduce the trauma associated with the insertion, newly constructed microtacks were recently developed and successfully tested in long-term observations (Taneri et al. 1999). A second disadvantage of tacks penetrating the retina, choroid, and sclera is the secondary formation of a capsule around the tack itself as well as proliferations sub-, intra-, and epiretinally close to the point of insertion. These secondary proliferations, although very limited, may be sufficient to dislocate the implant beyond a critical limit.

To achieve a much less traumatic fixation, especially for the implant area bearing microcontact electrodes, we and others have tested different kinds of bioadhesives (Bollmann et al. 1999; Gerding et al. 1998; Margalit et al. 2000). As a result of research in this field, biocompatible standardized procedures for the microapplication and induced binding of fibrin sealant to the internal limiting membrane were developed. This new technique was successfully tested in a series of microcontact implantations that were stabilized for the long term primarily by the application of sealant and secondarily by proliferation being limited to the edges of microcontacts foils.

7.4 Functional Testing of Retina Implants and Microelectrodes

The above-mentioned evidence of surviving ganglion cell neurons in the retinae of patients with diseases like retinitis pigmentosa that were demonstrated to convey electrically evoked perception is an essential but insufficient prerequisite for the successful rehabilitative application of retinal implants in humans. There are several qualitative and quantitative aspects of electrical stimulation of the retina that have to be explored in further detail:

1. The optimal temporal parameters of stimulation using final version microelectrodes.
2. The precise current threshold at different locations, with single microelectrodes positioned on the internal limiting membrane of the retina in nonhuman primates as well as healthy and diseased humans.
3. The quality of perception and temporal and spatial resolution that can be elicited with complex electrode arrays contacting the retina in humans.
4. Functional analyses of electrically active implants in long-term in vivo-experiments.

So far, preliminary results addressing the first three of these key questions are available. Several authors have determined thresholds for the elucidation of evoked cortical responses using epiretinal electrodes driven by balanced bipolar rectangular impulse series in rabbits (Humayun et al. 1994; Nadig 1999; Walter and Heimann 2000). The threshold of stimulation for the detection of electrically evoked potentials (EEP) was determined in these experiments to be in the range of 10 μA–50 μA with short half-wave pulses (75 μs–400 μs). The charge density applied by the electrodes at threshold was in the range of 8.9 μC/cm^2–30 μC/cm^2 working with electrodes 75 μm–500 μm in size. The same threshold range (40 μC/cm^2) was evaluated in stimulation experiments in macaque monkeys (Gerding et al. 2000a). Much lower current thresholds (1.7 μA for salamander and 16 μA for rabbit) were observed in stimulation experiments with smaller electrodes, but the delivered charge density was higher in these experiments than in the above-mentioned (Grumet et al. 1998; Rizzo et al. 1997). As with any kind of electrode use for neuronal tissue stimulation, the limits of charge injection at which adverse effects such as dissolution, oxidation/reduction of electrodes, or even gas bubbles are produced have to be evaluated critically. The acceptable upper limit for platinum electrodes in the cited experimental series was 100 μC/cm^2 (Roblee and Rose 1990) for long-term use. The results reported so far clearly show that minimalization of electrode diameter, which would be desirable for high spatial resolution, is critically limited by the increasing charge:area ratio resulting from the nonlinear charge:electrode area ratio. New materials, for example activated iridium oxide electrodes, allow a much higher limit of safe charge injection (1000 μC/cm^2) (Beebe and Rose 1988) and seem to be a promising option for future development.

Results documented so far on retinal threshold stimuli necessary to yield EEP responses have to be interpreted as a frame delineating safe ranges of stimulation. They definitely do not characterize stimuli useful for the perception of single image pixels. This question has been addressed in stimulations performed with epiretinal electrodes in humans with retinitis pigmentosa (Humayun et al. 1996, 1999a). The evaluated thresholds for the perception of „evoked lights“ in these experiments were beyond the upper limit of the safe charge density known for platinum electrodes. The given information that the implanted electrodes in these experiments were not directly in contact with the internal limiting membrane suggests that it will be possible to obtain positive perceptions with smaller stimuli. The fact that EEPs in macaques (Gerding et al. 2000a) could be recorded at much lower levels of stimulation within a safe range of charge transfer favor this assumption. Regarding all the other aspects of evaluated stimulation in humans using epiretinally implanted microelectrodes, i.e., the correspondence of „evoked lights,“ the position of the stimulation electrodes and first evaluations of two-point resolutions (Humayun et al. 1996, 1999a; Rizzo et al. 2000) suggest that the successful development of epiretinal prostheses is a realistic aim despite the many problems to be solved.

7.5 Implants Stimulating the Optic Nerve

Surviving ganglion cells in retinal diseases may be contacted following the idea of a retinal bypass either directly on the retinal surface (epiretinal retina implant concept) or using optic nerve stimulators. According to the concept developed by a Belgian group (Veraart et al. 1998, 1999) it was intended to develop flexible cuff structures bearing a small number of stimulating electrodes that could be placed on and wrapped around the optic nerve. These researchers demonstrated the first results after transcranial implantation and long-term observation of such an electrode in one patient. They provided evidence for the long-term stability of the electrodes as tested in repetitive stimulation procedures. It seems that basic anatomical and physiological parameters (small number of electrodes, topographic relation of electrodes, and axonal anatomy) are severe limitations of this system regarding the accessible resolution of transformed images.

7.6 Cortical Implants

The concept of visual rehabilitation using electrodes placed on the surface of the visual cortex has been under investigation by several groups and goes back to the historic approach of Brindley and others in the late 1960s (Brindley 1973, 1982; Brindley and Lewin 1968; Dobelle and Mladejovsky 1974; Dobelle et al. 1974, 1976;). Their investigations showed that it is possible to elicit occipital phosphenes, potentially useful for the restoration of basic orientation in blind people. Stimulation experiments in humans revealed several problems which set limits on the approach, i.e., the need to inject relatively high electrical currents (1 mA–2 mA), interactions of phosphenes elicited simultaneously at distant points of stimulation, flickering of phosphenes, and in some cases the persistence of visual sensations after discontinuing the application of stimuli (Brindley 1973, 1982; Brindley and Lewin 1968; Dobelle and Mladejovsky 1974; Dobelle et al. 1976). These aftersensations may be an indicator of neuronal activity such as that seen in epileptiform afterdischarges (BAK et al. 1990). These problems and the necessity of a rather invasive surgical procedure led to the discontinuation of attempts using epicortical electrodes. Recently, new data appeared on one of the patients who received epicortical electrode implants more than 20 years ago (DOBELLE 2000) which were now driven by a newly designed computerized video decoder and stimulator. It is not yet clear whether this concept might overcome the previously documented and above-mentioned principal problems of epicortical devices.

The idea of a visual cortex implant bypassing the afferent visual system has been reevolving during the past few years (NORMAN et al. 1996), initiated by the observation that *intra*cortical stimulation using penetrating electrodes yields detectable visual sensations in nonhuman primates at much lower currents (1 μA–5 μA) than in epicortical trials (BARTLETT and DOTY 1980). The threshold for punctate visual sensation in the human visual cortex was evaluated to be as low as 20 μA–200 μA. SCHMIDT et al. (1996) recently reported a 4-month trial of an intracortical implant based on these new microelectrodes in a volunteer who was blind from glaucoma. Their results clearly demonstrated a higher spatial resolution (with separation of electrodes by 500 μm) and much lower current threshold (from 1.9 μA, mainly <25 μA) in comparison to the early epicortical implants.

7.7 Hybrid Implants

Retinal and optic nerve implants are intended to bypass retinal diseases primarily located distally to the ganglion cell layer. These concepts depend on and are limited to diseases that preserve a sufficient number of retinal ganglion cells. A wide range of epidemiologically important, potentially blinding diseases (glaucoma, optic nerve trauma) cannot be targeted with these distal contact systems. There are two conceptual approaches to overcome this limitation by placing a more centrally located visual bypass system. These are: (1) hybrid (retina/optic nerve) implants and (2) cortical visual prostheses (see above). The hybrid system (Yagi et al. 1999) is intended to combine the implantation of an intraocular stimulator and the transplantation of an optic nerve graft that should contact the lateral geniculate nucleus (LGN). The technological and biomedical challenge of this project needs solutions to several major problems: (1) technical development of a biocompatible and stable intraocular implant, (2) development of a long-term stable contact between implant and optic nerve graft, (3) survival of the optic nerve graft, and (4) achievement of a neuronal contact between the optic nerve graft and LGN that permits the transduction of useful image processing.

References

Ando F, Kondo J (1983) A plastic tack for the treatment of retinal detachment with giant retinal tear. Am J Ophthalmol 95:260–261

Ando F, Kondo J (1986) Surgical techniques for giant retinal tears with retinal tacks. Ophthalmic Surg 17:408–411

Bak M, Girvin JP, Hambrecht FT, Kufta CV, Loeb GE, Schmidt EM (1990) Visual sensations produced by intracortical microstimulation of the human occipital cortex. Med Biol Eng Comput 28:257–259

Bartlett JR, Doty RW (1980) An exploration of the ability of macaques to detect microstimulation of striate cortex. Acta Neurobiol Exp 40:713–727

Beebe X, Rose TL (1988) Charge injection limits of activated iridium oxide electrodes with 0.2 ms pulses in bicarbonate buffered saline. IEEE Trans Biomed Eng 35:494–495

Bollmann FP, Taneri S, Uhlig CE, Paulus W, Gerding H (1999) The retina implant project: Epiretinal implant fixation with electrochemically adhesive sealant. Invest Ophthalmol Vis Sci 40:S782

Brindley GS (1973) Sensory effects of electrical stimulation of the visual and paravisual cortex in man. In: Jung R (ed) Handbook of sensory physiology. Vol 7. Springer, New York, pp 583–594

Brindley GS (1982) Visual prostheses. Human neurobiol 1:281–283

Brindley GS, Lewin W (1968) The sensations produced by electrical stimulation of the visual cortex. J Physiol (Lond) 196:479–493

Chow AY (1991a) Artificial retina device. United States Patent No. 5,016,633 issued May 21, 1991

Chow AY (1991b) Artificial retina device. United States Patent No. 5,024,223 issued June 18, 1991

Chow AY (1993) Electrical stimulation of the rabbit retina with subretinal electrodes and high density microphotodiodes array implants. Invest Ophthalmol Vis Sci 34:S835

Chow AY, Chow V (1995) Independent photoelectric artificial retina device and method using same. United States Patent No. 5,397,350 issued March 14, 1995

Chow AY, Chow VY (1997) Subretinal electrical stimulation of the rabbit retina. Neurosci Lett 225:13–16

Curcio CA, Allen KA (1990) Topography of ganglion cells in human retina. J Comp Neurol 300:5

Dobelle WMH (2000) Artificial vision for the blind by connecting a television camera to the visual cortex. ASAIO J 46:3–9

Dobelle WH, Mladejovsky MG (1974) Artificial vision for the blind: Electrical stimulation of visual cortex offers hope for a functional prosthesis. Science 183:440–444

Dobelle WH, Mladejovsky MG, Grivin JP (1974) Phosphenes produced by electrical stimulation of human occipital cortex and their application to the development of a prosthesis for the blind. J Physiol 243:553-576

Dobelle WH, Mladejovsky MG, Evans JK, Roberts TS, Girvin JP (1976) „Braille" reading by a blind volunteer by visual cortex stimulation. Nature 259:111-112

Eckmiller R (1997) Learning Retina Implants with Epiretinal Conracts. Ophthalmic Res 29:281-289

Gerding H, Uhlig C, Thelen U (1998) The retina implant project: Development of techniques for implantation and epiretinal fixation of stimulators. Invest Ophthalmol Vis Sci 39:S991

Gerding H, Taneri S, Bollmann FP, Kupich S, Uhlig CE (1999) The Retina Implant Project: Implantation and fixation of combined systems with an anterior intraocular receiver and a posterior epiretinal stimulator pad. Invest Ophthalmol Vis Sci 40:S783

Gerding H, Hornig R, Köhler C, Taneri S, Benner FP, Niggemann B, Uhlig CE, Stieglitz T, Meyer JU, Eckmiller R (2000a) Electrically evoked response (EER) from the visual cortex of M. fascicularis after epiretinal implantation of retina stimulators. Invest Ophthalmol Vis Sci 41:S860

Gerding H, Taneri S, Benner FP, Meyer JU, Stieglitz T, Kupich S, Uhlig CE (2000b) 13. Kongress der Deutschsprachigen Gesellschaft für Intrakokularlinsen-Implantation und refraktive Chirurgie. Biermann, Cologne, pp 349-355

Grumet A (1994) Extracellular electrical stimulation of retinal ganglion cells. Master's thesis. Massachussetts Institute of Technology, Cambridge

Grumet AE, Wyatt JL, Rizzo JF (1998) Multi-electrode recording and stimulation of the salamander retina in vitro. Invest Ophthalmol Vis Sci 39: S565

Humayun M, Probst R, De Juan E, McCormick K, Hickingbotham D (1994) Bipolar surface electrical stimulation of the vertebrate retina. Arch Ophthalmol 112:110-116

Humayun M, Sato Y, Probst R, De Juan E (1995) Can potentials from the visual cortex be elicited electrically despite severe retinal degeneration and a markedly reduced electroretinogram? German J Ophthalmol 4:57-64

Humayun MS, De Juan E, Dagneli G, Greenberg RJ, Propst RH, Phillips DH (1996) Visual perception elicited by electrical stimulation of retina in blind humans. Arch Ophthalmol 114:40-46

Humayun MS, De Juan E, Weiland JD, Dagnelie G, Katona S, Greenberg R, Suzuki S (1999a) Pattern electrical stimulation of the human retina. Vision Res 39:2569-2576

Humayun MS, Prince M, De Juan E, Barron Y, Moskowitz M, Klock IB, Milam AH (1999b) Morphometric analysis of the extramacular retina from postmortem eyes with retinitis pigmentosa. Invest Ophthalmol Vis Sci 40:143-148

Kolb H, Linberg KA, Fischer SK (1992) Neurons of the human retina: A Golgi study. J Comp Neurol 138:147

Margalit E, Fujii G, Lai JC, Gupta P, Chen SJ, Weiland JD, De Juan E (2000) Bioadhesives for intraocular use. Invest Ophthalmol Vis Sci 41:S746

Majji AB, Humayun MS, Weiland JD, Suzuki S, D'Anna SA, De Juan E (1999) Long-term histological and electrophysiological results of an inactive epiretinal electrode array implantation in dogs. Invest Ophthalmol Vis Sci 40:2073-2081

Nadig MN (1999) Development of a silicon retinal implant: Cortical evoked potentials following focal stimulation of the rabbit retina with light and electricity. Clin Neurophys 110:1545-1553

Norman RA, Maynard EM, Guillory KS, Warren DJ (1996) Cortical implants for the blind. IEEE Spectrum 33:54-59

Rizzo JF, Wyatt J (1997) Prospectus for a visual prosthesis. The Neuroscientist 3:251-262

Rizzo JF, Wyatt JL (1999) Retinal prosthesis. In: Berger JW, Fine SL, Maguire MG (eds) Age-related macular degeneration. Mosby, St. Louis, pp 413-432

Rizzo JF, Grumet AE, Edell DJ, Wyatt JL, Jensen RJ (1997) Single-unit recordings following extracellular stimulation of retinal ganglion cell axons in rabbits. Invest Ophthalmol Vis Sci 38:S40

Rizzo JF, Wyatt J, Loewenstein J, Kelly S (2000) Acute intraocular retinal stimulation in normal and blind humans. Invest Ophthalmol Vis Sci 41:S102

Roblee LS, Rose TL (1990) Electrochemical guidelines for selection of protocols and electrode materials for neural stimulation. In: Agnew WF, McGreery DB (eds) Neural prosthesis fundamental studies. Prentice Hall Int. Coop, Englewood Cliffs, pp 26-66

Santos A, Humayun MS, De Juan E, Greenburg RJ, Marsh MJ, Klock IB, Milam AH (1997) Preservation of the inner retina in retinitis pigmentosa. Arch Ophthalmol 115:511-515

Schein S (1988) Anatomy of macaque fovea and spatial densities of neurons in foveal representation. J Com Neurol 269:479-505

Schmidt EM, Bak MJ, Hambrecht FT, Kufta CV, O'Rourke DK, Vallabhanath P (1996) Feasibility of a visual prosthesis for the blind based on intracortical microstimulation of the visual cortex. Brain 119:507-522

Schwahn HN, Gekeler F, Sachs HG, Kobuch K, Koehler M, Jakob W, Gabel VP, Zrenner E (2000) Evoked cortical responses following multifocal electrical stimulation in the subretinal space of rabbit and minipig. Invest Ophthalmol Vis Sci 41:S102

Stone JL, Barlow WE, Humayun MS, De Juan E, Milam AH (1992) Morphometric analysis of macular photoreceptors and ganglion cells in retinas with retinitis pigmentosa. Arch Ophthalmol 110:1634-1639

Taneri S, Bollmann FP, Uhlig CE, Thelen U, Gerding H (1999) The retina implant project: in vitro and in vivo testing of different tack types for intraocular fixation of retina implants. Invest Ophthalmol Vis Sci 40:S733

Veraart CG, Delbeke J, Wanet-Defalque MC, Vanlierde A, Legat JD, Trullemans C (1999) Chronic electrical stimulation of the optic nerve in a retinitis pigmentosa blind volunteer. Invest Ophthalmol Vis Sci 40:S783

Veraart C, Raftopoulos C, Mortimer JT, Delbeke J, Pins D, Michaux G, Vanlierde A, Parrini S, Wanet-Defalque MC (1998) Visual Sensations produced by optic nerve stimulation using an implanted self-sizing spiral cuff electrode. Brain Res 813:181-186

Vobig MA, Berk H, Marzella GM, Walter P (2000) Long-term results following implantation of an inactive compound retinal prosthesis in rabbits. Invest Ophthalmol Vis Sci 41:S859

Walter P, Heimann K (2000) Evoked cortical potentials after electrical stimulation of the inner retina in rabbits. Arch Klein Exp Ophthalmol 238:315-318

Walter P, Szurman P, Vobig M, Berk H, Lüdtke-Handjery HC, Richter H, Mittermayer C, Heimann K, Sellhaus B (1999) Successful long-term implantation of electrically inactive epiretinal microelectrode arrays in rabbits. Retina 19:546-552

Wyatt J, Rizzo J (1996) Ocular implants for the blind. IEEE Spectrum 33:47-53

Yagi T, Ito Y, Kanda Y, Tanaka S, Watanabe M, Uchikawa Y (1999) A prototype of a micro-electrode array for hybrid retinal implant. Invest Ophthalmol Vis Sci 40:S:732

Zrenner E, Miliczek KD, Gabel VP, Graf HG, Guenther E, Haemmerle H, Hoefflinger B, Kohler K, Nisch W, Schubert M, Stett A, Weiss S (1997) The development of subretinal microphotodiodes for replacement of degenerated photoreceptors. Ophthalmic Res 29:269–280

Zrenner E, Stett A, Weiss S, Aramant RB, Guenter E, Kohler K, Miliczek KD, Seiler MJ, Haemmerle H (1999) Can subretinal microphotodiodes successfully replace degenerated photoreceptors? Vision Res 39:2555–2567

8 Transplantation of Retinal Pigment Epithelial Cells

MONIKA VALTINK, JUDITH WEICHEL, GISBERT RICHARD, and KATRIN ENGELMANN

CONTENTS

8.1 Introduction

Transplantations of retinal pigment epithelial (RPE) cells into the subretinal space in animal models of age-related macular degeneration (ARMD) have demonstrated that degenerative processes can be prevented, and much hope is pinned on this therapeutic approach. During the past 2 decades, intra- or subretinal transplantation of retinal cells or tissues was extensively studied using various animal models. The most common animal used is the Royal College of Surgeons (RCS) rat, which develops postpartal RPE degeneration. Successful RPE transplantation is based on gaining functional cells as a sheet, in suspension or after multiplication. Maintenance of differentiated morphology and of typical functions of the RPE cells during serial passaging is – besides propagation of the cells – the main task of successful cell culturing in order to provide functional RPE cell transplants. This requires the adaptation and optimization of culture methods with regard to the ocular material available. After transplantation, the cells should be capable of phagocytosing shed rod outer segments, supplying the photoreceptor cells with nutrients, and participating in the retinoid cycle. This implies that function and differentiation of the cells are maintained during cell culture, e.g., measurement of membrane currents is to date the most sensitive method of evaluating the differentiation status of a cell. Based upon this experience, we compared standard culture media with our optimized growth medium $F99_{RPE}$.

Even if the anatomic success of RPE cell transplantation has been demonstrated, there are still problems to overcome, e.g., cell adhesion on Bruch's membrane, cell density and polarity at the transplant site, and integration of the cells into the recipient tissue. Moreover, long-term survival of the graft is impeded when xenotransplantation is performed. Immunologic processes that influence graft survival are not fully understood, in particular the role of the immune privilege of the subretinal space. This chapter presents an overview of the different attempts and results of RPE transplantation projects and discusses possibilities and limitations.

M. VALTINK, Dipl.-Ing. FH Biotechnology
Department of Ophthalmology, University of Hamburg, Martinistrasse 52, 20246 Hamburg, Germany
J. WEICHEL, Veterinary Surgeon
Department of Ophthalmology, University of Hamburg, Martinistrasse 52, 20246 Hamburg, Germany
G. RICHARD, MD
Professor, Department of Ophthalmology, University of Hamburg, Martinistrasse 52, 20246 Hamburg, Germany
K. ENGELMANN, MD
Professor, Department of Ophthalmology, University of Hamburg, Martinistrasse 52, 20246 Hamburg, Germany

8.2 RPE Cell Culture

8.2.1 Culture Methods

In the past three decades, several reports on the in vitro cultivation of RPE cells have been published.

Albert et al. (1972) described the in vitro behavior of explants of the choroid in culture. Since then different methods of isolating the cells and different culture conditions have been examined. Success of culturing is influenced by – among other things – postmortem time, and with increasing postmortem time the number of viable cells is considerably reduced. Therefore, the aim of many studies was the optimization of cell culture methods to obtain as many viable cells as possible out of a specimen with longer post mortem times and to cover their specific needs for nutrients to help isolated cells start proliferation. Previous studies demonstrated that the choice of enzyme for isolating cells has a major influence on starting primary cell cultures of RPE. The methods described for the isolation of RPE cells include repeated trypsinization of choroidal sheets (Baumgartner et al. 1989) or of the eyecups (Flood et al. 1980) and the use of other enzymes such as pronase (Zavazava et al. 1991) or dispase (Pfeffer 1991). While trypsin, a nonselective protease, cleaves proteins, including membrane proteins, rapidly and aggressively and thus reduces viability of the cells, mild proteases like dispase or pronase have been shown to be less effective in isolating a sufficient number of cells. Our own studies demonstrated that a mixture of collagenases is most effective in isolating high cell numbers from donor eyes with long postmortem times without reducing their viability (Sobottka Ventura et al. 1996).

The method described here was established at our laboratory and was designed especially for donor eyes with postmortem times longer than 24 h. After enucleation, the corneoscleral disc is dissected according to standardized methods established for corneal organ culture, as described by Böhnke (1991). Subsequently, RPE cells are isolated according to the method of Baumgartner et al. (1989) modified by Sobottka Ventura et al. (1996): the choroidal sheets are carefully prepared off the sclera with scissors and forceps and incubated in 2 ml of a collagenase solution[1] for 16 h in a humidified atmosphere of 5% CO_2 and 95% air at 37° C to loosen RPE cells. This technique yields sufficient viable RPE cells to establish cell cultures for transplantation studies, HLA typing, and other experiments involving RPE cells. Nevertheless, multiplication of the cells after the successful establishment of primary cultures is, in most cases, required for further studies.

A varying number of standard media have been used to culture RPE cells, including RPMI 1640, EMEM, DMEM, Ham's F10 (Albert et al. 1972; Baumgartner et al. 1989; Flood et al. 1980; Ho and Del Priore 1997; Mannagh et al. 1972; Zavazava et al. 1991). None of these culture media or methods was designed specially or proven for its growth-promoting efficiency. In contrast, a very detailed study to evaluate the growth behavior of RPE cells was presented by Pfeffer (1991). He developed a special culture medium for RPE cells which can be used in two modifications: depending on the calcium concentration, the medium can be used to promote either proliferation or differentiation of the cells. One reason that this very well designed medium was not used by other groups may be its detailed and more complicated recipe. Nevertheless, our own studies demonstrated the importance of defining the nutrient needs of highly differentiated human cells (Engelmann et al. 1988; Engelmann and Friedl 1989). Prevention of deadaptation or dedifferentiation of primary cells during cell culture is possible by definition of the nutritional environment, thus preventing loss of typical characteristics and functions. Therefore, the aim of our studies was to design a refined medium for RPE cells followed by evaluation of special functions (membrane currents) and characteristics (MHC antigen expression).

The proceedings at our laboratory involve the use of a specially designed RPE growth medium called $F99_{RPE}$, which was developed by Sobottka Ventura et al. (1996) specifically to cover the nutrient needs of adult human RPE cells isolated after long postmortem times. $F99_{RPE}$ is based on F99, which is more suitable for culturing RPE cells than other basal media. It is supplemented with 10% FCS, 1 mM sodium pyruvate, 1 µg insulin/ml, antibiotics, and – most importantly – 15% choroid-conditioned medium. Conditioned medium is produced by incubating the remnants of the choroidal sheets in F99 plus 1% FCS for 4 days after collagenase treatment. The content of the conditioned medium is unknown, but its beneficial effect was proven (Sobottka Ventura et al.1996; Valtink et al. 1999). It is likely that hormones and growth factors secreted by residual cells during the conditioning process are responsible for growth promotion (MacDonald 1994). This has also been described for other cell types (Astaldi 1983; Hoshi and McKeehan 1984). For further information on the topic of culture media and medium design, see Ham and McKeehan (1979). Isolated RPE cells are cultured with $F99_{RPE}$ until the cultures become confluent and are monitored by phase con-

Collagenase solution consists of a 1+1 mixture of collagenase types IA and IV in basal medium F99 at a final concentration of 0.5 mg collagenase/ml. Basal medium F99 consists of a 1+1 mixture of Medium 199 and Ham's F12.

trast microscopy. Contaminating cells like choroidal melanocytes can be easily distinguished from RPE cells by their different morphologic appearance. They are only sparsely seen and usually do not survive in medium $F99_{RPE}$. However, such contaminated cell cultures should not be used for transplantation studies.

Like other primary cells, RPE cells in culture undergo morphologic changes described as dedifferentiation (MacDonald 1994). Cells of a later passage and greater age correspond to a more fibroblastoid phenotype. Alteration of cell morphology towards a more mesenchymal and contractile phenotype has also been described (Grisanti et al. 1997). Current studies in the field of RPE culturing deal mainly with the preparation and attachment of the cells for subsequent cell transplantation (Giordano et al. 1997; Tezel and Del Priore 1997; Tezel et al. 1997). Only a few studies focus on proliferation and differentiation of the cells, cell function, and alteration during subculture in vitro: Grisanti et al. (1997) examined the growth factor-mediated stimulation of matrix contraction by cultured RPE cells, Bost et al. (1994) examined the density-dependent expression of bFGF and clarified the underlying cellular mechanisms, and Strauss et al. (1994a, b, 1997) examined differentiation processes by evidence of altered membrane currents in RPE cells grown under different culture conditions. Membrane current patterns, which can be abducted from the cell surface after stimulation, are specific for the type of cell as well as the species from which the cell was derived, as reported by Ueda and Steinberg (1993, 1995) and Wen et al. (1994). The results from experiments with freshly isolated RPE cells were confirmed by experiments using primary cell cultures (Botchkin and Matthews 1993; Strauss and Wienrich 1994a, b; Strauss et al. 1997). Wen et al. (1994) demonstrated that pigmented cells in culture are capable of drastic changes in their electrophysiologic features toward a neuronal cell type after serial passaging. Our studies revealed that first-passage cells as well as cryopreserved and recultivated cells express a certain type of voltage-dependent Ca^{2+} channel, characteristic for freshly isolated RPE cells only, when improved culture conditions are employed (Valtink et al. 1999) (Fig. 8.1).

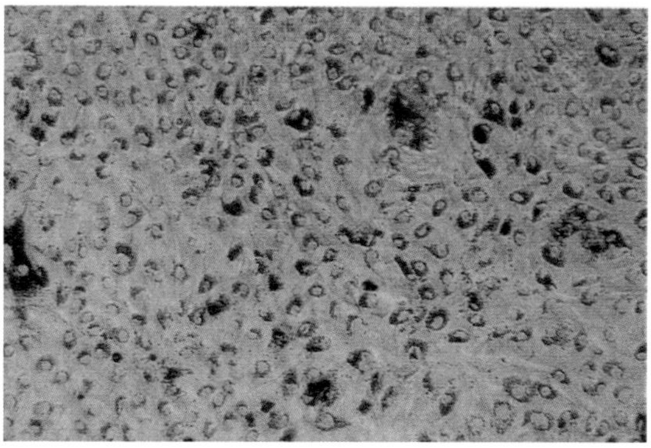

Fig. 8.1. Cultured RPE cells of early passages show an epithelioid morphology and heavy pigmentation

8.2.2 RPE Cell Bank

Like other epithelia, RPE cells express MHC antigens (see Sect. 3.5). It can therefore be assumed that immunologic reactions are likely to occur after cell transplantation. One possible way of overcoming immunologic graft rejection is to transplant histocompatible cells that are stored in a cell bank until a patient with matching HLA type has been found. Donor eyes can serve as a source of corneas for keratoplasty and also of RPE cells. Human leukocyte antigen typing of RPE cell cultures has led to more typed corneas used for keratoplasty in high-risk patients and also to typed RPE cell cultures for patients suffering from RPE degeneration. The cornea bank in Hamburg, established in 1985, receives donor eyes from the Institutes of Pathology and Forensic Medicine at the University Hospital Hamburg-Eppendorf. The average annual quantity amounts to 300–320 pairs of donor eyes. Consent for organ donation is obtained according to statutory principles. Since 1996, RPE cell cultures isolated from donor eyes are stored cryopreserved in a cell bank. The cell bank contains 106 cell cultures for transplantation from 502 isolated cell cultures. We could not detect any relation between culture success and age of donor or postmortem time (up to 106 h). Nevertheless, a tendency towards successfully culturing of differentiated, highly proliferative cultures derived from donors aged 50 or more can be observed. The average age of the donors of the cryopreserved cell cultures is 54.2±12.3 years; average postmortem time before isolation of the cells is 40.4±13.4 h. Cultures that retain some of their original pigmentation display a differentiated epithelioid-to-fusiform morphology during expanding and are fully HLA-typed are provided for subsequent transplantation studies (Table 8.1).

Table 8.1. Statistical data of the Hamburg RPE cell bank from 1996 to the present

Performance	Total
Isolated cell cultures	502
Experimental use/thrown	337
Fully HLA-typed	155
Cryopreserved for patients	106
Patient registration	42
Transplantations performed	11

For cryopreservation, confluent primary RPE cell cultures of passage P0 are trypsinized, and the cell number is determined with a Coulter counter. Half of the cell suspension is pelleted, resuspended in 1 ml FCS containing 7% DMSO, and frozen to -80°C at an approximate freezing rate of -1°C/min. The frozen cells are transferred into liquid nitrogen and stored until further use. The other half of the suspension is subcultured for HLA typing and MHC antigen expression is induced by incubating the cells with 1000 IU of interferon-g/ml in medium F99 supplemented with 10% FCS. After 24 h, the cells are trypsinized and typed. The HLA class-I typing is performed by rabbit complement-mediated cytotoxic antibody testing on RPE cells using HLA allele-specific monoclonal antibodies. HLA class II is analyzed by locus-specific polymerase chain reaction (PCR) amplification using biotinylated primers and subsequent hybridization to allele specific oligonucleotide probes according to ERLICH et al. (1991). A cell culture that matches the HLA type of a patient (correspondence on at least four MHC gene loci with preference for DRB1, A, and B, in that order) is thawed and cultured until confluence as described in Sect. 2.1 (omitting choroid-conditioned medium as a supplement). Sterility of the culture and morphology are monitored and documented. Prior to transplantation, the cells are trypsinized and centrifuged and the pellet is resuspended in basal medium F99. Membrane integrity and cell number are determined by trypan blue dye exclusion test.

8.3 RPE Cell Transplantation

8.3.1 Transplantation Studies in Various Animal Models

Retinal pigment epithelial cell transplantation has been performed in primates, rabbits, miniature pigs, and rats. The rabbit is a common animal model for studying methods of RPE cell transplantation (EL DIRINI et al. 1992). YAMAGUCHI et al. (1992), WONGPICHEDCHAI et al. (1992), and HE et al. (1993) studied methods and techniques to implant and visualize RPE cells in the rabbit subretinal space. In contrast to LOPEZ et al. (1987), who observed reattachment of the retina 24–48 h after RPE grafting, WONGPICHEDCHAI et al. (1992) observed atrophy of RPE cells caused by long-term retinal detachment (up to 1 week).

The most frequently used animal model is the Royal College of Surgeons (RCS) rat. Compared to other animal models like rabbit (SHENG et al. 1995), monkey (GOURAS et al. 1985; VALENTINO et al. 1995), or pig (LANE et al. 1989), RCS rats develop a uniform, slow, postpartal retinal degeneration which originates in the RPE, suiting them as a model for acquired or inherited retinal diseases such as ARMD, Stargardt's disease, or vitelliform macular dystrophy (LITCHFIELD et al. 1997). The retinal dystrophy of RCS rats allows scientists to study not only acceptance of the graft but also graft function, as reported in recent studies by COFFEY et al. (1989), WHITELEY et al. (1996), and SAUVE et al. (1996).

Because of the small size of the rodent eye, LUND et al. (1997) and LITCHFIELD et al. (1997) suggested choosing other animal models like dogs to compare the transplantation of cell suspensions with embedded cell sheets. To help form an opinion, surgical approaches and transplantation techniques are presented in Sect. 3.3.

8.3.2 Transplantation in Humans

The first RPE transplantation in humans was reported by PEYMAN et al. (1991), who treated one patient with an autologous pedicle graft and one with a homologous RPE–choroid patch derived from an adult donor after enucleation. The first patient had subfoveal neovascularization, subretinal hemorrhage, disciform scar formation, and RPE degeneration. After pars plana vitrectomy and scar removal, the patient received a pedicle RPE transplant as a narrow sheet of RPE cells from the normal RPE adjacent to the submacular scar area. Visual acuity improved from counting fingers at 5 feet (ca. 154 cm) to 20/400 during the next 14 months. The second patient was diagnosed with subfoveal neovascularization, disciform scar formation, and degeneration and was deemed unamenable to photocoagulation. The surgical procedure resembled that of the first case, but the transplant was derived from a donor who had to undergo enucleation due to a traumatic eye injury. The transplant, a sheet of RPE with underlying choroid, was taken from an intact area of the injured eye and transplanted without further processing. After 10 months, the transplanted RPE was proliferating and the graft was surrounded by fibrocytes without vascularization. The patient's visual acuity remained stable at the preoperative level of counting fingers at 2 feet (ca. 62 cm). Encapsulation of the graft was ascribed to the thickness of the transplant or a possible tissue incompatibility reaction.

Algvere et al. (1994, 1997) reported the transplantation of patches of fetal human RPE into five patients after removal of subfoveal fibrovascular membranes and into four patients with dry geographic atrophy, and transplantation of suspensions of fetal human RPE cells into four patients with nonexudative AMD. In cases of disciform lesions, the transplants developed macular edema accompanied by fluorescein leakage and visual impairment approximately 3 months after surgery. Patients with geographic atrophy or nonexudative AMD showed no significant fluorescein leakage, edema, or morphologic changes in the grafts except for one transplant that was no longer discernible 8 months after surgery. Three of the patients who had large numbers of soft and confluent drusen preoperatively had only a few, if any, drusen 3–4 months later. While patients with disciform lesions had a gradual loss of visual acuity over 12 months after surgery, patients with nonexudative ARMD retained stable visual acuity close to preoperative levels. A decrease in visual function concomitant with retinal edema and fluorescein leakage in patients with disciform lesions was considered a result of chronic host-graft rejection

In 1998, an ongoing clinical trial to transplant human adult RPE cells in patients suffering from juvenile macular degeneration, ARMD (drusen, dry form), subretinal neovascularization, or chorioretinal dystrophy was approved by the ethics committee of the German Physician's Society according to national laws and regulations. Inclusion criteria are the size of macular degeneration or hyperfluorescent area and preoperative visual acuity. The initial symptoms may not date back longer than 9 months. Exclusion criteria are: concomitant diseases, diabetic retinopathy, retinal occlusion, advanced cataract or glaucoma, extended macular hemorrhages, preceding laser coagulation, and previous organ or tissue transplantation. Patients indicated for RPE cell transplantations are registered on a waiting list. Cell transplantation is performed when histocompatibility between donor cells and recipient has been proven (see Sect. 2.2). At present, 42 patients are registered. The average age of the registered patients is 58±17.2 years (range 17–88 years). An RPE cell transplantation is considered when at least four HLA loci of the donor cell culture match the patient, with emphasis on the loci DRB, A, and B. To date, 11 transplantations have been performed successfully without any clinical signs of immunologic failure, but long-term results are yet to be evaluated. The results will be published separately after a longer observation period.

8.3.3 Surgical Approaches and Transplantation Techniques

Application of RPE cells can occur via a transvitreal (anterior) or trans-scleral (posterior) approach to the subretinal space. The anterior approach, which is suitable for animals with large eyes and also for humans, includes a pars plana access through the vitreous (Fig. 8.2). In brief, after penetration of the

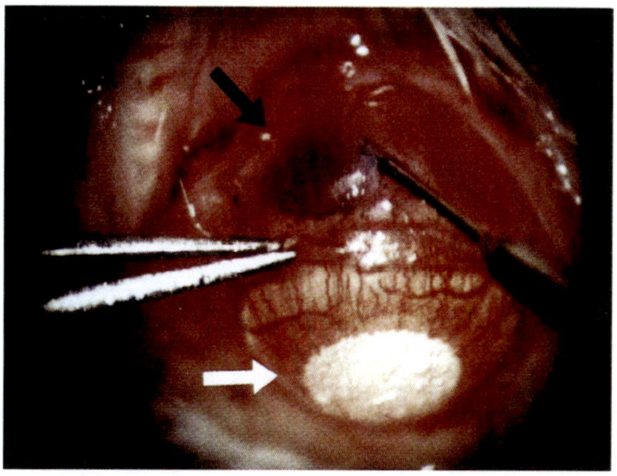

Fig. 8.2. Trans-scleral transplantation of an RPE cell suspension into the subretinal space of an RCS rat. Dorsal aspect onto the transplantation site through an operating microscope. *Black arrow* subretinal bleb, *white arrow* cornea

different layers of the eye, the transplantation instrument, usually a cannula, is directed transvitreally alongside the lens towards the retina. A retinotomy is made, the instrument is placed underneath the retina into the subretinal space, and the cells are released. El Dirini et al. (1992) improved this method by creating a second pars plana access and removing the vitreous, thus minimizing the risk of evoking proliferative vitreoretinopathy (PVR). Yamaguchi et al. (1992) described the transvitreal approach as advantageous because it allows visual control of intraoperative manipulations in the eye, the application of gas to facilitate reattachment of the retina, and the use of endocautery to minimize retinal trauma and postoperative inflammation of the eye. Another important criterion is the possibility of transferring the method to the human eye.

The trans-scleral approach occurs via laminar sclerotomy. The choroid and Bruch's membrane must be penetrated to place the graft into the subretinal space (Li and Turner 1988; Sheedlo et al. 1989). This method has the advantage of reducing loss of donor cells across the scleral lesion because, once the cannula has been removed, the tangential cut of the penetration wound functions as a seal. Furthermore, the acute angle of the injection spares the tissue immediately adjacent to the transplantation site by separating the injection site from the transplantation site (Wongpichedchai et al. 1992). As long as the retina is not penetrated, graft cells cannot migrate into the vitreous. Serious disadvantages of the trans-scleral approach are the lack of visual control of intraoperative manipulations and the destruction of the blood–retina barrier, which may initiate resorptive and inflammatory processes or immunologic complications (Lahiri-Munir 1995).

Transplantation of RPE cells can occur by simply injecting a cell suspension. This method allows the cells to spread in the subretinal space and form a cell layer that can be fragmentary, complete, or multilayered, according to the situation and density of the injected suspension (Fig. 8.3). Algvere et al. (1997) describe the transplantation of a cell suspension as advantageous because it provides an atraumatic way of distributing the cells, enables the covering of a larger area of the macula including the fovea, and requires a smaller retinotomy which self-seals and prevents reflux of the injected cells. There is a slight chance that cells may be lost due to reflux into the vitreous or through the injection channel. Furthermore, suspended cells can stick together in clumps, fail to adhere to the host Bruch's membrane, or orientate themselves in a wrong basal-apical direction.

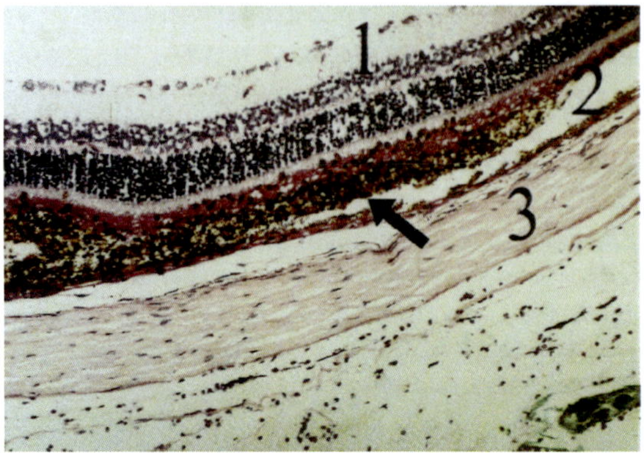

Fig. 8.3. Light microscopic illustration of an RCS rat eye 1 day after transplantation of human RPE cells showing retina (*1*), subretinal space (*2*), sclera (*3*), and transplanted, heavily pigmented RPE cells (*arrow*). PAS staining, 180+

Therefore, many investigators use cell sheets instead of suspensions to overcome these problems (Bhatt et al. 1994; Seiler and Aramant 1998; Sheng et al. 1995). These sheets consist of either gel-embedded cells or cells that are transplanted and cultured onto matrices, e.g., Descemet's membrane or lens capsule, in vitro (Hartmann et al. 1999; Thumann et al. 1997).

Sheets have the advantage that orientation and adhesion of cells are fixed and clumping or reflux cannot occur. But the use of sheets can be problematic as well. They tend to curl up when transplanted into the host's eye and thus aggravate correct placement under the retina, causing failure of recently described methods. Special instruments are needed to place a sheet underneath the retina, such as a broader pipette (Algvere et al. 1997) or a spatula with a vacuum device to prevent the sheet from floating during surgery (Steinhorst et al. 1999). In addition, the sheet must be designed in such a way that it can adhere to the host's Bruch's membrane. However, implantation (and curling) of sheets thickens the matrix between RPE and choroid and may impede diffusion of nutrients and metabolic waste between retina and choroid, contributing to retinal destruction.

At our laboratory, we established the RCS rat model for experimental transplantation of suspensions of adult human cells from the RPE cell bank. Application of the cells is performed via the trans-scleral approach described above. The primary aim of the studies was to develop a method of injecting cells that is less traumatic for the recipient tissue as well as for the donor cells (Weichel et al. 1999). Cells are applied with an oil-hydraulic microinjection pump instead of a manually controlled syringe to minimize iatrogenic damage which can be produced by the cannula used or the injection pressure (Fig. 8.4) exerted. The hydraulic pump has been shown to be more practical because it is operated by an assistant, so the hand of the surgeon is not forced to manipulate a syringe while moving the cannula into the subretinal space of the recipient eye. We ascribe a further beneficial effect to the slow and controlled build-up of injection pressure of with-the hydraulic instrument. The risk of tissue damage directly correlates with the pressure produced by the injection system. However, a residual risk of iatrogenic retinal perforation remains, due to factors that are not technically remediable, such as lack of visual control of the depth of needle insertion during transscleral surgery.

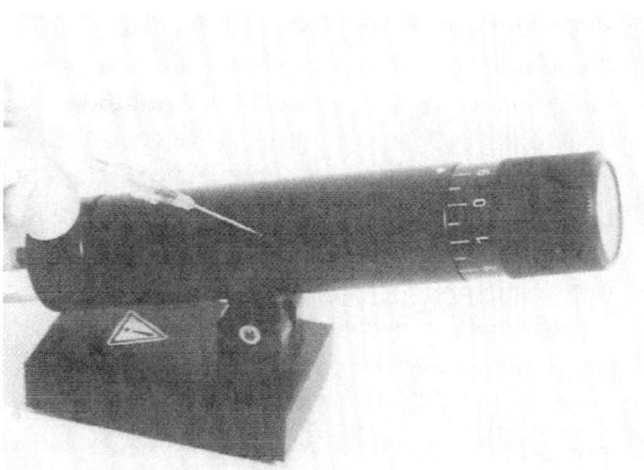

Fig. 8.4. Oil-hydraulic microinjection pump (Eppendorf-Netheler-Hinz GmbH, Germany)

8.3.4 Limitations of RPE Cell Transplantation

Despite promising results in transplantation studies involving various animal models, a complete and long-lasting rescue of photoreceptors from degeneration could not be achieved. This is mainly ascribed to incomplete concentration and adhesion of donor cells caused by inadequate surgical techniques and deficient long-term survival of the grafted cells. Other factors that limit transplantation success are mostly cell-related, e.g., dedifferentiation or loss of polarization of cells can occur during cell culture before transplantation, or cells can be falsely orientated after transplantation. Such problems are well known to occur when cells are cultured in vitro and can negatively affect any subsequent propagation and cell transplantation.

Li and Turner (1988) and La Vail et al. (1992) observed a reduction of photoreceptor degeneration after transplantation of RPE cells, but this beneficial effect did not extend to the transplant site. It became evident that larger areas need to be covered with donor cells to prolong the rescue effect. This can be achieved by injecting cell suspensions instead of transplanting cell sheets (Algvere et al. 1997). But the dynamic micromilieu of the subretinal space also plays a key role in RPE cell transplantation because fluid streams and intraocular pressure promote dispersion of injected cells, as reported by Seiler et al. (1998) and Lane et al. (1989).

Lopez et al. (1987) and Del Priore et al. (1993) held destruction of the host matrix by surgery responsible for insufficient and incomplete adhesion of the transplants. Lopez et al. (1987) found that grafted cells were integrated in only 25% of the transplanted animals. They considered failed transplantation from destruction or incomplete clearance of the Bruch's membrane from the host RPE to be caused by an inadequate transplantation technique. Blair et al. (1990), Del Priore et al. (1993), and Valentino et al. (1995) stated that saving Bruch's membrane, which is the physiologic foundation for RPE cells and has a major influence on survival of the grafts and development of a cell monolayer, must be ensured by appropriate and sensitive surgical techniques. Tezel and Del Priore (1997) showed in vitro that preventing adhesion of RPE cells to a substrate induces apoptosis. In their opinion, improving the conditions for adhesion of the cells must be the subject of further investigations. Lane et al. (1989) point out that trauma and bleeding evoke inflammatory reactions that disturb cell adhesion and must be prevented. This statement is supported by Seiler et al. (1998), who state that iatrogenic trauma of the blood–brain barrier and Bruch's membrane initializes immunologic defense reactions.

Current studies focus on the whereabouts of the donor cells months or years after transplantation. Gabrielian et al. (1999) hold cytokines that are released due to surgical trauma responsible for evoking phagocytosis or degeneration of donor cells. Six months after allogenic cell transplantation into rabbits, Crafoord et al. (1999) observed infiltration of the graft with glial cells and macrophages as well as cells with intracytoplasmatic melanin granules in the neural retina. These findings were, in part, accompanied by destruction of photoreceptor and donor cells. The cause of glial and phagocytic invasion of the transplant after both allogenic and xenogenic cell transplantation remains to be elucidated. Loss or degeneration of donor cells may be based upon immunologic reactions or nonspecific inflammation. Because immunologic reactions in the immune privileged subretinal space (see Sect. 3.5) have not been defined in full detail, some investigators classify edema as graft rejection, others the invasion of mononucleate cells or fibrosis. It is therefore necessary to study immunologic processes following a strict time course and with labeled donor cells in which the labeling may not destroy donor cells or host tissue intra vitam or change the physiologic environment of the subretinal space during the experiment.

8.3.5 Immunologic Aspects

A healthy CNS is in an immunologically privileged position: it is capable of excluding components of the immune system by means of the blood–brain barrier, thus evading direct immune reaction. In cases of diseases accompanied by destruction of the blood–brain barrier, e.g., viral encephalitis or multiple sclerosis, T cell invasion of brain tissue can be observed. How extensively the CNS and immunologic defense systems communicate in such cases is the topic of current studies (Fabry et al. 1994). In the eye, the blood–brain barrier is represented by Bruch's membrane and the RPE monolayer.

The immune privilege of the eye, also termed anterior chamber-associated immune deviation (ACAID), as described by Streilein (1990, 1997), has been discovered and studied predominantly for the anterior part of the eye. The mechanism of ACAID is that local expression of immunogenic responses is limited during exposure to a foreign antigen. Systemic response is characterized by lack of T cell mediators of delayed hypersensitivity. These T lymphocytes suppress immunogenic inflammation and retain immune mediators of concomitant immunity. A similar mechanism is considered for the subretinal space and has been described by Jiang et al. (1993, 1994). Furthermore Jörgensen et al. (1998) discussed RPE cell-induced apoptosis of activated T cells by Fas ligand expression of RPE cells, which suppresses immunologic reactions in the eye.

It remains unknown how far this immune privilege prevents rejection of allogenic or xenogenic RPE cell transplants. Liversidge et al. (1988) demonstrated that RPE cells can function as antigen-representing cells capable of evoking immune responses or inflammation processes. The RPE cells express MHC antigens completely, and in vitro cultured RPE cells can be used to determine the tissue type of the donor (Baumgartner et al. 1989; Sobottka Ventura et al. 1996; Valtink et al. 1999). The question remains whether observed postoperative invasion of the transplant site by macrophages or the „disappearance" of transplanted cells can be considered a chronic immunologic process.

Grisanti et al. (1997) and Enzmann et al. (1998) demonstrated that the local immune privilege of the eye is not absolute. RPE cells that have been stimulated to express fully MHC class I and class II antigens prior to transplantation evoked inflammation at the transplant site, depending on the number of cells injected. Furthermore, it could be demonstrated that RPE cells express autoantigens after syngenic transplantation into conventional sites such as the subconjunctival space. According to Grisanti et al. (1997), it remains to be elucidated if the RPE-specific ACAID phenomenon represents a permanent state or can be erased by the presence of an immune factor.

Many groups performed allogenic transplantation of RPE cells in RCS rats to study interaction of graft and host tissue. Gouras et al. (1989) transplanted RPE cells of nondystrophic, pigmented RCS rats into dystrophic, albinotic RCS rats without immune suppression. The authors demonstrated a delay of photoreceptor degeneration and phagocytic activity of the transplanted cells for as long as 3 months and observed no signs of immunologic processes. Li and Turner (1991) observed retardation of photoreceptor degeneration up to 1 year after RPE transplantation under similar experimental conditions. An outstanding result of their work was the long-term survival of the grafted cells by using young and healthy donor cells (donor age 6–9 days post natum) and early transplantation (postnatal day 17). Li and Turner (1991), Lopez et al. (1989), and Yamamoto et al. (1993) failed to document graft rejection in cases of allogenic RPE cell transplantation in RCS rats. Another allogenic transplantation study performed by Zhang and Bok (1998) revealed a less effective rescue of photoreceptors when donor cells and host displayed mismatches in MHC class I and class II antigens than when only incompatibility of MHC class II antigens was present. They evaluated reduced rescue of photoreceptors by the transplanted cells as a sign of chronic graft rejection.

Positive long-term outcome of allogenic transplantation experiments without immune suppression led scientists to study transplantation of xenogenic donor material into the subretinal space of RCS rats. Little et al. (1996) transplanted sheets of fetal human RPE with underlying choroid under immune suppression with cyclosporin A. After 1 month, morphologic analysis of the grafted eyes revealed rescue of photoreceptors and no signs of immune responses in the form of macrophage invasion. Ophthalmoscopic examination of the fundi of the grafted eyes revealed no redness, swelling, or edema. Castillo et al. (1997) transplanted adult human RPE cell suspensions under immune suppression. They could demonstrate that the transplanted cells were integrated into the host tissue after 1 month and the loss of photoreceptors could be reduced. Although these studies show that no acute immune response can be expected under immune suppression when xenogenic material is transplanted, Kohen et al. (1997) postulate a chronic immune reaction after transplantation of xenogenic RPE cells.

Long-term xenogenic transplantation experiments with and without immune suppression are due to establish the possibility of recording and defining immunologic processes in the subretinal space of host animals. Some authors defined edema and others defined invasion of mononucleate cells or fibrosis as immune responses, although these reactions may be assigned to resorptive inflammation in the framework of repair processes of the operative trauma and can be found histologically at every operation site. To date, only indirect parameters have been taken into consideration to describe immunologic reactions; direct parameters have not been examined. In future studies, emphasis must be placed on a clear distinction between immunologic reactions and inflammatory processes of different origin, especially in xenogenic transplantation.

8.4 Conclusion

It has become evident that retinal diseases originating in RPE atrophy, such as Stargardt's disease, vitelliform macular dystrophy, or dry forms of age-related macular degeneration, are treatable by RPE cell transplantation, and this therapeutic option should be pursued. Despite the difficulties and problems, many investigators of RPE cell transplantation in animal models reported morphologic and – to a lesser degree – functional success of RPE cell transplantation. Allograft transplantation in the RCS rat demonstrated survival of the graft for up to 1 year and a delay of retinal dystrophy at the transplant site. The integration of grafted cells into the host tissue up to 3 months after transplantation was also observed. Furthermore, it could be shown that transplanted cells are capable of phagocytosing shed rod outer segments, and a physiologic phagocytic rate of photoreceptor debris by transplanted RPE cells could be determined.

A more difficult task is the determination of cell function after transplantation. A normal function of photoreceptor cells after RPE cell transplantation has been proven by determination of opsin localization and distribution of membrane-bound Na-K-ATPase. Weak impulses of ganglion cells underneath the transplant and restoration of retinal functions were demonstrated by electroretinogram recording. Improvements in pupillary reflexes, field of vision, and recognition of patterns of grafted RCS rats were also reported.

Nevertheless, more critical aspects of the results of RPE cell transplantation have been pointed out by some investigators. Cell concentration and cell adherence seem insufficient, and vital function of the cells after transplantation has not been proven. In addition, discrimination between donor and recipient cells or other pigmented cells, e.g., macrophages that are secondarily pigmented by phagocytosing nonviable RPE cells, has to be studied in detail.

For these reasons, more basic and detailed research is needed to improve both cell culture and surgical methods. In the field of RPE cell culture, basic aspects to be examined are modulation of differentiation and maintenance of typical characteristics to obtain polarized and functional transplants. Regarding surgical techniques, instruments and practices for applying cells in the subretinal space must be modified to obtain better control over adhesion and orientation of the grafted cells. In our laboratory, research has started into possible improvement of RPE cell culture techniques, which have been demonstrated to improve the differentiation of the cells by recording of membrane currents using the whole-cell version of the patch-clamp technique. Moreover, we improved the surgical technique for cell transplantation into the subretinal space of RCS rats with minimization of donor cell and recipient tissue damage by using an oil-damped hydraulic microinjection pump.

Future studies must first clarify the immunologic conditions in animal experiments. Clinical trials involving patients should proceed after careful evaluation of current clinical trials and new results from animal studies. The aim is to improve the situation for both the patient and the surgeon.

References

Albert DM, Tso MOM, Rabson AS (1972) In vitro growth of pure cultures of retinal pigment epithelium. Arch Ophthalmol 88:63–69

Algvere PV, Berglin L, Gouras P et al (1994) Transplantation of fetal retinal pigment epithelium in age-related macular degeneration with subfoveal neovascularization. Graefes Arch Clin Exp Ophthalmol 232:707–716

Algvere PV, Berglin L, Gouras P et al (1997) Transplantation of RPE in age-related macular degeneration: observations in disciform lesions and dry RPE atrophy. Graefes Arch Clin Exp Ophthalmol 235:149–158

Astaldi GCB (1983) Use of human endothelial cell supernatant (HECS) as a growth factor for hybridomas. In: Langone JJ, van Vunakis H (eds) Methods in Enzymology Vol 92. Academic Press, New York, pp 39–46

Baumgartner I, Huber-Spitzy V, Grabner G et al (1989) HLA-typing from human donor eyes. Graefes Arch Clin Exp Ophthalmol 227:541–543

Bhatt NS, Newsome DA, Fenech T et al (1994) Experimental transplantation of human retinal pigment epithelial cells on collagen substrates. Am J Ophthalmol 117:214–221

Blair JR, Gaur V, Laedtke TW et al (1990) In oculo transplantation studies involving the neural retina and its pigment epitelium. Prog Ret Res 10:69–88

Böhnke M (1991) Corneal preservation in organ culture. Curr Opin Ophthalmol 2:432–442

Bost LM, Aotaki-Keen AE, Hjelmeland LM (1994) Cellular adhesion regulates bFGF gene expression in pigment epithelial cells. Exp Eye Res 58:545–552

Botchkin LM, Matthews G (1993) Chloride current activated by swelling in retinal pigment epithelium cells. Am J Physiol 265:C1037–C1045

Castillo BV, del Cerro M, White RM et al (1997) Efficacy of nonfetal human RPE for photoreceptor rescue: a study in dystrophic RCS rats. Exp Neurol 146:1–9

Coffey PJ, Lund RD, Rawlins JNP (1989) Retinal transplant-mediated learning in a conditioned suppression task in rats. Proc Natl Acad Sci USA 86:7248–7249

Crafoord S, Algvere PV, Seregard S et al (1999) Long-term outcome of RPE allografts to the subretinal space of rabbits. Acta Ophthalmol Scand 77:247–54

Del Priore L, Kaplan H, Silverman M et al (1993) Experimental and surgical aspects of retinal pigment epithelial cell transplantation. Eur J Implant Ref Surg 5:128–132

El Dirini AA, Wang H, Ogden TE et al (1992) Retinal pigment epithelium implantation in the rabbit: technique and morphology. Graefes Arch Clin Exp Ophthalmol 230:292–300

Engelmann K, Böhnke M, Friedl P (1988) Isolation and long-term cultivation of human corneal endothelial cells. Invest Ophthalmol Vis Sci 29:1656–1662

Engelmann K, Friedl P (1989) Optimization of culture conditions for human corneal endothelial cells. In Vitro Cell Dev Biol 25:1065–1072

Erlich H, Bugawan T, Begovich AB et al (1991) HLA-DR, DQ, and DP typing using PCR amplification and immobilized probes. Eur J Immunogen 18:33–55

Fabry Z, Raine CS, Hart MN (1994) Nervous tissue as an immune compartment: the dialect of the immune response in the CNS. Immunol Today 15:218–224

Flood MT, Gouras P, Kjeldbye H (1980) Growth characteristics and ultrastructure of human retinal pigment epithelium. Ophthalmol Vis Sci 19:1309–1320

Gabrielian K, Oganesian A, Patel SC et al (1999) Cellular response in rabbit eyes after human fetal RPE cell transplantation. Graefes Arch Clin Exp Ophthalmol 237:326–335

Giordano GG, Thomson RC, Ishaug SL et al (1997) Retinal pigment epithelium cells cultured on synthetic biodegradable polymers. J Biomed Mat Res 34:87–93

Gouras P, Flood MT, Kjeldbye H et al (1985) Transplantation of cultured human retinal pigment epithelium to Bruch's membrane of the owl monkey eye. Curr Eye Res 4:253–265

Gouras P, Lopez R, Kjeldbye H et al (1989) Transplantation of retinal pigment epithelium prevents photoreceptor degeneration in the RCS rat. In: Inherited and environmentally induced retinal degeneration. Liss, New York, pp 659–671

Griffith TS, Brunner T, Fletcher SM et al (1995) Fas ligand-induced apoptosis as a mechanism of immune privilege. Science 270:1189–1192

Grisanti S, Esser P, Schraermeyer U (1997) Retinal pigment epithelial cells: Autocrine and paracrine stimulation of extracellular matrix contraction. Graefes Arch Clin Exp Ophthalmol 235:587–598

Ham RG, McKeehan WL (1979) Media and growth requirements. In: Methods in enzymology, vol LVIII. Academic Press, New York, pp 44–93

Hartmann U, Sistani F, Steinhorst UH (1999) Human and porcine anterior lens capsule as support for growing and grafting retinal pigment epithelium and iris pigment epithelium. Graefes Arch Clin Exp Ophthalmol 237:940–945

He S, Wang HM, Ogden TE et al (1993) Transplantation of cultured human retinal pigment epithelium into rabbit subretina. Graefes Arch Clin Exp Ophthalmol 231:737–742

Ho TC, Del Priore LV (1997) Reattachment of cultured human retinal pigment epithelium to extracellular matrix and human Bruch's membrane. Invest Ophthalmol Vis Sci 38:1110–1117

Hoshi H, McKeehan WL (1984) Brain and liver cell-derived factors are required for growth of human endothelial cells in serum free culture. Proc Natl Acad Sci USA 81:6413–6417

Jiang LQ, Jorquera M, Streilein JW (1993) Subretinal space and vitreous cavity as immunologically privileged sites for retinal allografts. Invest Ophthalmol Vis Sci 34:3347–3354

Jiang LQ, Jorquera M, Streilein JW (1994) Immunologic consequences of intraocular implantation of retinal pigment epithelial allografts. Exp Eye Res 58:719–728

Jörgensen A, Wiencke AK, la Cor M et al (1998) Human retinal pigment epithelial cell-induced apoptosis in activated T cells. Invest Ophthalmol Vis Sci 39:1590–1599

Kohen L, Enzmann V, Faude F et al (1997) Mechanisms of graft rejection in the transplantation of retinal pigment epithelial cells. Ophthalmic Res 29:298–304

La Vail MM, Li L, Turner JE et al (1992) Retinal pigment epithelial cell transplantation in RCS rats: normal metabolism in rescued photoreceptors. Exp Eye Res 55:555–562

Lahiri-Munir D (1995) Retinal pigment epithelial transplantation. Springer, Berlin Heidelberg New York

Lane C, Boulton M, Marshall J (1989) Transplantation of retinal pigment epithelium using a pars plana approach. Eye 3:27–32
Li L, Turner JE (1988) Transplantation of retinal pigment epithelium cell to immature and adult rat hosts. Short-term and long-term survival characteristics. Exp Eye Res 47:771–785
Li L, Turner JE (1991) Optimal conditions for long-term photoreceptor cell rescue in RCS rats: the necessity for healthy RPE transplants. Exp Eye Res 52:669–679
Litchfield TM, Whiteley SJ, Lund RD (1997) Transplantation of retinal pigment epithelial, photoreceptor, and other cells as treatment for retinal degeneration. Exp Eye Res 64:655–666
Little CW, Castillo B, DiLoreto DA et al (1996) Transplantation of human fetal retinal pigment epithelium rescues photoreceptor cells from degeneration in the Royal College of Surgeons rat retina. Invest Ophthalmol Vis Sci 37:204–211
Liversidge JM, Sewell HF, Forrester JV (1988) Human retinal pigment epithelial cells differentially express MHC class II (HLA DP, DR, and DQ) antigens in response to in vitro stimulation with lymphokine or purified IFN-gamma. Clin Exp Immunol 73:489–494
Lopez R, Gouras P, Brittis M et al (1987) Transplantation of cultured rabbit retinal epithelium to rabbit retina using a closed-eye method. Invest Ophthalmol Vis Sci 28:1131–1137
Lopez R, Gouras P, Kjeldbye H et al (1989) Transplanted retinal pigment epithelium modifies the retinal degeneration in the RCS rat. Invest Ophthalmol Vis Sci 30:586–588
Lund RD, Coffey PJ, Sauve Y et al (1997) Intraretinal transplantation to prevent photoreceptor degeneration. Ophthalmic Res 29:305–319
MacDonald C (1994) Primary culture and the establishment of cell lines. In: Davis JM (ed) Basic cell culture: a practical approach. IRL Press, Oxford, pp 149–180
Mannagh J, Arya DV, Irvine AR Jr (1972) Tissue culture of human retinal pigment epithelium. Invest Ophthalmol 12:52–64
Peyman GA, Blinder KJ, Paris CL et al (1991) A technique for retinal pigment epithelium transplantation for age-related macular degeneration secondary to extensive subfoveal scarring. Ophthalmic Surg 22:102–108
Pfeffer BA (1991) Improved methodology for cell culture of human and monkey retinal pigment epithelium. Prog Ret Res 10:251–291
Sauve Y, Klassen H, Whiteley SJO et al (1996) Retinotopic analysis of response parameters in the superior colliculus of RCS rats following retinal pigment epithelial cell transplantation. Soc Neurosci Abstr 22:1978
Seiler MJ, Aramant RB (1998) Intact sheets of fetal retina transplanted to restore damaged rat retina. Invest Ophthalmol Vis Sci 39:2121–2131
Sheedlo HL, Li L, Turner JE (1989) Functional and structural characteristics of photoreceptor cells rescued in RPE-cell grafted retinas of RCS dystrophic rats. Exp Eye Res 48:841–854
Sheng Y, Gouras P, Cao H et al (1995) Patch transplants of human fetal retinal pigment epithelium in rabbit and monkey retina. Invest Ophthalmol Vis Sci 36:381–390
Sobottka Ventura AC, Böhnke M, Löliger C et al (1996) HLA-Typisierung von Spenderhornhäuten mit hohen post-mortem-Zeiten. Ophthalmologe 93:262–267
Steinhorst UH, Wichmann U, Kastern T et al (1999) Subretinal transplantation of confluent pigment epithelium: a novel device for nontraumatic tissue handling. Klin Monatsschr Augenheilkd 214:103–106
Strauss O, Wienrich M (1994a) Ca2+ conductances in cultured rat retinal pigment epithelial cells. J Cell Physiol 160:89–96
Strauss O, Wienrich M (1994b) Extracellular matrix proteins as substrate modulate the pattern of calcium channel expression in cultured rat retinal epithelial cells. Pflugers Arch 429:137–139
Strauss O, Mergler S, Wiederholt M (1997) regulation of L-type calcium channels by tyrosine kinase (PTK) and protein kinase C (PKC) in cultured rat and human retinal pigment epithelial cells. FASEB J 11:859–867
Streilein JW (1990) Anterior chamber associated immune deviation: The privilege of immunity in the eye. Surv Ophthalmol 35:67–73
Streilein JW (1997) Regulation of ocular immune responses. Eye 11:171–175
Tezel TH, Del Priore LV (1997) Reattachment to a substrate prevents apoptosis of human retinal pigment epithelial cells. Graefes Arch Clin Exp Ophthalmol 235:41–47
Tezel TH, Del Priore LV, Kaplan HJ (1997) Harvest and storage of adult human retinal pigment epithelial sheets. Curr Eye Res 16:802–809
Thumann G, Schraermeyer U, Bartz-Schmidt KU et al (1997) Descemet's membrane as membraneous support in RPE/IPE transplantation. Curr Eye Res 16:1236–1238
Ueda Y, Steinberg RH (1993) Voltage-operated calcium channels in fresh and cultured rat retinal pigment epithelial cells. Invest Ophthalmol Vis Sci 34:3408–3418
Ueda Y, Steinberg RH (1995) Dihydropyridine-sensitive calcium currents in freshly isolated human and monkey retinal pigment epithelial cells. Invest Ophthalmol Vis Sci 36:373–380
Valentino TL, Kaplan HJ, Del Priore LV et al (1995) Retinal pigment epithelial repopulation in monkeys after submacular surgery. Arch Ophthalmol 113:932–938
Valtink M, Engelmann K, Strauß O et al (1999) Physiological features of primary cultures and subcultures of human retinal epithelial cells prior to and following cryopreservation for cell transplantation. Graefes Arch Clin Exp Ophthalmol 237:1001–1006
Weichel J, Valtink M, Richard G, Engelmann K (1999) Optimization of a surgical approach for transplanting adult human retinal pigment epithelial cells into the subretinal space of RCS rats [ARVO Abstract]. Invest Ophthalmol Vis Sci 40 (4):S727. Abstract nr 3841
Wen R, Liu GM, Steinberg RH (1994) Expression of a tetrodotoxin-sensitive Na^+ current in cultured human retinal pigment epithelial cells. J Physiol 476:187–196
Whiteley SJO, Litchfield TM, Coffey PJ et al (1996) Improvement of the pupillary reflex of Royal College of Surgeons rats following RPE cell grafts. Exp Neurol 140:100–104
Wongpichedchai S, Weiter JJ, Weber P et al (1992) Comparison of external and internal approaches for transplantation of autologous retinal pigment epithelium. Invest Ophthalmol Vis Sci 33:3341–3352
Yamaguchi K, Yamaguchi K, Young RW et al (1992) Vitreoret-

inal surgical technique for transplanting retinal pigment epithelium in rabbit retina. Jpn J Ophthalmol 36:142–150
Yamamoto S, Du J, Gouras P et al (1993) Retinal pigment epithelial transplants and retinal function in RCS rats. Invest Ophthalmol Vis Sci 34:3068–3075
Zavazava N, Halene M, Westphal E et al (1991) Expression of MHC class I and II molecules by cadaver retinal pigment epithelium cells: optimization of postmortem HLA typing. Clin Exp Immunol 84:163–166
Zhang X, Bok D (1998) Transplantation of retinal pigment epithelial cells and immune response in the subretinal space. Invest Ophthalmol Vis Sci 39:1021–1027

Radiotherapy of Age-Related Macular Degeneration (ARMD) – Long-Term Results

9 Radiation Biology of Choroidal Neovascularisation of Age-Related Macular Degeneration

USHA CHAKRAVARTHY and SUSAN B. KLEIN

CONTENTS

9.1 Age-Related Macular Degeneration

Age-related macular degeneration (AMD) is a disorder of older people where there is progressive deterioration of central vision due to degenerative changes within the macula of the eye. The wet form of this disease is present in only one tenth of the individuals with AMD although it accounts for over 90% of those who suffer severe central visual loss (Ferris 1983). In the subgroup with wet AMD, the degenerative process results in the breakdown of the barrier between the choroid and the retina in the macular region and provokes growth of new vessels originating from the choriocapillaris (GASS 1967). These new vessels invade the sub-pigment epithelial and sub-retinal spaces and are accompanied by inflammatory cells, detached retinal pigment epithelial cells and fibroblasts. The new vessels are incompetent and leak fluid and blood, which are inimical to the health of the retinal pigment epithelium (RPE) and the photoreceptors. Fibrosis within the choroidal neovascularisation (CNV) leads to distortion of the RPE and photoreceptor architecture and is incompatible with normal central visual function.

Thermal laser photocoagulation has been used to destroy the CNV and has been the mainstay of treatment for wet AMD. However, randomised controlled clinical trials have shown that laser treatment is effective only when delivered to carefully selected cases (where the new vessels can be clearly delineated and where they lie outside the foveal avascular zone) in an optimised manner (MACULAR PHOTOCOAGULATION STUDY GROUP 1986a, b, 1991, 1994). However, these criteria are fulfilled in fewer than 15% of all cases of wet AMD. Furthermore, even after optimal and effective ablation of CNV, recurrence is common, and thus the visual outlook is uniformly poor (YANUZZI 1994). Although AMD does not result in total blindness, the loss of critical central visual function severely impacts on the quality of life of our rapidly ageing population. Thus, the search for new and more effective treatment modalities has been ongoing.

9.2 Angiogenesis

The use of ionising radiation for the treatment of CNV of AMD has captured the interest of ophthalmologists, radiation oncologists, and radiobiologists primarily because eight decades of radiation oncology have demonstrated its profound antiangiogenic effect. Angiogenesis is the term used to describe the growth of new blood capillaries. For angiogenesis to occur, there must be degradation of the basement membrane of the pre-existing capillaries and migration of the component cells (endothelial cells and pericytes), followed by proliferation of these cells to form solid tubes. Canalisation of solid tubes results in the formation of the lumen, new basement membrane synthesis and the commencement of perfusion within these vessels. Angiogenesis may be physiological and normal, for example in fetal tissues, or pathological, as in a corneal pannus or CNV.

U. CHAKRAVARTHY, MD
Professor of Vision Science and Consultant Ophthalmologist, Queen's University of Belfast, Royal Victoria Hospital, Belfast, BT12 6BA, Northern Ireland, UK
S.B. KLEIN, MD
Indiana University Cyclotron Facility, 2401 Milo B. Sampson Lane, Bloomington, IN 47408, USA

9.3 Radiosensitivity of the Vascular Endothelium

Vascular endothelial cells appear to be inherently more radiosensitive than other mesenchymal cell types such as vascular smooth muscle cells and fibroblasts (JOHNSON et al. 1982). The D_0 values (the dose that reduces cell survival by 1/e) for cultured endothelial cells range from 0.94 Gy to 1.65 Gy. These values fall within the lower half of experimentally obtained D_0 values for normal cultured human cells (RHEE et al. 1986; FUKS et al. 1992; HEI et al. 1987; MARTIN and FISHER 1984). The reasons for the increased radiosensitivity of endothelial cells are not fully understood. However, in general, cell radiosensitivity increases with active proliferation, the proportion of cells at the sensitive phase of the cell cycle, reduction in cytoplasmic organelles, and increased chromosome volume. Endothelial cells in culture exhibit many of these attributes, depending upon culture conditions. Following irradiation, protein synthesis and gene expression may be changed and some of the reported changes include altered enzymic activity (GERRITSEN et al. 1993; VERHEIJ et al. 1994), increased permeability (PHILLIPS et al. 1966), and modification of the levels of expression of adhesion molecules and attachment filaments (HIRSCH et al. 1983). In vivo and in vitro studies of the radiosensitivity of endothelial cells yield remarkably similar $D_0\theta$ values. Some of the earliest quantitative histological in vivo studies of radiosensitivity in irradiated vascular endothelium demonstrate a D_0 of 1.0 Gy, similar to that obtained in vitro (RHEINHOLD and BUISMAN 1973). However, irradiation in vivo may cause viable endothelial cells to lose contact with their basement membrane and become dislodged into the vascular lumen. Tritiated thymidine uptake following irradiation indicates that endothelial tissue begins new DNA synthesis earlier and to a greater extent than the surrounding tissues (HIRST et al. 1980). This has been interpreted as a healing response to replace cells lost through radiation damage. Although some cells may have been viable at the time of shedding, this effect is considered to contribute to the radiosensitivity of the tissue. Because irradiation causes upregulation of growth factors and cytokines in endothelial cells (WITTE et al. 1989; WILSON et al. 1993), inflammatory cells are recruited to the site of the damaged vascular tissue. These cells secrete additional cytokines, which interfere with endothelial function, destabilise endothelial metabolism, and weaken vessel wall structure (AUBIN et al. 1983). How the various pathological changes contribute to endothelial injury and impact upon cell survival and replication and, ultimately, radiosensitivity are as yet unclear.

Many synergistic biological mechanisms have been identified which also contribute to the overall pathological vascular tissue response to radiation exposure. Firstly, radiation causes swelling of endothelial cytoplasm, resulting in mechanical obstruction to flow, particularly within small vessels such as capillaries (ADAMSON et al. 1983). The resulting relatively anoxic conditions weaken the downstream cells. Secondly, radiation acts to alter blood flow within vessels through modified release of vasoactive substances, leading to thrombosis, vessel closure, endothelial activation and expression of injury (DONLON 1988). Thirdly, radiation results in the expression of adhesion molecules and recruitment of inflammatory cells with increased release of cytokines, with additional tissue damage (HIRSCH et al. 1983). Thus, the overall picture following exposure to radiation is one of endothelial damage within a procoagulant vasospastic environment.

Within the vasculature itself, there appears to be differential radiosensitivity in the components of large and small vessels (DIMITRIEVICH et al. 1984). Many studies have shown that new capillary growth is inhibited by extremely low doses of ionising radiation. TAKAHASHI (1930) found that new capillaries are more sensitive to radiation than larger vessels or fibroblasts. One mechanism accounting for the increased radiosensitivity of capillaries is the greater proportion of cycling endothelial cells than with more established, larger vessels (GILLETTE et al. 1975). Later studies revealed that the radiosensitivity of capillaries was due to a specific subpopulation of the endothelial cells' experiencing short cell cycle times (HIRST et al. 1980). Other reasons may include altered expression of growth factors in basement membranes in different vessel types. For example, basic fibroblastic growth factor (bFGF), an important angiogenic survival factor, is present in the basement membranes of blood vessels, but capillaries exhibit diminished immunoreactivity, compared with larger vessels (CORDON-CARDO et al. 1990). Exogenously added bFGF reduced the occurrence of in situ terminal transferase labelling in irradiated lung microvascular endothelial cells, indicating a reduction of radiation-induced apoptosis (FUKS et al. 1994).

9.4 Radiation Retinopathy

The radiosensitivity of the retina is due principally to the damage sustained by the retinal microvasculature, and there is a substantial body of literature on the pathogenesis of the clinical condition known as radiation retinopathy (GUNDUZ et al. 1999; TAKAHASHI et al. 1998; KINYOUN et al. 1996). A significant proportion of our knowledge on the response of the retina to ionising radiation is based on clinical observations in vivo and histopathological studies of enucleated eyes. Usually, enucleation has followed failed radiotherapy for intraocular neoplasms or when the eye has been damaged either directly or gratuitously through inclusion in the radiation field during treatment of tumours of adjacent tissues. However, when the total dose to the eye is less than 40 Gy and the fraction size has been kept below 1.8 Gy, radiation retinopathy is relatively uncommon (HARRIS and LEVENE 1976; GUNDUZ et al. 1999; PARSONS et al. 1994).

Experimental studies have shown that proliferating fibrovascular intraocular membranes in the animal model of a posterior perforating ocular injury can be inhibited by the application of a radioactive plaque to the site of perforation (CHAKRAVARTHY et al. 1989a, b) In these studies, the formation of granulation tissue between the opposing margins of an ocular wound was inhibited and delayed. It was particularly noteworthy that the inflammatory component was attenuated and that endothelial buds were sparse within the granulation tissue of irradiated wounds. Continuous irradiation of the wound using the radioactive plaque resulted in a total radiation dose between 6 Gy and 16 Gy. Doses in excess of 9.5 Gy were more effective in containing granulation tissue formation, with maximal inhibition at the highest dose of 16 Gy. The investigators also noted that the adjacent retinal neuropile, normal choroidal vasculature, and retinal pigment epithelium which were unaffected by the perforating injury appeared histologically intact, suggesting that, in the short term at least, these tissues were unaffected by radiation exposure in doses below 16 Gy. The cellular composition of the granulation tissue in the wound-healing response is not dissimilar to that seen in CNV (GROSSNIKLAUS et al. 1992). These observations led Chakravarthy et al. to suggest that low-dose ionising radiation may be useful for inducing the regression of CNV of AMD (CHAKRAVARTHY et al. 1993).

Clinical studies have shown that CNV of AMD grows rapidly, implying that the endothelial cells of the new vessels are mitotically more active than those of the established vasculature (KLEIN et al. 1989). As it is conventional wisdom that cycling cells exhibit increased radiation sensitivity, this attribute may be used to create a therapeutic advantage in terms of sparing healthy tissue.

9.5 Radiotherapy in Choroidal Neovascularisation of Age-Related Macular Degeneration

Based on the above rationale, a number of phase I and phase II clinical trials have been performed investigating the potential for low-dose radiation therapy for CNV of AMD using total doses between 10 and 15 Gy (CHAKRAVARTHY et al. 1993; HART et al. 1996; BERSON et al. 1996; BRADY et al. 1997; SPAIDE et al. 1998; STALMANS et al. 1998). While the majority of these studies suggested that radiotherapy was associated with less scarring and a better visual outcome than could be expected if no treatment were given, two studies have suggested that visual outcome in terms of natural history may be worse in radiotherapy-treated patients (SPAIDE et al. 1998; STALMANS et al. 1998). However, all the above studies lack prospective, concurrently recruited controls and thus cannot be viewed as conclusive evidence for or against treatment.

All of the above-mentioned phase I radiotherapy studies for CNV of AMD have used conventional fractionated teletherapy regimes with fraction sizes below 3 Gy and total doses below 15 Gy. However, a few have used nonstandard, large-fraction teletherapy regimes or brachytherapy (BERGINK et al. 1995; YONEMOTO et al. 1996; JAAKKOLA et al. 1998; FINGER et al. 1999). In cancer therapy, it is normal to use a large number of small fractions of radiation, as time-dose fractionation exploits the differences between the dose responses of cancerous and normal tissues. Cells in normal tissues are able to repair DNA damage and proliferate during the intervals between radiotherapy. However, when the target is non-neoplastic vascular malformations or blood vessels of benign tumours, significantly improved involution is seen following smaller total doses but larger fraction sizes of radiation (LUNSFORD et al. 1991; STEINER et al. 1992). Intuitively, the vessels comprising the choroidal neovascular membrane are more likely to resemble normal vasculature than blood vessels of cancerous tissue. Thus, it may be argued that larger fraction sizes may be more appropriate for the purposes of inducing vascular injury in non-neoplastic tissue. Nonetheless, a multicentre pooled analysis of phase I data on radiotherapy for CNV of AMD revealed no additional benefit from larger fraction sizes (Chakravarthy and Mackenzie 2000). More recent data from two small randomised controlled trials, however, do suggest a visual benefit following radiotherapy, and in both these trials fraction sizes in excess of 4 Gy were used (Bergink et al. 1998; Char et al. 1999).

Substantial controversy exists regarding the initiation, maintenance and regression of CNV of AMD. Natural history studies suggest that there is an initial period of expansion and leakage from the CNV which is followed by involution, closure of the vessels and scar formation (Stevens et al. 1997). The anti-angiogenic properties of ionising radiation suggest that it is likely to be useful in inducing and hastening neovascular regression while minimising scar formation. Ultimately, however, radiotherapy for CNV of AMD can only be used as a therapeutic measure if clinical effectiveness can be proved in terms of maintained visual function. The many ongoing, randomised, controlled clinical trials should answer this question in the near future.

Acknowledgements. These studies were partly supported by Strategic Project Grant G9404235 from the Medical Research Council, UK to Professor Chakravarthy and a travelling fellowship to Dr. S. Klein and Professor Chakravarthy from the Wellcome Burroughs Foundation, USA.

References

Adamson IYR, Bowden DH (1983) Endothelial injury and repair in radiation-induced pulmonary fibrosis. Am J Pathol 12:224–230

Aubin JE, Alders E, Heersche JN (1983) A primary role for microfilaments, but not microtubules, in hormone-induced cytoplasmic retraction. Exp Cell Res 43:439–450

Bergink GJ, Deutman AF, van den Broek JE, van Daal WA, van der Maazen RM (1995) Radiation therapy for age-related subfoveal choroidal neovascular membranes. A pilot study. Doc Ophthalmol 90:67–74

Bergink GJ, Hoyng CB, van der Maazen RWM, Vingerling JR, van Daal WAJ, Deutman AF (1998) A randomized controlled clinical trial on the efficacy of radiation therapy in the control of subfoveal choridal neovascularization in age-related macular degeneration: radiation versus observation. Graefes Arch Clin Exp Ophthalmol 236:321–325

Berson A, Finger PT, Sherr DL, Emery R, Alfieri A, Bosworth JL (1996) Radiotherapy for age-related macular degeneration: Preliminary results of a potentially new treatment. Int J Radiat Oncol Biol Phys 36:861–865

Brady LW, Freire JE, Longton WA, et al. (1997) Radiation therapy for macular degeneration: Technical considerations and preliminary results. Int J Radiat Oncol Biol Phys 39:945–948

Chakravarthy U, Biggart JH, Gardiner TA, Archer DB, Maguire CJF (1989a) Focal irradiation of perforating eye injuries with iodine-125 plaques. Curr Eye Res 8:1241–1250

Chakravarthy U, Gardiner TA, Archer DB, Maguire CJF (1989b) A light microscopic and autoradiographic study of irradiated ocular wounds. Curr Eye Res 8:337–347

Chakravarthy U, Houston RF, Archer DB (1993) Treatment of age-related subfoveal neovascular membranes by teletherapy: A pilot study. Brit J Ophthalmol 77:265–273

Chakravarthy U, Mackenzie G. External Beam Radiotherapy for Age-related macular degeneration. Brit J Ophthalmol 2000; 73:305–313

Char DH, Irvine AI, Posner MD, Quivey J, Phillips TL, Kroll S (1999) Randomized trial of radiation for age-related macular degeneration. Am J Ophthalmol 127:574–578

Cordon-Cardo C, Vlodavsky I, Haimovitz-Freedman A, Hicklin D, Fuks Z (1990) Expression of basic fibroblast growth factor in normal human tissues. Lab Invest 63:832–840

Dimitrievich GS, Fischer-Dzoga K, Griem ML (1984) Radiosensitivity of vascular tissue. I. Differential radiosensitivity of capillaries: A quantitative in vivo study. Radiat Res 99:511–535

Donlon MA (1988) Role of mast cell mediators in radiation injury and protection. Pharmacol Ther 39:373–377

Ferris FL III (1983) Senile macular degeneration: A review of epidemiologic features. Am J Epidemiol 118:132–151

Finger PT, Berson AM, Tracy NG, Szechter A (1999) Ophthalmic plaque radiotherapy for age-related macular degeneration associated with subretinal neovascularization. Am J Ophthalmol 127:170–177

Fuks Z, Vlodavsky I, Andreeff M, McLoughlin M, Haimovitz-Friedman A (1992) Effects of extracellular matrix on the response of endothelial cells to radiation in vitro. Eur J Cancer 28/A:725

Gass JDM (1967) Pathogenesis of disciform detachment of the neuroepithelium. III. Senile disciform macular degeneration. Am J Ophthalmol 63:617

Gerritsen ME, Bloor CM (1993) Endothelial cell gene expression in response to injury. FASEB J 7:523–532

Gillette EL, Maurer GD, Severin GA (1975) Endothelial repair of radiation damage following beta irradiation.Radiology 16:175–177

Grossniklaus HE, Martinez JA, Brown VB, Lambert HM, Sternberg P, Capone A, Aaberg T, Lopez PF (1992) Immunohistochemical and histochemical properties of surgically excised subretinal neovascular membranes in age-related macular degeneration. Am J Ophthalmol 114:464–472

Gunduz K, Shields CL, Shields JA, Cater J, Freire JE, Brady L W (1999) Radiation retinopathy following plaque radiotherapy for posterior uveal melanoma. Arch Ophthalmol 117:609–614

Harris JR, Levene MB (1976) Visual complications following irradiation for pituitary adenomas and craniopharyngiomas. Radiology 120:167–171

Hart PM, Chakravarthy U, Mackenzie G, Archer DB, Houston RF (1996) Teletherapy for subfoveal choroidal neovascularization of age-related macular degeneration: Results of follow-up in a nonrandomized study. Brit J Ophthalmol 80:1046–1050

Hei TK, Marchese MJ, Hall EJ (1987) Radiosensitivity and sublethal damage repair in human umbilical cord vein endothelial cells. Int J Radiat Oncol Biol Phys 13:879–884

Hirsch EZ, Chisolm GM, White HM (1983) Re-endothelialization and maintenance of endothelial integrity in longitudinal denuded tracks in the tracks of the aorta of rats. Atherosclerosis 46:287–307

Hirst DG, Denekamp J, Hobson B (1980) Proliferation studies of the endothelial and smooth muscle cells of the mouse mesentery after irradiation. Cell Tissue Kinet 13 91–104

Jaakkola A, Heikkonen J, Tommila P, Laatikainen L, Immonen I (1998) Strontium plaque irradiation of subfoveal neovascular membranes in age-related macular degeneration. Graefes Arch Clin Exp Ophthalmol 236:24–30

Johnson LK, Longenecker JP, Fajardo LF (1982) Differential radiation response of cultured endothelial cells and smooth myocytes. Anal Quant Cytol 4:188–198

Kinyoun JL, Lawrence BS, Barlow WE (1996) Proliferative radiation retinopathy. Arch Ophthalmol 114:1097–1100

Klein ML, Jorizzo PA, Watzke RC (1989) Growth features of choroidal neovascular membranes in age-related macular degeneration. Ophthalmology. 96:1416–1419

Lunsford LD, Kondziolka D, Flickinger, et al (1991) Stereotactic radiosurgery for arteriovenous malformations of the brain. J Neurosurg 75:512–524

Macular Photocoagulation Study Group (1986a) Argon laser photocoagulation for neovascular maculopathy. Three-year results from randomised clinical trials. Arch Ophthalmol 104:694–701

Macular Photocoagulation Study Group (1986b) Recurrent choroidal neovascularisation after argon laser photocoagulation for neovascular maculopathy. Arch Ophthalmol 104:503–512

Macular Photocoagulation Study Group (1991) Laser photocoagulation of subfoveal neovascular lesions in age-related macular degeneration. Arch Ophthalmol 109:1220–1231

Macular Photocoagulation Study Group (1994) Visual outcome after laser photocoagulation for subfoveal choroidal neovascularisation secondary to age-related macular degeneration. The influence of initial lesion size and initial visual acuity. Arch Ophthalmol 112:480–488

Martin DF, Fisher JJ (1984) Radiation sensitivity of cultured rabbit aortic endothelial cells. Int J Radiat Oncol Biol Phys 10:1903–1906

Parsons JT, Bova FJ, Fitzgerald CR, Mendenhall WM, Million RR (1994) Radiation retinopathy after external-beam irradiation: Analysis of time-dose factors. Int J Radiat Oncol Biol Phys 30: 765–773

Phillips TL (1966) An ultrastructural study of the development of radiation injury in the lung.Radiology 87:49–54

Reinhold HS and Buisman GH. (1973) Radiosensitivity of capillary endothelium. Br J Radiol 46:54-57

Rhee JG, Lee I, Song CW (1986) The clonogenic response of bovine aortic endothelial cells in culture to radiation.Radiat Res 106:182–189

Spaide RF, Guyer DR, McCormick B, et al (1998) External beam radiotherapy for choroidal neovascularisation. Ophthalmology 105:24–30

Stalmans P, Leys A, et al (1998) External beam radiotherapy fails to control the growth of chroidal neovascularisation in age-related macular degeneration. A review of 111 cases. Retina 17:481–492

Steiner L, Lindquist C, Adler JR, Torner JC et al (1992) Clinical outcome of radiosurgery for cerebral arteriovenous malformations. J Neurosurg 77:1–8

Stevens TS, Bressler NM, Maguire MG, et al (1997) Occult choroidal neovascularization in age-related macular degeneration. Arch Ophthalmol 15:345–350

Takahashi K, Kishi S, Muraoka K, Tanaka T, Shimizu K (1998) Radiation choroidopathy with remodeling of the choroidal venous system. Am J Ophthalmol 125:367–373

Takahashi T (1930) The action of radium upon the formation of blood capillaries and connective tissue. Br J Radiol 3:439

Verheij M, Koomen GC, van Mourik JA, Dewitt L (1994) Radiation-reduced cyclo-oxygenase activity in cultured human endothelial cells at low doses. Prostaglandins 48:351–366

Wilson RE, Taylor SL, Atherton GT, Johnson D, Waters CM, Norton JD (1993) Early response gene signaling cascades activated by ionizing radiation in primary human B cells. Oncogene 8:3229–3237

Witte L, Fuks Z, Haimovitz-Friedman A, Vlodavsky I, Goodman D S, Eldor A (1989) Effects of irradiation on the release of growth factors from bovine, porcine, and human endothelial cells. Cancer Res 49:5066–5072

Yanuzzi L (1994) A new standard of care for laser photocoagulation of subfoveal choroidal neovascularisation secondary to age-related macular degeneration. Arch Ophthalmol 112:462–464

Yonemoto LT, Slater JD, Friedrichsen EJ et al (1996) Phase I/II study of proton beam irradiation for the treatment of subfoveal choroidal neovascularization in age-related macular degeneration: treatment techniques and preliminary results. Int J Radiat Oncol Biol Phys 36:867–871

10 Principles and Technique of Radiotherapy of Age-Related Macular Degeneration

Ulrike Höller and Winfried E. Alberti

CONTENTS

10.1 Introduction

This chapter gives the reader not familiar with radiotherapy an introduction to the principles and techniques of irradiation of the eye.

Since the discovery of X-rays, radiation therapy has been employed in the management of benign conditions. Roentgen therapy was used for retinal diseases with newly formed vessels as early as 1948, and long-term treatment results of age-related macular degeneration (AMD) were reported in 1975 (Guyton and Reese 1948; Sautter and Utermann 1975). Experimental studies and recent favorable clinical results have renewed interest in the potential benefit of radiotherapy for AMD-related subfoveolar choroidal neovascularization (CNV) (Chakravarthy et al. 1993). To date, a variety of treatment techniques and dose fractionation regimens have been developed.

10.2 Rationale of Radiotherapy for Age-Related Macular Degeneration

The radiosensitivity of capillary endothelium has long been recognized. Radiotherapy is effective in choroidal hemangiomas (Alberti 1986; Scott et al. 1991). Doses of 20 Gy induced the resorption of subretinal exudation (Schilling et al. 1996).

The interaction of radiation with tissue is complex. On a molecular level, the main target is DNA. Ionizing radiation can cause double-strand breaks that result in immediate or reproductive cell death and ultimately in cell depletion. Less extensive lesions, so-called sublethal damage, can be repaired so that the cell recovers from the radiation injury (Raicu et al. 1993; Withers and McBride 1997). Further observed mechanisms of radiation include a decrease in cell replication and reduction of prostacyclin production (Hosoi et al. 1993; Rubin et al. 1996). Radiation also increases cell permeability and cell adhesion molecule expression and induces apoptosis of microvascular cells in vitro (Gaugler et al. 1997; Heckmann et al. 1998; Langley et al. 1997; Waters et al. 1996).

The rationale for radiotherapy of AMD-associated CNV is the observation that the radiosensitivity of vascular endothelium is high due to the high proliferation rate of capillary endothelial cells (Chakravarthy et al. 1989a; De Gowin et al. 1976; Johnson et al. 1982). The goal of irradiation is to inhibit further pathologic endothelial cell proliferation. Furthermore, radiotherapy possibly suppresses the inflammatory and exudative component of AMD (Archambeau et al. 1998; Chakravarthy et al. 1989a). All of these features were demonstrated in experimental choroidal neovascularization in rabbit eyes (Miya-

U. Höller, MD
W. E. Alberti, MD
Professor, Department of Radiotherapy and Radio-Oncology, University Hospital Hamburg, Martinistrasse 52, 20246 Hamburg, Germany

MOTO et al. 1999). The degenerative process itself and the persistence of the stimuli that upregulate the growth factors and angiogenesis are probably not altered by radiotherapy (SPAIDE et al. 1998).

10.3 Techniques of Radiotherapy

Ideally, the target volume, i.e., the macula region, is irradiated while sparing the adjacent normal tissue. The most radiosensitive structures are the lens, retina, and optic nerve of the treated and the fellow eye. Frequently, the tolerance dose of these organs at risk is similar to or even lower than the effective treatment dose, thus limiting it. Therefore, the goal of treatment technique is twofold: homogeneous, sufficiently high dose distribution within the target and a steep dose gradient to the surrounding structures. In modern radiotherapy, a wide array of ionizing beams with given physical properties is available. Each method has specific characteristics that offer specific advantages. In the planning procedure, beam quality, field arrangement, and beam modifiers are chosen for optimal dose delivery.

10.3.1 External Beam Radiotherapy

The term external beam therapy or teletherapy denotes radiation delivered at the large distance of 80–120 cm from the patient. Most commonly, photon beams of 4–8 MeV energy generated by a linear accelerator are employed.

10.3.1.1 Planning and Treatment Procedures

In the following the procedures of treatment preparation and delivery frequently used in radiotherapy are outlined. Treatment planning refers to the design of treatment portals that hit the target volume and spare the volume at risk and is achieved with a simulator. This is a machine with a diagnostic X-ray tube attached to a gantry that is positioned exactly like the treatment machine around the patient. It provides a high-quality image of the treatment portal in relation to the patient's anatomy so that the optimal treatment portal can be identified and marked on the patient or on a positioning device. Due to the small volume of the target and the proximity of critical structures prohibiting large safety margins, more sophisticated treatment techniques are sometimes used, especially if higher doses are aimed for. Such treatments are designed with computer-assisted planning on a computed tomogram of the patient's head fixed in treatment position. Cross-sectional anatomy and modern three-dimensional planning facilities allow optimization including the choice of multiple portals, gantry rotation, and beam modifiers.

For the planning procedures and therapy, the patient is placed comfortably in supine position on the table. The head is immobilized with an individual face mask of thermoplastic material to ensure setup accuracy (Fig. 10.1). Thus, day-to-day setup deviations during a 2- to 4-week treatment course may be limited to a range of 2–5 mm (SWEENEY et al. 1998; VAKAET et al. 1998). A cutout in the region of the eye allows the patient's gaze angle to be monitored during simulation and treatment.

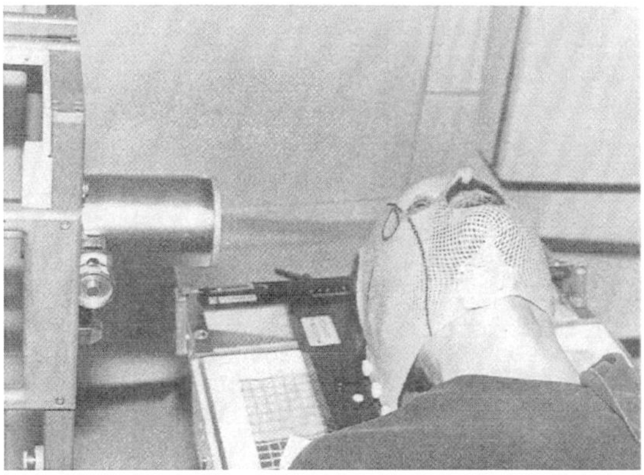

Fig. 10.1. Treatment setup in the accelerator room. The treatment portal is marked on the head mask

10.3.1.2 Dosimetry

Radiotherapy is best described by isodose distributions superimposed on cross-sectional anatomy on computed tomograms.

Frequently a half-beam technique is used. The anterior beam edge is placed a few millimeters posteriorly to the lens and the gantry is angled 5–10° posteriorly to avoid irradiating the lenses. An absorber in the shape of a D corresponding to the form of the eye globe may be added to protect surrounding structures

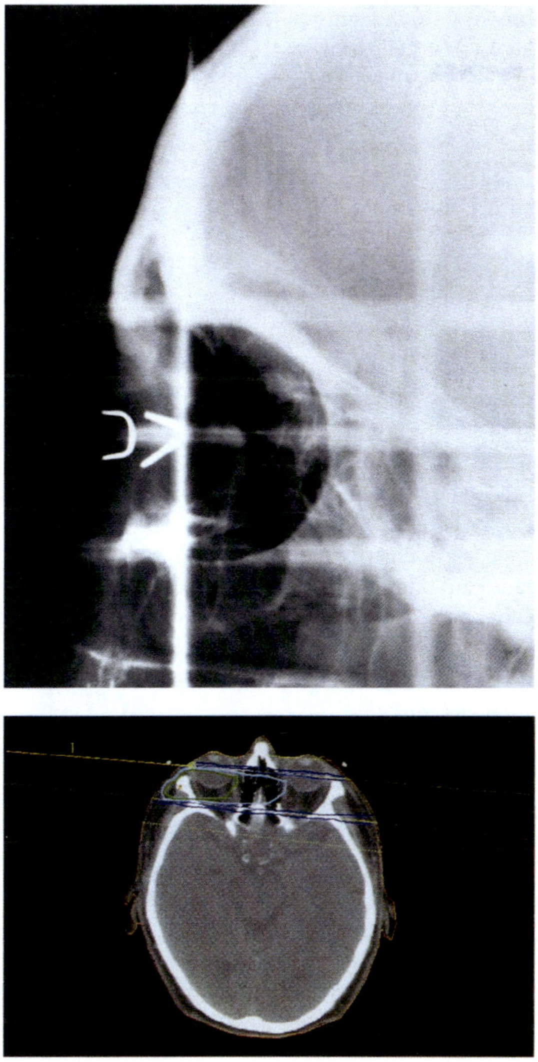

a

b

Fig. 10.2. a Simulation of a lateral oblique treatment portal D-shaped by a tungsten absorber. **b** Corresponding axial CT scan of the eye with superimposed isodoses (95%–80%–50%–20%). The macula is encompassed by the 95% isodose

(Fig. 10.2). Furthermore, the beam may be angled caudally to exclude the contralateral eye completely; this frequently requires the use of wedge filters. A beam's eye view reconstructs the patients anatomy as seen from the treatment portal and is most helpful when the beams are angled noncoplanar (Fig. 10.3).

Various other techniques have been described and are discussed elsewhere in this book. For example, BERGINK et al. (1994) chose two very small anterior fields of 1 cm (Fig. 10.4). Rotational techniques with an external collimator of very small diameter have been introduced (MAUGET-FAYSSE et al. 1999).

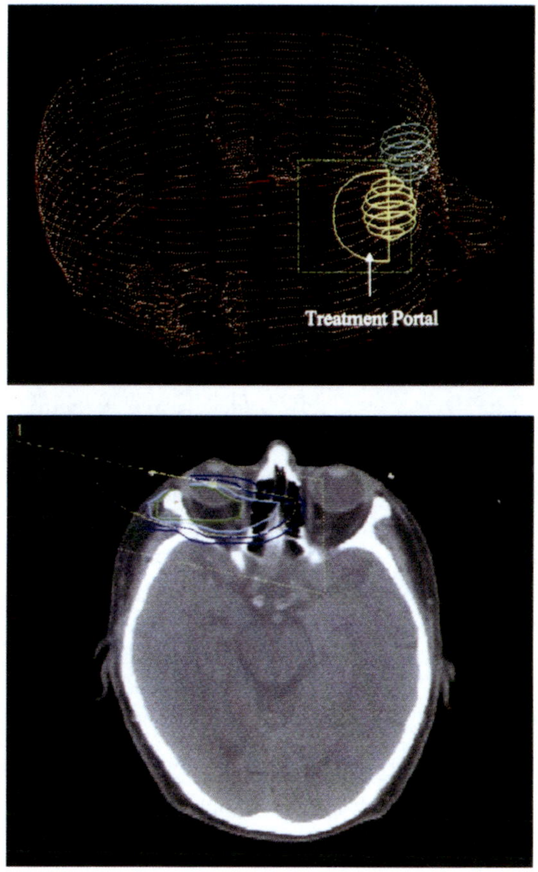

a

b

Fig. 10.3. a Beam's eye view. The right eye is treated by a lateral portal angled in the craniocaudal direction, thus avoiding the contralateral eye. **b** Corresponding axial CT scan

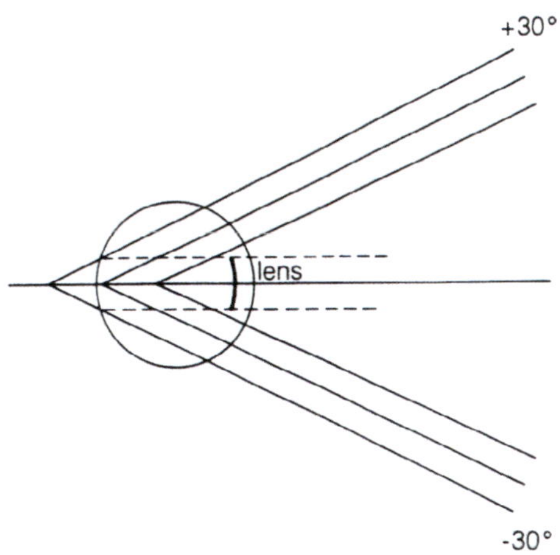

Fig. 10.4. Lens-sparing technique. The beams are directed 30° from the optical axis, field size 1 cm² (BERGINK et al. 1994)

10.3.1.3
Stereotactically Guided Radiotherapy

Stereotactically guided radiotherapy is a high-precision technique that delivers radiation to a small volume of 0.5–3 cm diameter with a very steep dose gradient of a few millimeters to the periphery so that the surrounding structures are well spared. It is performed with a dedicated linac or a Gamma knife, a machine mounted with approximately 200 small cobalt sources focused on the isocenter. Linacs are equipped with additional collimators of 0.5–2 cm diameter made of tungsten or micromultileaf absorbers to achieve conformal field shaping. For treatment planning and setup, individually defined stereotactic coordinates are used. This technique requires utmost immobilization of the patient's head with an individually fabricated special head mask or bite block. Repositioning accuracy of the head mask has been reported in the range of 1–3 mm (Delannes et al. 1991; Gill et al. 1991; Schlegel et al. 1992). During treatment of the eye, the patient can be asked to fixate a light signal throughout treatment to ensure correct alignment of the eye (Debus et al. 1997; Eter et al. 1998).

These labor- and time-intensive procedures are intended for the delivery of high doses in critical areas, e.g., curative treatment of melanoma (Debus et al. 1997). In view of the usually low and well-tolerated doses prescribed, few centers have used stereotactic techniques in the treatment of AMD (Holz et al. 1997).

10.3.2
Brachytherapy

Brachytherapy refers to radiation delivered at a very short distance to the patient by an applicator in contact with the surface of the target tissue. The resulting dose distribution is characterized by a high surface dose, a high but inhomogeneous dose within the target, and a steep gradient toward the inner ocular tissues and the optic nerve. The radioisotopes differ in their characteristic dose distribution in depth and dose rate, i.e., dose delivered per unit of time. For CNV, sealed radioactive plaques loaded with the β-ray-emitting radioisotope strontium-90 at a dose rate of 1.79 cGy/s or γ-ray-emitting palladium-103 at a rate of 1.071 cGy/h have been used (Finger et al. 1999; Jaakkola et al. 1998).

The applicator is sutured to the sclera beneath the macula and remains in place until the appropriate dose has been absorbed after 1 or 28 hours (strontium-90 or palladium-103, respectively). In comparison to external beam radiotherapy, this is a more invasive procedure available at few centers.

10.3.3
Proton Therapy

Protons are particles with a positive charge that travel through the tissue depositing little energy along the path until near the end of the track. Here the protons slow down and produce more ionization so that the dose rapidly rises to a maximum. In the peak region, the dose substantially exceeds that in the more superficial tissues (Hendee and Ibbott 1996). The resulting dose distribution is depicted by a graph of dose versus depth in tissue and displays the characteristic Bragg peak (Fig. 10.5). In comparison to X-rays, electrons, and photons, the unique advantage of protons is the steep falloff after a well-defined penetration depth in tissue, delivering relatively high doses at the chosen depth and low doses en route and beyond the target tissue.

The radiobiologic properties of the proton beam are comparable to those of X-rays. The relative biologic effectiveness (RBE) is assumed to be 1.1 relative to cobalt-60. The dose is prescribed as cobalt Gray equivalent (cGe), i.e., the absorbed dose multiplied by RBE 1.1 (Hendee and Ibbott 1996; Joiner 1993).

In a comparison of the dosimetry of photon and proton beam therapy, the contralateral eye is clearly better protected with the latter technique (Mazal et

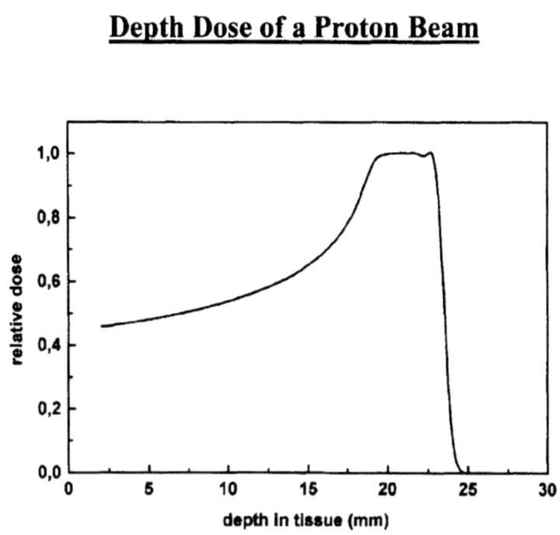

Fig. 10.5. Depth-dose curve of a proton beam depicting the Bragg peak. (Proton Therapy Facility, Hahn-Meitner Institute, Berlin)

al. 1998). However, due to the very steep dose gradient, a high-precision setup procedure is necessary to avoid geographic miss.

Unfortunately, the cyclotrons or synchrotrons that generate proton beams are very expensive, so that there are only few machines available throughout the world.

10.4 Fractionation

The effect of radiotherapy is determined by the physical dose distribution and by the fractionation schedule. The latter comprises total dose, dose per fraction, overall treatment time, time per fraction (i.e., dose rate), and interval between fractions.

The dose-response relationship for radiotherapy is typically described by a sigmoid curve, with a large variability in steepness from one study and tissue to another (BENTZEN 1994). Higher doses of irradiation are more effective in (tumor) growth control but also increase damage to normal tissue. The dose to normal tissue should, therefore, be reduced as much as possible by the treatment technique. A further differential effect on target tissue and normal tissue can be achieved by dose fractionation schedules making use of the different mechanisms of recovery of normal and target tissue to radiation injury. In fractionated radiotherapy, surviving cells are able to repair injury, proliferate, and replace lost cells. The reactions of tissue have been described by the 5 R's of radiotherapy – recruitment of cells from the quiescent G0 phase into the cell cycle, reoxygenation of hypoxic tumors, repair of the molecular injury, repopulation of depleted cells by (accelerated) proliferation of stem cells, and intrinsic radiosensitivity (WITHERS and MCBRIDE 1997). The contribution of each mechanism to the radiation effect varies considerably from tissue to tissue. Increasing the dose per fraction puts late-reacting tissues such as the retina, optic nerve, and lens at a higher risk of toxicity than applying the same total dose applied in smaller fractions (AMOAKU et al. 1992; HARRIS and LEVENE 1976; PARSONS et al. 1994a, b). Therefore, in order to minimize side effects of a given therapeutic total dose, radiotherapy is conventionally fractionated in daily doses of 1.8–2 Gy five times per week.

However, hypofractionated or single-fraction radiation may be appropriate for CNV. In a benign disease of larger vessels, intracranial arteriovenous malformation, single-dose radiation with 15–25 Gy proved more effective than fractionated therapy (ENGENHART et al. 1994; GLANZMANN 1978; MAKOSKI et al. 1989). To date, the most encouraging results with irradiation of CNV have been achieved with fairly high total and fractional doses, suggesting a small therapeutic window (BERGINK et al., MAUGET-FAYSSE et al., and YONEMOTO et al. in this edition). The linear-quadratic model (also termed LQ or α/β model) is a mathematical description of biological response to radiation. It can be used to compare the biological effectiveness of differing fractionation regimes and to estimate biological isoeffect doses (BED). The dose of 4×6 Gy (BERGINK et al. 1998) is assumed to be isoeffective to 32 Gy in highly proliferative tissue (α/β value 10 Gy) and to 48 Gy in optical nerve or retina (α/β value 2 Gy) applied with conventional 2 Gy fractions. So far, the α/β value for CNV has not been determined, but it probably resembles that for proliferating tissue.

10.5 Clinical Studies

10.5.1 Nonrandomized Studies of External Beam Radiotherapy

In 1993, Chakravarthy and coworkers reported a series of 19 patients treated with external beam irradiation at doses of 10, 12 or 15 Gy in fractions of 2 or 3 Gy. After 1 year, visual acuity stabilized or improved in 63% of patients and significant regression of the membrane was measured in 77% (CHAKRAVARTHY et al. 1993). In a control group of six patients who refused treatment, visual acuity deteriorated in all patients but one and the membrane enlarged in all. In a later report of 41 patients treated with 10, 12 or 15 Gy, the mean change in visual acuity was less than 1 line, in contrast to the control group, which lost a mean of 3.5 lines at 12 months (HART et al. 1996). The difference between treated and untreated patients was significant ($p<0.03$).

These results suggested that radiation can maintain vision and encouraged numerous prospective studies (Table 10.1). A comparison of these studies is limited by the heterogeneity of patient groups: classic CNV may indicate a more rapid loss of vision, and patients with good baseline visual acuity experience a greater loss of vision because they already „have a lot to lose."Furthermore, the definitions of endpoint, i.e., the point of stabilized visual acuity, vary from

Table 10.1. Radiotherapy of AMD: summary of peer-reviewed studies

Study	Dose	*N* patients or eyes	Control group	Follow-up (months)*	Vision stable at 1 year	Endpoint loss of VA	Comments
Pöstgens 1997	2 Gy/0.5 Gy×4	67	Untreated *n*=96	84	–	–	No difference between groups
Spaide 1997	10 Gy/ 2 Gy×5	91	Historical *n*=119	12 (90% of patients)	51% vs. 62%, NS	≤-2 lines	
Hollick 1966	11 Gy–12.5 Gy/5F	19	None	Minimum 12	53%		
Prettenhofer 1998	14.4 Gy/1.8 Gy×8	40	None	Minimum 12	15%	≤-2 lines	Classic CNV size 500%–700% of baseline
Hart 1996	10 Gy/2 Gy×5 12 Gy/2 Gy×6 15 Gy/3 Gy×5	41	Patients refusing treatment, *n*=13	24 treated, 55 untreated	Worsening 12% of baseline vs. 75% at 24 months		
Staar 1999	16 Gy/ 2 Gy×8	73	Untreated, *n*=18	Median 13, minimum 11	37%	≤0 lines	No difference to untreated patients in matched pair analysis
RAD 1999	16 Gy/ 2 Gy×8	101	Randomized sham irradiation, *n*=104	12 (89% of patients)	48% (treated) vs. 49% (sham treated), NS	≤-3 lines	Refer also to chapter Bellmann et al. this book
Stalmans 1997	20 Gy/2 Gy×10	111	None	Minimum 12	20%	≤-2 lines	CNV median size 134% and 264% of baseline (occult/classic)
Sasai 1997	10 Gy/2 Gy×5 20 Gy/2 Gy×10	18 18	Historical, *n*=18 Median 15	Median 24	55% in both dose groups vs. 35%, NS	≤-2 lines	More frequent decrease in membrane size in 20 Gy group (p<0.05)
Thölen 1999	10 Gy/2 Gy×5 36 Gy/2 Gy×18	16 16	Randomized observed patients, *n*=19	12 (80% of patients)	Classic CNV: -5.4 to -6 vs. -8 lines (p<0.05), occult CNV: no differ.		4/16 eyes retinopathy in 36 Gy group
Mauget-Faysse 1999	20 Gy/4 Gy×4 16–20 Gy/4 or 5F	212	None	12 (50% of patients)	34% improvement	≥+2 lines	No difference between groups, 47% decrease in membrane size
Char 1999	7.5 Gy×1	14	Randomized observed patients, *n*=13	Mean 15	78% vs. 38% control, p<0.04	≤-3 lines	
Bergink 1994	8 Gy×1 12 Gy/6 Gy×2 18 Gy/6 Gy×3 24 Gy/6 Gy×4	40	None	Mean 24 Mean 14 Mean 11 Mean 6	40% 70% 60% 80%	≤-2 lines	No difference between groups
Bergink 1998	24 Gy/6 Gy×4	32	Randomized observed patients, *n*=36	12 (95% of patients)	52% (treated) vs. 32% (observed), p=0.03	≤-2 lines	Refer also to Bergink et al. in this book
Finger 1999	Brachytherapy 12.5 Gy–23.6 Gy×1	23	None	Mean 19	9/13	≤-3 lines	Refer also to Finger et al. in this book
Yonemoto 2000	Proton therapy 8 CGE 14 CGE	 21 27	None	Mean 21	 36% 89%	≤-2 lines	Significant response in high-dose group, minor retinopathy, refer also to Yonemoto et al. in this book

VA, visual acuity; F, fractions. *Only studies with mean or minimum follow-up of approximately 1 year are included.

losses of 0 to 3 lines. Some studies include control groups of patients who refused treatment. However, most results are compared with the natural course of disease or the outcome of the Macular Photocoagulation Study observation group. This may be misleading because the radiation studies do not reflect the strict entry criteria of that study.

SPAIDE et al. (1998) reported a loss of 3 lines or more in 49% of 83 patients 1 year after treatment with 10 Gy in five fractions. There was no significant difference from a historical control group of observed patients from a randomized study investigating interferon.

STAAR et al. (1999) treated patients with exclusively classic CNV with 16 Gy (2 Gy per fraction). After a minimum follow-up of 11 months, visual acuity stabilized or improved in 37% of 73 patients. In a matched pair analysis with patients who refused treatment, radiotherapy proved ineffective.

Radiotherapy with 20 Gy in ten fractions was also ineffective in a group of 111 patients followed up for a minimum of 12 months (STALMANS et al. 1997). Twenty percent of patients had improved or stable vision and CNV growth was usually similar to that in the untreated eyes and sometimes even worse.

Low-dose radiation similar to that used in treatment of inflammatory diseases has also been evaluated; in a retrospective study, the outcome of 4×0.5 Gy for 67 patients with well- or ill-defined CNV was similar to the natural course in a historical control group after 1–10 years (PÖSTGENS et al. 1997).

Few dose-finding studies have been performed. A dose-response relationship has not yet been well established, probably due to the small number of patients. In the study of HART et al. (1996), there was no difference in results between 10, 12 and 15 Gy.

In another study, 10 or 20 Gy was administered in two consecutive groups of 18 patients each; at 12 months, vision was maintained in 55% of patients in both treated groups, compared to 35% in a historical control group (SASAI et al. 1997). However, the patients in the 20-Gy group showed a significant decrease in membrane size as opposed to the patients in the 10-Gy and control groups.

A randomized phase II study compared 10 Gy and 36 Gy (2 Gy per fraction) to observation. After 12 and 18 months, visual acuity of patients with classic CNV declined by 1.7–2.1 and 5.4–6 lines, respectively in the treated group versus 6.5 and 8 lines in the observation group ($p<0.05$). With respect to visual acuity, a dose of 36 Gy was no more effective than 10 Gy, whereas membrane growth was better controlled by the higher dose. However, the study was closed early due to unexpected retinopathy which presented with cotton wool exudates, hemorrhages, and microaneurysms in four of 16 patients but did not impair visual acuity (THÖLEN et al. 1998).

Hypofractionated therapy may be more effective than conventional fractionation. In a dose escalation study, groups of ten patients were treated with a single fraction of 8 Gy or with 12, 18 and 24 Gy, respectively, in fractions of 6 Gy using small fields (BERGINK et al. 1994). Forty percent of the patients treated with 8 Gy retained their vision, compared to 60–80% of those treated with higher doses. However, the mean follow-up ranged from 21 to 6 months in the 8-Gy and 24-Gy groups, respectively. The authors concluded that radiation therapy with a total dose of 12 Gy or more has a beneficial effect and initiated a randomized study employing 24 Gy.

Radiotherapy with 16–20 Gy in fractions of 4 Gy applied with a lateral beam or arc technique was promising: visual acuity improved in 34% of the patients and membrane size decreased in 47% of the eyes. However, late side effects occurred in a substantial number of patients (MAUGET-FAYSSE et al. 1999).

In a randomized study by CHAR et al. (1999), 27 patients were either treated with a single fraction of 7.5 Gy or observed. After a mean follow-up of 15 months, the loss of visual acuity was slightly less in the treated group, a finding of borderline significance ($p<0.046$).

10.5.2 Randomized Studies of External Beam Radiotherapy

As the potential of radiotherapy can only be determined by randomized trials, several trials were initiated in 1996 to study conventional therapy with 12–16 Gy low-dose radiation (4×0.25 Gy versus 4×2 Gy or 4×4 Gy) or hypofractionated therapy with 4×6 Gy.

Two studies have been published and are discussed in detail in this volume. Briefly, radiotherapy with a conventional fractionation of 8×2 Gy was ineffective in a double-blind study randomizing patients to irradiation or sham treatment (RAD 1999; HOLZ et al. in this volume). The double-blind design was chosen because the measurement of outcome variables is influenced by subjective factors such as enthusiasm and performance of patients and personnel.

In contrast, in the Nijmegen study, patients who received 24 Gy in fractions of 6 Gy had significantly less frequent and less severe loss of vision than untreated patients (Bergink et al. 1998). Retinopathy or optic neuropathy was not observed, perhaps due to the very small field of 1 cm^2.

10.6 Conclusion

Radiation therapy is considered an experimental treatment for AMD-related CNV. In vitro and in vivo radiosensitivity of the retinal epithelium and choriocapillaris has been demonstrated. In clinical experience, radiotherapy is well tolerated in the range of 20–30 Gy. Randomized studies have proven conventional treatment with 16 Gy to be ineffective in preserving vision after 2 years. The optimal fractionation and dose of radiotherapy and the role of macula-sparing techniques are still to be defined. Randomized, controlled trials are necessary to determine if a therapeutic window exists.

References

Alberti W (1986) Radiotherapy of choroidal hemangioma. Int J Radiat Oncol Biol Phys 12:122

Amoaku WMK, Mahon GJ, Gardiner TA et al (1992) Late ultrastructural changes in the retina of the rat following low-dose x-irradiation. Graefes Arch Clin Exp Ophthalmol 230:569–574

Archambeau JO, Mao XW, Yonemoto LT et al (1998) What is the role of radiation in the treatment of subfoveal membranes. Review of radiobiologic, pathologic, and other considerations to initiate a multimodality discussion. Int J Radiat Oncol Biol Phys 40:1125–1136

Bentzen, SM (1994) Radiobiological considerations in the design of clinical trials. Radiother Oncol 32:1–11

Bergink GJ, Deutman AF, Van den Broek JFCM et al (1994) Radiation therapy for subfoveal choroidal neovascular membranes in age-related macular degeneration. Graefes Arch Clin Exp Ophthalmol 232:591–598

Bergink GJ, Hoyng CB, Van der Maazen RWM et al (1998) A randomized controlled clinical trial on the efficacy of radiation therapy in the control of subfoveal choroidal neovascularization in age-related macular degeneration: Radiation versus observation. Graefes Arch Clin Exp Ophthlamol 236:321–325

Chakravarthy U, Biggart JH, Gardiner TA et al (1989a) Focal irradiation of perforating eye injuries: Minimum effective dose and optimum time of irradiation. Curr Eye Res 8:1241–1250

Chakravarthy U, Houston RF, Archer DB (1993) Treatment of age-related subfoveal neovascular membranes by teletherapy: A pilot study. Br J Ophthalmol 77:265–273

Char, DH, Irvine AI, Posner MD et al (1999) Randomized trial of radiation for age-related macular degeneration. Am J Ophthalmol 127:574–578

Debus J, Engenhart-Cabillic R, Holz FG et al (1997) Stereotactic precision radiotherapy in the treatment of intraocular malignancies with a micro-multileaf collimator. Front Radiat Ther Oncol 30:39–46

De Gowin RL, Lewis LJ, Hoak JC et al (1976) Radiosensitivity of human endothelial cells in culture. J Lab Clin Med 81:42–48

Delannes M, Daly N, Bonnet J et al (1991) Fractionated radiotherapy of small inoperable lesions of the brain using a non-invasive stereotactic frame. Int J Radiat Oncol Biol Phys 21:749–755

Engenhart R, Wowra B, Debus J, Kimmig BN et al (1994) The role of high-dose, single fraction irradiation in small and large intracranial arteriovenous malformations. Int J Radiat Oncol Biol Phys 30:521–529

Eter N, Schüller H, Spitznas M et al (1998) Fixation monitoring during radiation therapy for subfoveal neovascularization. Graefes Arch Clin Exp Opthalmol 236:806–810

Finger P, Berson A, Tracy NG et al (1999) Ophthalmic plaque radiotherapy for age-related macular degeneration asssociated with subretinal neovascularization. Am J Ophthalmol 127:170–177

Gaugler, MH, Squiban C, Van der Meeren A et al (1997) Late and persistent up-regulation of intercellular adhesion molecule-1 (ICAM-1) expression by ionizing radiation in human endothelial cells in vitro. Int J Radiat Biol 72:201–209

Gill SS, Thomas DGT, Warrington AP et al (1991) Relocatable frame for stereotactic external beam radiotherapy. Int J Radiat Oncol Biol Phys 20:599–603

Glanzmann C (1978) Zerebrale arteriovenöse Mißbildungen: Verlauf bei 18 Fällen nach Radiotherapie. Strahlenther Onkol 154: 305–308

Guyton, JS, Reese AB (1948) Use of roentgen therapy for retinal diseases characterized by new-formed blood vessels. Arch Ophthalmol 40: 389–412

Harris JR, Levene MR (1976) Visual complications following irradiation for pituitary adenomas and craniopharygiomas. Radiology 120:167–171

Hart PM, Chakravarthy U, MacKenzie G et al (1996) Teletherapy for subfoveal choroidal neovascularisation of age-related macular degeneration: results of follow up in a non-randomised study. Br J Ophthalmol 80:1046–1050

Heckmann M, Douwes K, Peter R, Degitz K (1998) Vascular activation of adhesion molecule mRNA and cell surface expression by ionizing radiation. Exp Cell Res 238:148–154

Hendee WR and Ibbott GS (1996) Radiation therapy physics, 2nd edn. Mosby, St. Louis, pp 508–512

Hollick EJ, Goble RR, Knowles PJ et al (1996) Radiotherapy treatment of age-related subfoveal membranes in patients with good vision. Eye 10:609–616

Holz FG, Engenhart-Cabillic R, Bellmann C et al (1997) Stereotactic radiation therapy for subfoveal choroidal neovascularization secondary to age-related macular degeneration. Front Radiat Ther Oncol 30:238–246

Hosoi Y, Yamamoto Y, Ono T, Sakamoto K (1993) Prostacyclin production in cultured endothelial cells is highly sensitive to low doses of ionizing radiation. Int J Radiat Oncol Biol Phys 63:631–638

Jaakkola A, Heikkonen J, Tommila P et al (1998) Strontium plaque irradiation of subfoveal neovascular membranes in age-related macular degeneration. Graefes Arch Clin Exp Ophthalmol 236:24–30

Johnson LK, Longenecker JP, Fajardo LF (1982) Differential radiation response of cultured endothelial cells and smooth myocytes. Anal Quant Cytol 4:188

Joiner M (1993) Particle beams in radiotherapy. In: Steele G (ed) Basic clinical radiobiology. Arnold, London, pp 139–141

Langley RE, Bump EA, Quartuccion SG, Medeiros D et al (1997) Radiation-induced apoptosis in microvascular endothelial cells. Br J Cancer 75:666–672

Makoski H-BR, Zeilstra DJ, Bettag W (1989) Die Strahlenbehandlung intrakranieller arteriovaskulärer Malformationen – Erfahrungen mit semi-stereotaktischer Technik. Radiobiol Radiother 30:213–218

Mauget-Faysse M, Chiquet C, Milea D et al (1999) Long term results of radiotherapy for subfoveal choroidal neovasculariztion in age related macular degeneration. Br J Ophthalmol 83:923–928

Mazal A, Schwartz L, Lacroix F et al (1998) A preliminary comparative treatment planning study for radiotherapy of age-related maculopathy. Radiother Oncol 47:91–98

Miyamoto H, Kimura T, Honda Y et al (1999) Effect of focal x-ray irradiation on experimental choroidal neovascularization. Invest Ophthalmol Vis Sci 40:1496–1502

Parsons JT, Bova FJ, Fitzgerald C et al (1994a) Radiation optic neuropathy after megavoltage external-beam irradiation: Analysis of time-dose factors. Int J Radiat Oncol Biol Phys 30:755–763

Parsons JT, Bova FJ, Fitzgerald C et al (1994b) Radiation retinopathy after megavoltage external-beam irradiation: Analysis of time-dose factors. Int J Radiat Oncol Biol Phys 30:765–773

Pöstgens H, Bodanowitz S, Kroll P (1997) Low dose radiation therapy for age-related macular degeneration. Graefes Arch Clin Exp Ophthalmol 235:656–661

Prettenhofer U, Haas A, Mayer R et al (1998) Photonentherapie der subfovealen choroidalen Neovaskularisation bei altersabhängiger Makuladegeneration. Strahlenther Onkol 174:613–617

RAD (1999) A prospective, randomized, double-masked trial on radiation therapy for neovascular age-related degeneration (RAD Study). Radiation therapy for age-related macular degeneration. Ophthalmol 106:2239–2247

Raicu M, Vral A, Thierens H, De Ridder L (1993) Radiation damage to endothelial cells in vitro, as judged by the micronucleus assay. Mutagenesis 8:335–339

Rubin DB, Drab EA, Kang HJ et al (1996) WR 1065 and radioprotection of vascular endothelial cells. I. Cell proliferation, DNA synthesis and damage. Radiat Res 145:210–216

Sasai K, Murata R, Mandai M et al (1997) Radiaation therapy for ocular choroidal neovascularization (phase I/II study): Preliminary report. Int J Radiat Oncol Biol Phys 39:173–178

Sautter H, Uterman D (1975) Gesichtspunkte zur medikamentösen Behandlung der „senilen" Maculaaffektionen. In: Bericht über die 73. Zusammenkunft der Deutschen Ophthalmologischen Gesellschaft. J.F. Bergman, Heidelberg

Schilling H, Sauerwein W, Friedrichs W et al (1996) Long-term outcome of radiotherapy of choroid hemangioma. Ophthalmologe 93:154–157

Schlegel W, Pastyr O, Bortfeld T (1992) Computer systems and mechanical tools for sterotactically guided conformation therapy with linear accelerators. Int J Radiat Oncol Biol Phys 24:781–787

Scott TA, Augsburger JJ, Brady LW et al (1991) Low-dose ocular irradiation for diffuse choroidal hemangiomas associated with bullous nonrhegmatogenous retinal detachment. Retina 11:389

Spaide RF, Guyer DR, McCormick B et al (1998) External beam radiation therapy for choroidal neovascularization. Ophthalmology 105:24–30

Staar S, Krott R, Mueller R-P et al (1999) External beam radiotherapy for subretinal neovascularization in age-related macular degeneration: Is this treatment efficient? Int J Radiat Oncol Biol Phys 45:467–473

Stalmans P, Leys A, Van Limbergen E (1997) External beam radiotherapy (20 Gy, 2 fractions) fails to control the growth of choroidal neovascularization in age-related macular degeneration: A review of 111 cases. Retina 17:481–492

Sweeney R, Bale R, Vogele M et al (1998) Repositioning accuracy: Comparison of a noninvasive head holder with thermoplastic mask for fractionated radiotherapy and a case report. Int J Radiat Oncol Biol Phys 41:475–483

Thölen A, Meister A, Bernasconi PP et al (1998) Radiotherapie von subretinalen Neovaskularisationsmembranen bei altersabhängiger Makuladegeneration (AMD). Ophthalmologe 95:691–698

Vakaet L, Bate M-T, Fortan LG et al (1998) Off-line verification of the day-to-day three-dimensional table position variation for radiation treatments of the head and neck region using an immobilization mask. Radiother Oncol 47:49–52

Waters CM, Taylor JM, Molteni A, Ward WF (1996) Dose response effects of radiation on the permeability of endothelial cells in culture. Radiat Res 146: 321–328

Withers RH, McBride WH (1997) Biologic basis of radiation therapy. In: Perez CA, Brady LW (eds), Principles and practice of radiation oncology. Lippincott-Raven, Philadelphia, pp 79–118

Yonemoto LT, Slater JD, Blacharski PB et al (2000) Dose response in the treatment of subfoveal choroidal neovascularization in age-related macular degeneration: results of a phase I/II dose escalation study using proton radiotherapy. J Radiosurg 3:47–54

11 Radiation Effects on the Eye

LUTHER W. BRADY and THEODORE E. YAEGER

CONTENTS

11.1 Introduction

CHALUPECKY (1897) first described the effects of ionizing radiation on the eye. Subsequent studies by BIRCH-HIRSCHFELD (1908) identified the first case of radiation cataract. Definitive investigations on the effects of ionizing radiation on the eye began with ROHRSCHNEIDER (1929). This author described a gradient in radiosensitivity of the ocular structures extending from the lens (the most sensitive tissue) through the conjunctiva, cornea, uvea, and the retina to the least sensitive tissue – the sclera. POPPE (1942) further elucidated the work of Rohrschneider.

L.W. BRADY, MD
Hylda Hohn/American Cancer Society Professor of Clinical Oncology and Professor, Department of Radiation Oncology, Hahnemann University Hospital, Broad and Vine Streets, Mail Stop 200, Philadelphia, PA 19102, USA
T.E. YAEGER, MD
Department of Radiation Oncology, Halifax Medical Center, Daytona Beach, FL 32115, USA

This paper is directed toward summarizing the current available clinical and experimental data on the effects of radiation on the eye and ocular adnexa and to suggesting guidelines for radiation tolerance of normal ocular tissues.

Even though many clinicians have an almost morbid fear of the harmful effects of irradiating the eye and orbit, modern innovative radiation therapy technologies allow appropriate treatment programs to be administered with minimal complications. Table 11.1 illustrates the potential magnitude of the problem and Table 11.2 demonstrates the techniques and dosages generally used in radiation therapy of eye lesions (BIRCH-HIRSCHFELD 1908).

The presence of complications, whether functional or cosmetic, will vary depending upon a number of factors:

1. The cellular composition of the injured tissue (in the eye there is a broad diversity of types of cellular composition)
2. That tissue's functional reserve to withstand evolution of a clinically apparent complication
3. Other factors such as the vascular-nutritional integrity of the organ

These factors underlie a general scheme that can be applied to the eye and the orbital contents.

Table 11.1. Malignant tumors in or near the orbit in the USA

Site	Number of patients
Head and neck	29 800
Central nervous system	14 700
Eye	1 900
Skin	100 000
Other – rhabdomyosarcoma, lymphoma, etc.	3 000
Metastases	80 000

11.2 Acute Lesions

Acute lesions represent primary functional cell necroses affecting rapidly proliferating cells. Acute radiation-induced lesions may be defined as effects which

Table 11.2. Usual radiation dosages (Gy) in the treatment of eye diseases

Ocular lesions	90Sr radionuclide plaques, low-energy X-rays	Medium- and high-voltage X-rays, 60Co	Megavoltage X-rays high energy electrons
Non-neoplastic	30–60 in 2–6 weeks	25–40 in 2–4 weeks	25–40 in 2–4 weeks lesions
Malignant tumors of the eye	20–160 in 5 days to 12 weeks	40–60 in 2 weeks	35–75 in 3 -8 weeks
Malignant tumors of or involving the orbit	–	–	35–75 in 4–7 weeks

occur either during the course of fractionated radiation therapy or within several weeks following completion of the radiation therapy program. With proper medical management, recovery from these mild forms generally occurs within several weeks after completing the treatment program. Such lesions typically occur in the skin of the eyelid (blepharitis), in the conjunctiva (conjunctivitis), and in the corneal epithelium (keratitis). Subsequent cellular recovery may be followed by delayed lesions which are predominately stromal in pathogenesis. These lesions may consist of edema followed by interstitial fibrosis. Pathogenic mechanisms include endothelial damage in the microcirculation with passage of proteinaceous fluid into the interstitial spaces through the damaged vascular barrier.

Late effects may also occur coincidentally with permanent changes in arterioles and small arteries. Late tissue complications, particularly where there is a lack of rapidly proliferating cells, are thought to be due to the nutritional consequences of ischemic vascular damage. Typical delayed radiation-induced effects on the eye include cataract formation and radiation retinopathy. Such lesions commonly develop after a latent interval of at least several months, however, the latent period can vary from a few months to many years depending upon individual biologic factors and the total radiation dose delivered. In general, the higher the radiation dose employed, the earlier a particular response will be observed.

Factors influencing the probability of radiation injury may be divided into technical and nontechnical. Technical factors include human mistakes in the delivery of the radiation therapy and systematic errors such as those due to inaccurate initial adjustment of the equipment, incorrect procedures, or unrecognized deviation of a particular parameter with time. Estimates of the incidence and significance of mistakes in the delivery of radiation therapy programs range from 1% to 40% according to the type of treatment and the complexity of the treatment technique.

Strict attention to detail is mandatory in radiation therapy for tumors in or about the eye, since precise and proper control of the technical components of the treatment will significantly reduce the potential for radiation complications.

The important technical factors are fraction size, durationof the course of treatment, hyperfractionation, the type of radiation employed (beta, photon, electrons, neutrons, protons, etc.), the radiosensitivity of the tissue being irradiated, and the patient's age, among others.

Nontechnical factors which modify radiation tolerance include the presence of a concurrent disease which either compromises the tissue's arterial blood flow, such as diabetes mellitus or systemic hypertension, or increases the sensitivity of normal tissues to radiation damage, such as ataxia, telangiectasia, or simultaneous or sequential treatment with chemotherapeutic agents which may modify the radiation tolerance.

Merriam (1955), Merriam and Focht (1957, 1962), and Merriam et al. (1965) summarized the reported clinical complications according to the ocular tissue involved, the latent period, and the dose responsible for each effect.

11.3 Ocular Tissues and Their Response to Ionizing Radiation

11.3.1 Lid Skin

Erythema of the eyelids develops in a fashion similar to that in other areas of irradiated skin. It generally develops early, is transient in character, and disappears promptly after completion of the radiation therapy program. It is seen most commonly where basal cell or squamous cell carcinomas of the lid are irradiated definitively. Moist desquamation may be seen when higher doses are delivered, but even that heals promptly with proper local care. Time-dose relationships are critical for skin effects in terms of their severity and the rapidity with which they disappear after treatment (Table 11.3).

Table 11.3. Effects of radiation on the lid skin

Effect	Latent period		Dose (Gy)	
	Early	Late	Single	Divided
Erythema	2–4 weeks	–	6	$600t^{0.33}$daily schedule
Pigmentation	2–4 weeks	–	4–6	–
Depigmentation	–	6–12 months	–	40–50 in 4–5 weeks
Telangiectasia	–	2–5 years	–	30–60 in 3–6 weeks
Moist desquamation	2–8 weeks	–	–	50–60 in 5–6 weeks
Scarring	–	>6	–	80 in 3–8 weeks

Hyperpigmentation and depigmentation of the eyelid skin have both been described. Most commonly, these pigmentary changes occur as late complications of the treatment, usually becoming manifest 12 months or more after completion of definitive irradiation of the eyelid. Telangiectasia generally does not appear until 4–5 years after completion of the radiation therapy, producing no symptoms and representing essentially a cosmetic change. Ulceration of the skin is in direct relationship to fraction size, the total dose delivered, and the duration of the treatment program. This complication is rarely seen with contemporary techniques of radiation therapy. Lid edema may be seen as a late effect.

Rounding of the lid margins is another frequent complication of the treatment of eyelid tumors. It is seen in the treated area with loss of cilia, rounding of the margins, and some thinning. However, no functional loss is noted and the appearance is seldom a cosmetic problem. Ectropion or entropion are seldom seen with current dosage schedules. These abnormalities are usually associated with the extensive scarring of the lids and adjacent conjunctiva most commonly associated with prior surgical techniques.

11.3.2 Tarsus

This fibrous plate in the lids can undergo late atrophy and thinning when curative levels of radiation therapy are administered. It is most commonly seen in patients treated for basal cell or squamous cell carcinomas of the lid but produces no functional impairment and is essentially a clinical observation (Table 11.4).

11.3.3 Lid Margin

Eyelash loss may occur following therapeutic radiation therapy and is directly dependent upon the dose delivered to the hair follicles. It may be temporary or permanent, depending upon the total dose delivered to the volume being treated. Eyelash loss is generally not a significant cosmetic blemish, but regrowth can on occasion produce trichiasis, requiring treatment. Effective surgical techniques of management for in-turned lashes are presently available (Table 11.5).

11.3.4 Lacrimal Ducts

Radiation dosages at the curative level will cause obliteration of the puncta and usually the canaliculi. Symptoms associated with this radiation effect are generally minor in character; however, some patients develop bothersome epiphora following punctal and canalicular radiation damage.

Table 11.4. Effect of radiation on the tarsus

Effect	Latent period		Dose (Gy)	
	Early	Late	Single	Divided
Atrophy	–	>6 months	–	40–60 in 4–6 weeks

Table 11.5. Effects of radiation on the lid margin

Effect	Latent period		Dose (Gy)	
	Early	Late	Single	Divided
Epilation	1–5 weeks		10	20–30 in 2–3 weeks
Rounding of Ectropion	–	6–12 months	–	40–60 in 4–6 weeks
Entropion	–	>1 year	–	60–100 in 1 day to 10 weeks

11.3.5 Lacrimal Gland

When the lacrimal gland is included within the volume for treatment, atrophy of the gland and consequent reduction in the tear volume may occur. These effects are seen only at the higher dose levels used for curative treatment. Together with invasion or destruction of the gland by tumor, this can lessen the secretory ability of the gland and produce a dry eye. In most patients, symptoms related to radiation-induced dry eye can be managed adequately by the use of artificial tears (Table 11.6).

Table 11.6. Effect of radiation on the lacrimal gland

Effect	Latent period		Dose (Gy)	
	Early	Late	Single	Divided
Atrophy	–	>6 months	20	30–60 in 5–6 weeks

11.3.6 Conjunctiva

Conjunctival hyperemia commonly develops when shielding is not possible during the radiation therapy program and when conjunctival shields are not adequately coated with wax absorb low-energy secondary X-rays. It is a dose-related phenomenon and, at higher doses, can be associated with corneal complications and iritis. Conjunctival hyperemia may be a direct effect of the radiation therapy but also may be secondary to involvement of other ocular structures by the tumor (Table 11.7).

Conjunctivitis of varying severity may accompany hyperemia and on occasion be associated with secondary infection. In most patients, however, it responds well to topical cortical steroids and antibiotics. It occurs most frequently at higher dose levels and is dose-related. It usually subsides gradually with appropriate medical management some 2–4 weeks after completion of the treatment program.

Table 11.7. Effects of radiation on the conjunctiva

Effect	Latent period		Dose (Gy)	
	Early	Late	Single	Divided
Hyperemia	Immediate	–	–	>5
Conjunctivitis	1–3 weeks	–	–	50 in 4–5 weeks
Telangiectasis	–	2–5 years	–	30–60 in 3–6 weeks
Keratinization	–	>1 year	–	50–100 in 5–10 weeks
Symblepharon	–	>1 year	–	80–100 in 8 weeks

Conjunctival telangiectasia is a frequent late complication seen with higher dose levels. The incidence increases with dose ,and telangiectasia is most apt to develop with curative doses of radiation. It represents essentially a cosmetic problem, producing no symptoms.

Keratinization of the conjunctival epithelium, particularly the palpebral conjunctiva, has been observed with radiation dosages in excess of 50 Gy delivered in 5 weeks. In some instances it is asymptomatic. If the palpebral conjunctiva becomes keratinized, however, the patient may develop keratitis. This complication can usually be avoided by appropriate attention to total dose delivered and by adequate shielding.

Symblepharon represents a very severe radiation injury to the conjunctiva in which both the palpebral and bulbar conjunctiva are denuded of their epithelium and the opposing surfaces become adherent. This results in adhesion of the lids to the globe, with deformity of the lids and limitation of ocular motion. Surgical correction may be necessary to deal with this complication. However, it is rarely seen in contemporary radiation therapy practice.

11.3.7 Cornea

In many instances it is impossible to shield the cornea adequately during ocular radiation therapy (Table 11.8). Punctate keratitis is an acute radiation effect in which multiple small defects occur in the corneal epithelium within several weeks to months after treatment. Symptoms include irritation of the eye with varying amounts of tearing. The injury can be seen with low doses of radiation, in the range of 30–50 Gy, delivered within 4–5 weeks. In general, it will subside over a period of 4–6 weeks with appropriate management using topical corticosteroids and antibiotics. Proper attention to the radiation therapy technique, including proper coating of conjunctival shields with wax to protect the cornea, is critically important.

Stromal edema of the cornea has been observed with radiation dosages in the range of 40–50 Gy in 4–5 1/2 weeks. In general, this complication is transient, lasting only 2–4 weeks. In some patients, however, it may persist longer. Stromal edema is generally seen with doses greater than 50 Gy and most com-

Table 11. 8. Effects of radiation on the cornea

Effect	Latent period		Dose (Gy)	
	Early	Late	Single	Divided
Punctate keratitis	Several weeks	–	10	30–50 in 3–5 weeks
Edema	1–3 weeks	–	–	–
Mild ulceration	Several weeks	–	–	30–40 in 2–3 weeks
Chronic ulceration	–	Several months	20	>60 in 5–6 weeks
Perforation	–	4–12 months	–	>60 in 5–6 weeks
Thinning	–	Several months	–	30–50 in 3–5 weeks
Scarring	–	1 year	–	>60 in 5–6 weeks
Keratinization	–	1 year	–	>50 in 4–5 weeks
Vascularization	–	>1 year	–	>50 in 2–3 weeks
Lipid infiltration	–	>1 year	–	>70 in 5–7 weeks
Poor wound healing	–	–	–	>60

monly with those in the range of 70–80 Gy. Appropriate medical management with topical corticosteroids and antibiotics is indicated.

Corneal ulceration is a rare radiation-induced ocular tissue effect. In severe cases, the full thickness of the cornea may melt away, leaving the eye at risk of overwhelming infection (endophthalmitis or panophthalmitis). Corneal ulceration has been reported to occur most commonly with radiation doses exceeding 60 Gy in 6 weeks. Thinning and perforation of the cornea have been described at various dose levels but generally occur at higher levels. If perforation occurs, the eye is often lost. In some cases, however, the perforation and resulting tissue dehiscence are repaired by regeneration of the corneal epithelium. Unfortunately, considerable visual disturbance usually results from such a perforation. The likelihood of corneal ulceration can be diminished if care is taken to prevent corneal epithelial trauma and secondary infection.

Keratinization is a late corneal complication of radiation therapy and can result in severe visual loss. In general, it is more likely to develop when radiation exceeds 50 Gy within 4–5 weeks. It is often associated with varying degrees of scarring, thinning, and vascularization.

Corneal vascularization can occur as a late result of radiation therapy. It typically does not become manifest until several years after the treatment and can result from conventional clinical radiation dosages, but it generally occurs with dosages much larger than normal.

Lipid infiltration of the cornea has been reported as a late complication of ocular irradiation. This effect has usually been observed with corneal dosages exceeding 75 Gy. The effect on vision depends upon the location and the density of the lipid deposits.

11.3.8
Sclera

Thinning of the sclera has been reported with dosages ranging from 15 Gy to 20 Gy on the surface. Localized areas of scleral thinning following ocular irradiation usually do not require treatment. Perforation of the sclera rarely occurs, even with the high local dosages for malignant melanomas of the choroid and ciliary bodies using radioactive plaques. In some cases, a scleral perforation can be repaired successfully with a scleral patch graft. However, the incidence is rare and most frequently occurs at doses above 300 Gy–400 Gy and often with prior surgical trauma (Table 11.9).

Table 11. 9. Effect of radiation on the sclera

Effect	Latent period		Dose (Gy)	
	Early	Late	Single	Divided
Atrophy	–	Several years	–	200–300

11.3.9
Iris

Radiation therapy to the iris may produce iritis, an acute and usually transient dose-related inflammation. Radiation-induced iritis often occurs conjointly with keratitis or corneal ulceration. Affected patients are usually severely photophobic. The inflammation commonly leads to pigment deposition on the anterior capsule of the lens. Various degrees of iris atrophy can also occur. Atrophy of the iris is usually localized to a sector and has been seen most often following the use of beta irradiation. It is a late effect, typically becoming manifest several years after the radiation event, but is essentially asymptomatic and remains localized.

Trabecular meshwork glaucoma develops in some eyes in response to radiation therapy. This form of glaucoma is often quite resistant to medical or surgical therapy. It usually occurs as a consequence of intraocular inflammation, which acts by clogging the trabecular meshwork with inflammatory cells or debris or closing the filtration angle with posterior synechiae, or it leads to development of iris neovascularization (rubeosis iridis) (Table 11.10).

Table 11.10. Effects of radiation on the iris

Effect	Latent period		Dose (Gy)	
	Early	Late	Single	Divided
Iritis	Several days	–	20	>60 in 5–6 weeks
Rubeosis	-	Several months to several years	–	70–80 in 6–8 weeks
Atrophy	-	>3 years	–	>60

11.3.10 Lens

Radiation effects on the lens are those directly related to the production of cataract (Table 11.11). Animal work, clinical observation, and experience have identified the doses of various qualities of radiation that produce lens opacity and determine the manner in which the cataract develops, the time of onset, and the metabolic and pathologic changes that result (MERRIAM et al 1957). The amount of radiation given to the lens has an impact upon the degree of opacity, the time of onset of the cataract being directly dose-related. It is evident that the lens is the most radiosensitive structure in the eye. In overall consideration of a radiation therapy program, the acceptance of a radiation-induced cataract of the lens may be necessary for treating tumors in this area. It should be appreciated that a progressive cataract, when it develops with loss of vision, may be extracted as easily as a senile one, with restoration of vision provided the rest of the eye is unaffected. However, the interval between the radiation event and the extraction of the lens of the eye should be at least 1 year.

Table 11.11. Effects of radiation on the eye lens

Effect	Latent period		Dose (Gy)	
	Early	Late	Single	Divided
Cataract	–	>1 year	>2	CD50 4 Gy t0.17 daily schedule

11.3.11 Retina

Radiation injury to the retina occurs clinically in spite of the fact that the retina is quite radioresistant. Most radiation-induced retinal changes appear to occur based on retinal vascular damage. Clinical changes in the retina can be observed with radiation dosages as low as 35 Gy delivered within 3 weeks. With increasing dosage, there is an increased incidence of retinal changes. Effects on the retina have been observed in patients treated with external beam radiation as well as those treated with various radionuclide plaques for malignant tumors involving the eye. Initially, edema of the retina may be noted early in the course of radiation therapy. This acute retinal edema commonly subsides within several weeks. In some eyes, retinal edema recurs as a late complication of treatment, often in association with intraretinal or preretinal hemorrhages and exudates. These effects appear to be secondary to progressive radiation-induced obliteration of the retinal vessels. Optic papillitis, retinal microaneurysms, and macular exudates may simulate the picture of severe arteriosclerotic-hypertensive retinopathy. New vessel formation (neovascularization) may occur in an aberrant attempt to improve the local circulation. The fragile new vessels commonly bleed into the vitreous resulting in further visual impairment. The vitreous hemorrhage may become organized with retinitis proliferans, resulting in detachment of the retina. The entire retina occasionally becomes severely ischemic, with

Table 11.12. Effects of radiation on the retina

Effect	Latent period		Dose (Gy)	
	Early	Late	Single	Divided
Edema	Several months	–	–	20–35 in 2–4 weeks
Vascular occlusion	–	–	–	–
Telangiectasia	–	–	–	–
Hemorrhages	–	6 months to many years	–	30–60 in 3–6 weeks
Exudates	–	–	–	–
Degeneration	–	–	–	–
Atrophy	–	–	–	50–80 in 4–8 weeks

the ischemia leading in some eyes to ocular inflammation and neovascular glaucoma (Table 11.12).

11.3.12 Optic Nerve

The optic nerve can develop radiation-induced papillitis. This condition is characterized by hyperemic disc swelling, usually accompanied by circumpapillary exudates and profound visual loss. Optic nerve atrophy has also been observed in patients with severe retinal changes. This condition is characterized by disc pallor and severe visual loss. It is felt that this feature is generally secondary to retinal degeneration. However, the circulation to the nerve itself may be impaired and may result in optic atrophy.

11.3.13 Orbit

Radiation effects on the orbit are directly related to inhibition of the growth of bone (Table 11.13). When the radiation therapy is delivered in childhood, such treatment can result in marked facial deformities. The typical deformity is a hollowed-out appearance in the temporal region due to the failure of growth of the lateral wall of the orbit.

If the nasal bones are included in the field of treatment, their growth may also be impaired, resulting in a saddle nose deformity. In general, these changes occur at dosages exceeding 35 Gy delivered within 3-4 weeks in childhood.

The potential for the development of malignant tumors in the irradiated area is well-known and has been reported by many investigators (SAGERMAN et al. 1969). Here again, the critical factors are long survival with the tumor controlled and total dose delivered to normal tissue. There is a direct relationship between dose and incidence of second radiation-induced tumors. In general, the criteria set forth by CAHAN et al. (1948) for the diagnosis of a radiation-induced tumor must be met:

Table 11.13. Effects of radiation on the orbit

Effect	Latent period		Dose (Gy)	
	Early	Late	Single	Divided
Growth failure	–	Several years	–	30–70 in 3–7 weeks

1. The tumor must develop within the irradiated volume.
2. The tumor must be of a different histologic type from the original primary tumor.
3. The total radiation dose delivered to the normal tissues within the volume should be in excess of 60 Gy within 6–7 weeks.
4. The interval between the initial radiation event and the development of a second tumor should exceed 6–7 years.

The latent period has been reported to range from 4 to 30 years, with a mean of 11 years. When treating a malignant tumor, the possibility of a late radiation-induced cancer, as well as other radiation complications must be accepted as a calculated risk.

11.4 Conclusion

The frequency of radiation complications to the eye and orbital structures can be minimized with proper attention to careful design of treatment programs and precise attention to detail in their delivery. This includes specific attention to the type of radiation instrument to be employed, whether electron beam, photon beam, or radioactive plaques. In general, the critical factors influencing radiation complications from treatment to the eye and orbital structures are the age of the patient, coexisting medical conditions, the number of fractions in the treatment program, the total dose, and the time during which the radiation dose is delivered to the normal structures within the volume being treated.

References

Birch-Hirschfeld GVA (1908) Zur Wirkung der Röntgenstrahlen auf das menschliche Auge. Klin Monatsbl Augenheilkd 46:129

Cahan WG, Woodard HQ, Higinbotham NL, Stewart FW, Coley BL (1948) Sarcoma arising in irradiated bone. Report of eleven cases. Cancer 1:3–29

Chalupecky H (1897) Über die Wirkung der Röntgenstrahlen auf das Auge und die Haut. Zentralbl Augenheilkd 21:234–368

Merriam GR Jr (1955) Late effects of beta radiation on the eye. Arch Ophthalmol 53:708-717

Merriam GR Jr, Focht EF (1957) A clinical study of radiation cataracts and the relationship to dose. Am J Roentgenol 77:759

Merriam GR Jr, Focht EF (1962) A clinical and experimental study of the effect of single and divided doses of radiation on cataract production. Trans Am Ophthalmol Soc 60:35
Merriam GR Jr, Biavati BJ, Bateman JL, Rossi HH, Boud VP, Goodman L, Focht EF (1965) The dependence of RBE on the energy of fast neutrons. IV. Indication of lens opacities in mice. Radiat Res 25:123
Poppe E (1942) Experimental investigation of the effects of roentgen rays on the eye. Oslo. Thesis
Rohrschneider W (1929) Experimentelle Untersuchungen über die Veränderungen normaler Augengewebe nach Röntgenbestrahlung. III. Mitteilung. Veränderungen der Linse, der Netzhaut, und des Sehnerven nach Röntgenbestrahlung. Graefes Arch Ophthalmol 122:282
Sagerman RH, Cassady JR, Tretter P, Elsworth RM (1969) Radiation-induced neoplasia following external beam therapy for children with retinoblastoma. Am J Roentgenol 105:529-535

12 Long-Term Results of Radiotherapy for Age-Related Macular Degeneration

G.J. Bergink, C.B. Hoyng, R.W.M. van der Maazen, J.R. Vingerling, W.A.J. van Daal, and A.F. Deutman

CONTENTS

12.1 Introduction

As laser photocoagulation therapy leads to immediate and permanent visual loss in eyes with subfoveal choroidal neovascularisation (CNV) in age-related macular degeneration (ARMD), other treatment options are under investigation, including photodynamic therapy, pharmacological therapy, surgical therapy and radiotherapy.

Radiotherapy has been used experimentally for subfoveal CNV due to its potential to inhibit growth of vascular endothelial cells and cause obliteration of small vessels. Many pilot studies reported positive results on visual acuity using external beam radiotherapy for CNV in ARMD, including reduction in scar size after treatment (Hart et al. 1997; Chakravarthy et al. 1996). Radiotherapy is noninvasive and causes little inconvenience to patients; however, it is time-consuming and expensive.

12.2 Radiation Technique

The departments of Radiotherapy and Ophthalmology of Nijmegen University Hospital in The Netherlands developed a technique for treating the macular area with the total radiation dose and at the same time sparing the structures outside the macular area. To reduce dose to the lens, the beams were directed at an angle of 30° from the optical axis in the cranial/caudal direction and crossed the eye axis in the macular area (Fig. 12.1). With this lens-sparing technique, 16 MV photons were used on a 1 cm^2 section of the macular area. Outside the macular area, the dose was less than 50% of the total and the lens of

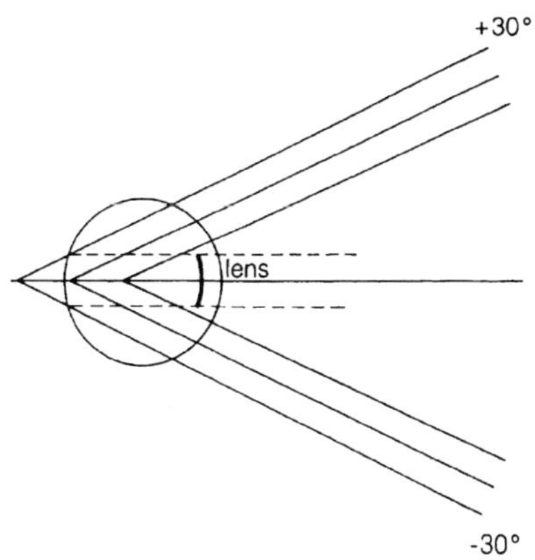

Fig. 12.1. Lens-sparing technique. The radiation beams are directed at an angle 30° from the optical axis. They intersect on the macular region

G.J. Bergink, MD
University Hospital Rotterdam, Park Arenberg 54a, 3731 ET De Bilt, The Netherlands
C.B. Hoyng, MD
Institute of Ophthalmology, P.O. Box 9101, 6500 Nijmegen, The Netherlands
R.W.M. van der Maazen, MD
Institute of Radiotherapy, University Hospital Nijmegen, P.O. Box 9101, 6500 Nijmegen, The Netherlands
J.R. Vingerling, MD
Institute of Ophthalmology, University Hospital Rotterdam, Rotterdam, The Netherlands
W.A.J. van Daal, MD
Institute of Radiotherapy, University Hospital Nijmegen, P.O. Box 9101, 6500 Nijmegen, The Netherlands
A.F. Deutman, MD
Professor and Chairman, Institute of Ophthalmology, University Hospital Nijmegen, P.O. Box 9101, 6500 Nijmegen, The Netherlands

the eye received less than 30%. Altogether, 24 Gy was given in four fractions of 6 Gy to the macular area over 3 weeks, which is biologically equivalent to 50 Gy in 25 fractions of 2 Gy. This provides a relatively high dose in the macular area without exceeding tolerance levels of the surrounding ocular tissues. The important difference between this technique and the lateral approach used by many other investigators, for example the Belfast study group, is that the treatment volume is small and therefore the maximum dose is not delivered beyond the macular area.

Table 12.1. Inclusion criteria

1. Recent drop in visual acuity
2. Best corrected Snellen visual acuity >0.1
3. Angiographically proven classic, occult, or mixed subfoveal CNV in ARMD
4. Informed consent
5. No previous laser photocoagulation in the macular area
6. No radiation treatment for brain or throat, nose, or ear disease
7. No diabetes mellitus

12.3 Results of a Randomised Trial at Two-Year Follow-Up

12.3.1 Introduction

In 1998 we published the results of a clinical trial comparing radiation and observation groups (Bergink et al. 1998). At 12-month follow-up, preservation of visual acuity was significantly better in the treatment group, (32.0% had reductions of three or more lines vs. 52.2% in the observation group) (p=0.03, log rank test). We present the results at 2-year follow-up of the same study population. The primary objective was to determine whether eyes with subfoveal CNV in ARMD benefit from radiotherapy to maintain central vision. The influence of radiotherapy on scar size was also evaluated.

12.3.2 Materials and Methods

The inclusion criteria are listed in Table 12.1. Patients were referred to the outpatient clinic of the University Hospital of Nijmegen by ophthalmologists throughout The Netherlands between 1995 and 1997. Patients who met the inclusion criteria were asked to participate in the trial and, after giving informed consent, they were assigned randomly to either radiotherapy or observation. The study protocol was approved by the institution's ethics committee.

Each patient underwent a complete ophthalmic examination including best-corrected distance Snellen visual acuity and Amsler grid testing, biomicroscopic slit-lamp examination of the lens, 35° colour fundus photographs and stereoscopic fluorescein angiography of the macular area and optic disc of both eyes angiography, was carried out 3, 6, 12, 18 and 24 months after randomisation. Fluorescein angiography (FA) was performed using a standard protocol with early, midvenous, and late frames. Cases of proven CNV on the FA were classified into three subgroups according to the Macular Photocoagulation Study Group (MPS) criteria:

1. Classic CNV with an area of bright, well-demarcated hyperfluorescence in the early phase of the angiogram, with progressive dye leakage into the overlying subsensory retinal space in the late phase.
2. Occult CNV, further divided into types I and II. Type I (group 2A) is a fibrovascular pigment epithelial detachment with areas of irregular elevation of the retinal pigment epithelium (speckled hyperfluorescence) within 1 min after dye injection, with persistent staining or leakage in the late phase after 10 min. Occult CNV type II (group 2B) is late leakage of an undetermined source not due to early hyperfluorescence.
3. Mixed CNV is CNV with both classic and occult components.

The angiograms were graded independently by different investigators (J.R.V., C.B.H.). Discrepancies were openly adjudicated by the same two readers, and those that could not be resolved were reviewed for final classification by a third ophthalmologist (G.J.B.). The readers were blinded for treatment status. The features graded included (1) type of CNV (classic, occult, or mixed) and (2) size of CNV membrane lesion, determined by superimposing a transparent sheet with printed standard MPS disc area circles (1, 2, 3, 3.5, 4, 6, 9, 12, and 16 times the disc area) over the entire macular lesion. Size doubling was scored when a lesion progressed, for example, from circle 1 to 2, from 2 to 4 or from 3 to 6. Size progression was scored when an increase to the next larger circle was observed.

Visual acuity was measured on a Snellen chart with a fixed unit under standard conditions. A visual loss of three lines on the chart represents a doubling of the minimum angle of resolution, e.g., a change from 20/100 to 20/200 in Snellen equivalents.

Patients randomised to the control group did not receive sham radiation treatment. Those randomised to the treatment group received a total dose of 24 Gy in the macular area of the affected eye in four fractions of 6 Gy over 3 weeks. Further details concerning the radiation technique can be found in Sect. 12.2.

Side effects were monitored during follow-up, including scoring of the development of posterior subcapsular radiation cataract and early angiographic signs of radiation retinopathy.

Sample size was estimated on the assumption that the proportion of eyes losing one or more Snellen lines of vision and ending up with visual acuity of <0.1 was expected to be 70% in the control group and 30% in the treatment group. A two-sided significance level of 0.05 and a power of 0.90 required 32 patients in each group. Anticipating a 10% rate of impossible follow-up and/or nonevaluable patients in each group, 36 patients were needed in each group and 72 would be randomised into the trial. Baseline characteristics of the study population are summarised in Table 12.2.

Differences in baseline characteristics were analysed using the *t*-test for comparing the means of independent samples. Visual acuity scores and CNV lesion size were subgrouped according to ordered variables. Comparison of ordered variables was performed using the chi-square test for trends on one degree of freedom. Endpoints for decline in visual acuity were defined as 3 or more lines and 6 or more lines . Other endpoints compared between treatment and observation groups were: visual acuity of less than 0.1 and doubling and enlargement of CNV size. Endpoints in the treatment groups were compared during follow-up using Kaplan-Meier curves and log rank test.

12.3.3 Results

Two-year follow-up was available for 63 of 74 patients; none had been lost to follow-up at the 1-year control. Patients in the treatment group were slightly younger than controls. Other baseline characteristics were very similar (Table 12.2).

Visual decline of three or more lines was observed more frequently in the observation group than in the treatment group. At 24 months, 78.1% of the observation group versus 51.2% of the irradiation group had lost 3 or more lines (p=0.001 log rank test). Furthermore, visual decline of six or more lines was observed in 54.0% of the observation group and 28.6% of the irradiation group (p=0.003) (Fig. 12.2). After 24 months, 60.9% of the observation group and 39.8% of the treatment group had lost visual acuity to levels below 0.1 (p=0.08 log rank test, p=0.01 log rank test stratified for baseline visual acuity) (Fig. 12.3). Additional subgroup analysis showed a small effect in the occult and mixed CNV subgroups and a more pronounced beneficial effect in the classic subgroup at 24 months.

Table 11.2. Baseline characteristics of the study population by treatment group. Values given as percentages in parentheses unless stated otherwise

Characteristics	Treatment group (n=36)	Observation group (n=32)	P*
Mean age in years	73.1 (5.8)	76.1 (5.8)	0.07
Gender (% women)	20 (55.6)	18 (56.3)	0.96
Composition of lesion			
Classic CNV	19 (52.8)	16 (50.0)	
Occult CNV	8 (22.2)	8 (25.0)	0.96
Mixed CNV	9 (25.0)	8 (25.0)	
Visual acuity			
>0.1–<0.3	13 (36.1)	15 (46.9)	0.51
>0.3	23 (63.9)	17 (53.1)	
Lesion size, MPS grid			
<1	13 (40.6)	15 (41.7)	
>1–<2	8 (25.0)	11 (30.6)	0.82
>2	11 (34.4)	10 (17.7)	

**P* values taken from chi-squared statistics for unordered variables, when applicable.

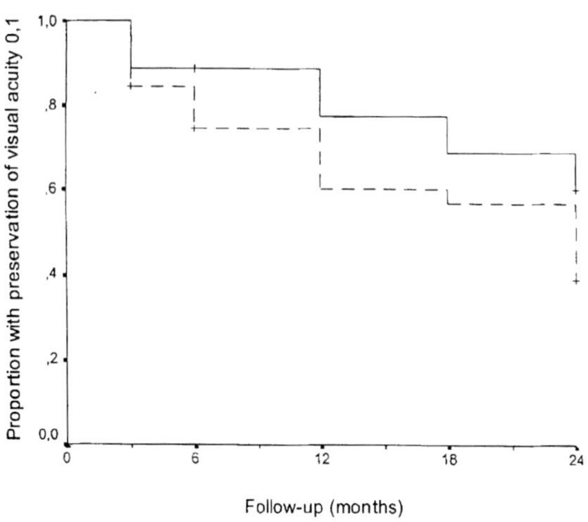

Fig. 12.2. Kaplan-Meier curve for the proportion of eyes with decreases in visual acuity of six lines or more from baseline to each follow-up examination. The *solid line* indicates irradiated group (*n*=36) and the *broken line* indicates observation group (*n*=32) (*p*=0.003, log rank test)

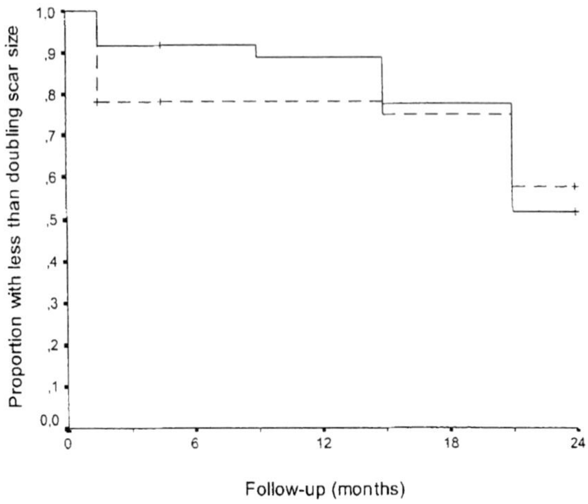

Fig. 12.3. Kaplan-Meier curve for the proportion of eyes with preserved visual acuity of 0.1 or more. The *solid line* indicates irradiated group (*n*=36) and the *broken line* indicates observation group (*n*=32) (*p*=0.001, log rank test stratified for visual acuity at baseline)

The CNV size doubled during 24 months in 42.2% of the observation group versus 48.5% in the treatment group (*p*=0.83 log rank test) (Fig. 12.4). At 24 months, 69.4% of treated and 78.4% of observation eyes showed CNV lesion size progression into a larger disc area compared with baseline (*p*=0.14).

12.3.4 Discussion

At 1-year follow-up, 52.2% of the observation group and 32.0% of the treatment group had lost three or more lines of vision (*p*=0.03) (Bergink et al. 1998). At 2 years, 78.1% of the observation group and 51.2% of the treatment group had lost three or more lines (*p*=0.001). The differences between the two groups concerning visual loss remain; however, visual decline continued in both observation and treatment groups between 1 and 2 years. The Snellen visual loss at 2 years in the observation group (78.1% losing three or more lines) corresponds to MPS and other data concerning the natural history of age-related subfoveal CNV using Early Treatment of Diabetic Retinopathy Study (ETDRS) charts (Macular Photocoagulation Study Group 1994).

Visual loss to levels below 0.1 was found in 39.6% of those in the observation group versus 20.0% in the treatment group at 1 year and 60.9% versus 39.8%, respectively, at 2 years. Even after stratification for baseline visual acuity, these results suggest a beneficial effect of irradiation at 2 years.

In contrast to the analysis at 12 months, subgroup analysis in classic and mixed/occult CNV suggests a more pronounced effect in the classic subgroup at 24 months. We do not have a full explanation for this change; however, it is partly due to the relatively small study population.

Doubling of the CNV area occurred in 25.2% of the observation group versus 20% of the treatment group at 12 months and in 42.2% versus 48.5% at 24 months. This leads to the conclusion that radiotherapy had no effect on CNV size doubling. Measuring CNV lesion size with an overlaid MPS sheet is not the most precise method; however, we chose it to allow accurate comparison with MPS data. Growth of CNV can occur within the limits of the baseline disc area, which can lead to the false conclusion that a CNV membrane has stabilised while in reality an increase has occurred. Furthermore, CNV size doubling is not an exact indication, because growth from disc area 2 into area 3 reflects a substantial membrane growth, but is not scored as scar size doubling in the data used by the MPS and in this study. Therefore, an additional analysis of the scar size data was performed. Growth of a CNV membrane from one disc area (baseline disc area) into a larger area at 24 months was found in 78.4% of the observation group and in 69.4% of the irradiation group; the difference was not significant. Eyes treated with radiotherapy did not develop scar size reduction compared with controls in our study.

In some of the treated eyes, we noticed angiographically proven CNV reactivation after a stable

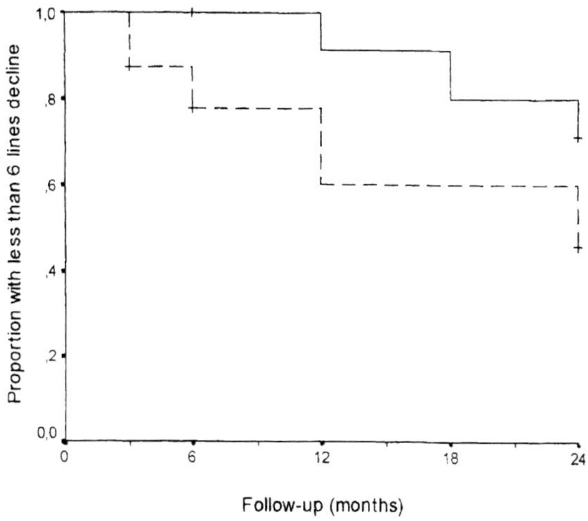

Fig. 12.4. Kaplan-Meier curve for the proportion of eyes with scar size less than doubled. The *solid line* indicates irradiated group (n=36) and the *broken line* indicates observation group (n=32) (p=0.83, log rank test)

period of at least 12 months, resulting in visual loss and scar size enlargement. The same is seen after laser therapy when the CNV is temporarily destroyed; however, recurrences take place because the stimuli for growth of the neovascular complex remain (SPAIDE et al. 1998). During their natural course, CNV lesions tend to leak and bleed repeatedly over many months or even years, even without treatment (AUGSBURGER et al. 1998).

How can we explain the significant effect of treatment on visual loss in the absence of a significant difference between the two groups in scar size? Perhaps the scar size is less important for visual function than the amount of subretinal macular fluid. Perhaps more photoreceptor cells survive after radiotherapy. Hypothetically, reduction of submacular fluid is caused by the reduced CNV vessel leakage in irradiated eyes.

Although slight changes in lens opacification cannot be ruled out, we did not observe the development of subcapsular posterior radiation cataract or radiation retinopathy at 24 months; however, we are aware of the longer lag time, up to 6 years, needed for these side effects to occur.

Concerning methodological points, as we already mentioned with 12-month follow-up, we do not think that the differences in visual outcome were caused by differences in baseline characteristics because, as can be seen in Table 12.2, these were very similar. We used strict entrance criteria in this trial, with close attention to the duration of the CNV membrane at inclusion, reflected in a baseline visual acuity of >0.3 in more than 50% of eyes in both observation and treatment groups (Table 12.2).

We believe that restricting our study population led to differences in results compared with other studies, for example that of STALMANS et al. (1997). They treated patients with 20 Gy in 2-Gy fractions and included many patients with a central vision of 20/200 or worse and those with prior macular laser treatment. Visual acuity remained relatively unchanged in a proportion of eyes with growth of CNV membranes definitely proven on fluorescein angiogram. The inclusion of many patients with poor acuity in the study of Stalmans et al. creates difficulties judging the influence of irradiation in eyes already worsened by the natural course of the disease.

SPAIDE et al. (1998) reported no effect of irradiation with external beam radiotherapy (10 Gy in 2-Gy fractions) after 1-year follow-up and concluded that patients should not be treated with this relatively low total dose. The Belfast Study Group stated that radiotherapy (12 Gy in 2-Gy fractions, 3+3 cm lateral port) resulted in stabilisation of visual acuity and smaller scar size over natural course eyes at 12- to 24-month follow-up (HART et al. 1996, 1997).

Using stereotactic radiotherapy (16 Gy, 2-Gy fractions), HOLZ et al. (1997) noted a stabilisation of visual acuity in 70% and a reduction in CNV scar size in 68% of patients at 6 months follow-up. Stereotactic radiotherapy minimises the field of exposure and the dose outside the target volume. FREIRE et al. (1997) observed that 90% of patients became visually stable 3 months after radiation therapy (14.4 Gy in 1.8-Gy fractions).

Recently, two studies were performed in France. Radiotherapy with lateral beams (20 Gy in 4-Gy fractions) resulted in stabilisation of visual and anatomical outcomes compared with natural history in newly diagnosed subfoveal CNV at 18 months (MAUGET-FAYSSE et al. 1999). External beam radiotherapy (16 Gy in 4-Gy fractions, n=28) for subfoveal occult CNV resulted in CNV size stabilisation in 93% of patients and visual acuity stabilisation in 87% at 6 months (DONATI et al. 1999).

A prospective study by CHAR et al. (1999) in 27 eyes with subfoveal CNV with a single fraction of 7.5 Gy resulted at 17-month follow-up in reduced visual loss in irradiated eyes (p<0.046, borderline significance), with no differences in angiographic characteristics between treated and observation eyes.

Important data are provided by the results of a double-blind, randomised trial by HOLZ et al. (1999) including 205 patients. Treated eyes received eight fractions of 2-Gy external beam lateral irradiation and control eyes received a sham treatment. At 1 year, 49% of treated eyes and 48% of controls had lost three or more lines of visual acuity. No difference in visual loss between treatment and observation groups was found with either classic or occult membranes. Radiotherapy with 16 Gy (2-Gy fractions) provided no benefit for subfoveal classic and occult CNV in ARMD.

Some of the publications cited above ended with considerations including the following: (1) Is stabilisation of visual acuity a permanent and long-lasting effect? (2) Does irradiation lead to reduced scar formation? and (3) What are the influences of total dose and fraction dose?

Concerning the first question, it is important to note that visual acuity in irradiated eyes deteriorated after a stable period of 12–18 months. This leads to the conclusion that even if stabilisation is present, it is not a permanent effect in treated eyes. The answer to the second question already discussed above is negative. In our data, no significant difference in scar size was observed at 12- month or 24-month follow-up. The third question cannot be answered before more data from other randomised trials become available. The technique used in our study limited the field of irradiation to the macular area, in contrast to the standard lateral approach used in other studies.

Furthermore, the questions of whether radiotherapy has a place in adjuvant treatment after laser photocoagulation or is an indication for treatment of CNV from other causes, such as high myopia, angioid streaks, POHS or idiopathic CNV, cannot be answered with the current data.

12.4 Overall Conclusions

In a recent article, Augsburger stated that the studies reported to date do not provide sufficient evidence of a substantial treatment benefit in a large enough proportion of patients to justify the expenditure required for a large-scale randomised clinical trial of this therapy (Augsburger 1998). We agree that results from small groups of selected patients must be interpreted with caution because of the multiple clinical variables in subfoveal age-related CNV. In this study, control and treatment groups did not differ in age, duration of visual symptoms, size of lesion, or visual acuity (Table 12.2). However, differences in associated drusen, clumping of macular pigment epithelium, and associated geographic atrophy were not monitored. We are aware of the small sample size and the absence of both sham treatment and ETDRS acuity measurement in our study.

We have previously stated that there is no proof that radiotherapy (24 Gy in 6-Gy fractions, small field) prevents visual loss in all patients with age-related subfoveal CNV at 1-year follow-up (Bergink et al. 1992, 1998). The results at 2 years confirm these findings. Nevertheless, there is a significant difference in visual loss at 24 months in favour of the treatment group, but without a subsequent difference in scar size. Long-term side effects remain possible but have not been encountered yet.

Without propagating radiotherapy as a proven treatment option, this outcome justifies further study on this subject. We agree that there is presently no place for radiotherapy in age-related subfoveal CNV outside the context of randomised controlled clinical trials (Augsburger et al. 1998; Finger et al. 1998). The results of a multicentre randomised trial of 12-Gy external beam radiation therapy in the UK have to be awaited.

References

Augsburger JJ (1998) External beam radiation therapy is not effective in the treatment of age-related macular degeneration. Arch Ophthalmol 116:1509–1511

Bergink GJ, Deutman AF, van Daal WAJ (1992) Radiation therapy for subfoveal choroidal neovascular membranes in age-related macular degeneration: A pilot study. Int Ophthalmol 16 [Suppl]:16

Bergink GJ, Hoyng CB, van der Maazen RWM et al (1998) A randomised controlled clinical trial on the efficacy of radiation therapy in the control of subfoveal choroidal neovascularisation in age-related macular degeneration. Radiation versus observation. Graefe's Arch Clin Exp Ophthalmol 236:321–325

Char DH, Irvine AI, Posner MD et al (1999) Randomized trial of radiation for age-related macular degeneration. Am J Ophthalmol 127:574–578

Ciullia TA, Danis RP, Harris A (1998) Age-related macular degeneration: A review of experimental treatments. Survey Ophthalmol 43:134–146

Donati G, Soubrane D, Quaranta et al (1999) Radiotherapy for isolated occult subfoveal neovascularisation in age-related macular degeneration: A pilot study. Br J Ophthalmol 83:646–651

Finger PT, Chakravarthy U (1998) External beam radiation therapy is effective in the treatment of age-related macular degeneration. Arch Ophthalmol 116:1507–1509

Finger PT, Berson A, Sherr D et al (1996) Radiation therapy for subretinal neovascularisation. Ophthalmology 103:878–889

Freire J, Longton WA, Miyamoto CT (1997) External radiotherapy in macular degeneration: Technique and preliminary subjective response. Front Radiat Ther Oncol 30:247–252

Hart PM, Chakravarthy U, MacKenzie G et al (1996) Teletherapy for subfoveal choroidal neovascularisation of age-related macular degeneration: Results of follow-up in a nonrandomised study. Br J Ophthalmol 80:1046–1050

Hart PM, Archer DB, Chakravarthy U (1997) Teletherapy in the management of patients with age-related macular degeneration complicated by subfoveal neovascularisation: An overview. Front Radiat Ther Oncol 30:229–237

Holz FG (1999) Results of a prospective, randomized, controlled, double blind, multicenter clinical trial on external beam radiation therapy for subfoveal choroidal neovascularization secondary to ARMD (RAD study). Abstract ICG-Angiography Symposium, Baden-Baden

Holz FG, Engenhart R, Bellmann C et al (1997) Stereotactic radiation therapy for subfoveal choroidal neovascularisation secondary to age-related macular degeneration. Front Radiat Ther Oncol 30:238–246

Macular Photocoagulation Study Group (1994) Visual outcome after laser photocoagulation for subfoveal choroidal neovascularisation secondary to age-related macular degeneration. Arch Ophthalmol 112:480–488

Mauget-Faysse M, Chiquet C, Milea D et al (1999) Long-term results of radiotherapy for subfoveal choroidal neovascularisation in age-related macular degeneration. Br J Ophthalmol 83:923–928

Spaide RF, Guyer DR, McCormick B et al (1998) External beam radiation therapy for choroidal neovascularisation. Ophthalmology 105:24–30

Stalmans P, Leys A, van Limbergen E (1997) External beam radiotherapy (20 Gy, 2 Gy fractions) fails to control the growth of choroidal neovascularisation in age-related macular degeneration. Retina 17:481–492

13 External Beam Radiation Therapy for Age Related Macular Degeneration: Two-Year Results

Robert H. Sagerman and Sri Gorty

CONTENTS

13.1 Introduction

Age-related macular degeneration (ARMD) is the leading cause of blindness in people older than 65 and the second most common cause for patients aged 45–64 years (Ganley and Roberts 1983; Leibowitz et al. 1980a, 1980b; Klein et al. 1992). There are approximately 200,000 new cases of ARMD each year, with over 100,000 people considered legally blind. The prevalence ranges from 0.1% in persons aged 43–54 years to 7.1% in those older than 75 (Klein et al. 1992; Mitchell et al. 1995; Vingerling et al. 1995).

The accepted therapy for choroidal neovascularization (CNV) is laser photocoagulation based on randomized studies performed by the Macular Photocoagulation Study Group (MPS 1982). The MPS demonstrated a delay in the worsening of visual acuity. Eyes with extrafoveal CNV and visual acuity of 20/200 or better were treated with laser photocoagulation and compared with the control arm. The incidence of severe visual loss at 18 months was 25% for treated eyes vs. 60% for untreated eyes. Visual acuity decreased by 6 or more lines in 46% of treated eyes and 64% of untreated eyes. However, over 50% of the treated eyes developed recurrent neovascularization.

R.H. Sagerman, MD, FACR
S. Gorty, MD
Department of Radiation Oncology, SUNY Upstate Medical University, 750 E. Adams Street, Syracuse, NY 13210, USA

Eyes with juxtafoveal and subfoveal CNV were also studied and demonstrated similar results, but the consequence of laser therapy for subfoveal lesions is an immediate and permanent decrease in visual acuity (MPS 1982b, 1991c, 1994a, 1994b). Unfortunately, the MPS criteria are strict and excluded many patients because they had occult CNV, large CNV, subretinal fibrosis, or severe loss of visual acuity.

Radiotherapy has long been known to affect the vascularity of an organ. Clinically, radiotherapy is very effective in controlling hemoptysis due to lung cancer and vaginal bleeding from cervical carcinomas. It has also been quite effective with benign tumors such as arteriovenous malformations (Colombo et al. 1989; Steiner et al. 1992) and choroidal hemangiomas (Alberti 1986; Plowman et al. 1986, 1997; Schilling et al. 1997). Radiation has also been used to modify healing of ocular wounds (Chakravarthy et al. 1989). This led Chakravarthy et al. (1993) to propose its use as an alternative to laser photocoagulation or when laser photocoagulation could not be used or was not acceptable to the patient because of the immediate decrease in acuity.

There is extensive literature regarding the effects of irradiation on the structures of the eye, both when the eye is the site of the lesion (e.g., retinoblastoma (Egbert et al. 1978; Gagnon et al. 1980), melanoma (Petrovich et al. 1993), hemangioma (Plowman and Harnett 1986, 1997; Schilling et al. 1997) or when it is radiated incidentally (e.g., in sinus cancer) (Parsons et al. 1988) and „safe doses“ have been defined for each structure (Egbert et al. 1978; Gagnon et al. 1980; Parsons et al. 1983, 1988; Petrovich et al. 1993).

13.2 Materials and Methods

After careful consideration of the number of patients and facilities required, the authors decided to undertake a prospective pilot study of low-dose irradiation for subfoveal CNV which began in June of 1996. All patients were seen and evaluated by a group of retinal/vitreous surgeons. Clinical evaluation included family history as well as the patient's ophthalmological history. A complete physical examination, including blood pressure and pulse rate, was performed. All medications were listed. Ophthalmological examination included intraocular pressure, indirect ophthalmoscopy, inspection of the macula with a 78D lens and/or Hruby contact lens, and visual acuity. Fluorescein angiography and/or indocyanine green angiography was carried out and patients were classified as having classic, occult, or strongly suspected subfoveal choroidal neovascularization. When it was concluded that laser photocoagulation would cause an immediate and significant loss of visual acuity, all alternative managements were reviewed with the patient. No patient was excluded by virtue of age, sex, or other general health criteria. In cases of symptomatic unilateral involvement, a careful description of the contralateral eye was recorded.

One hundred forty-five consecutive patients who elected to proceed with low-dose irradiation signed an informed consent, were registered, and were followed up for 6 months to 2 years. Complete reevaluation was accomplished at 1.5, 3, 6, 12, and 24 months.

The visual acuity data of the pilot study patients was compared with that of an age-matched population who represented the untreated control patients of the National Subfoveal Photocoagulation Study published in 1991. We acknowledge with gratitude the change in lines of visual acuity from baseline in these untreated patients supplied by the MPS. Visual acuity measurements were recorded as letter scores and also as LogMar or Snellen acuity. Visual acuity was measured according to the early treatment diabetic retinopathy study (ETDRS).

The mean age of the patients was 75 years, with a range of 49 to 90 years. The majority (56%) were between 71 and 80 years of age (Table 13.1). The mean age for the MPS control group was also 75 years. Sixty-two percent of the study population and 59% of the controls were female. The size of the neovascularization in both groups was less than 3.5 disc areas. In contrast to the MPS controls, the study group had a greater percentage of patients with better visual acuity (≤20/80) (32.4% vs. 15.2%) and with worse vision (<20/400) (16.6% vs. 0.5%). Twenty-six percent of the patients in our study had previous laser photocoagulation, while such patients were excluded from the MPS Studies. Forty-two percent of our treated patients were legally blind in the other eye vs. 20% in the MPS study.

Table 13.1. Age distribution of study patients

Age (years)	Percent
<60	2
61–70	16
71–80	56
>81	27

13.3 Technique

Radiation therapy began at varying times after ophthalmological evaluation, ranging from a few days to 1–2 months. This occurred for various patient-centered reasons and, although all patients were asked whether or not their vision had changed from the time of ophthalmological evaluation, visual acuity was not remeasured.

Radiation therapy was delivered with a Clinac 2100 C (Varian, Palo Alto, Ca, USA) employing 6-MV photons at 1-m target axis distance through a 10° left or right anterior oblique field after careful patient fixation. For the majority of patients, 1600 cGy was delivered in eight equal fractions of 200 cGy over a period of 9 days; time constraints (e.g., holidays) led to some patients receiving 1610 cGy in seven fractions of 230 cGy each over a period of 7–8 days. A half-field block technique was utilized, with the central axis being set just behind the limbus. Each treatment field was set visually after fixation of the head and with the patient focusing on a distant object.

13.4 Results

Through 12 months, irradiated patients had significantly better visual acuity than the MPS control patients. In both populations, the median visual acuity decreased over time but to a lesser degree in the irradiated patients (Fig. 13.1). At 3 months, the median loss in visual acuity was -0.6 lines in the study patients and -1.7 lines in the MPS control group. This difference persisted at 6 months (-1.2 vs. -2.8 lines), at 12 months (-2.3 vs. -4.8 lines), and at 24 months (-3.4 vs. -4.8 lines) (p=0.034).

In the MPS study, failure was measured as a loss of 6 lines on the ETDRS scale. When comparing our

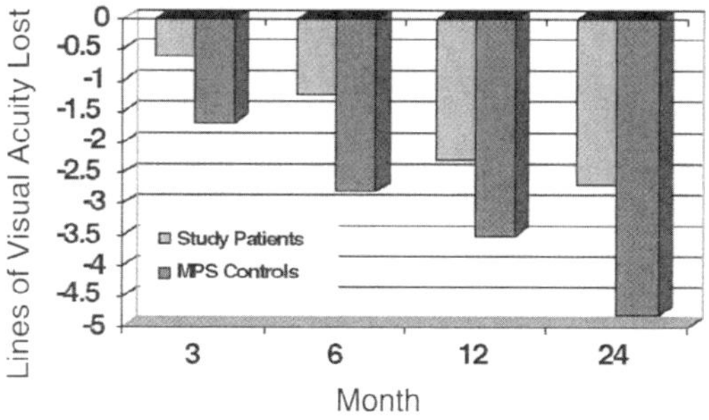

Fig. 13.1. Lines of visual loss with time

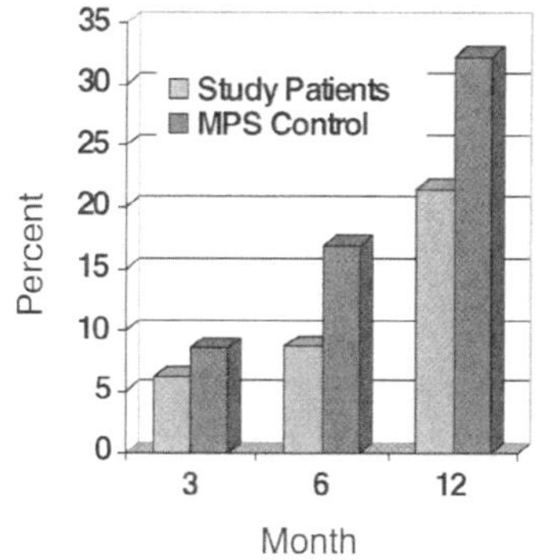

Fig. 13.2. Percent of patients showing 6-line visual loss

patients to the MPS control group, we found a significant difference (p=0.0002) in the 6-line failure rate at 12 months (Fig. 13.2). At 12 months, 21.5% of our patients had 6-line failure, compared to 32.3% in the MPS control group. This difference was noted again when comparing 3-line failures at 12 months (54.6% vs. 70.8%) (Fig. 13.3). Similar differences were seen at 3 and 6 months. The cumulative 6-line failure rate at 24 months was 45% vs. 53% (p=0.11) for the study and the control patients, respectively. Removing the 25 patients classified as „occult" did not alter the results significantly.

Patients were stratified by age (Fig. 13.4), and in each age group there was a difference in the 6-line failure rate in favor of the study group. Also, 6-line failure affected a greater percentage of those of 71–80 years than the other age groups.

Interestingly, patient eyes with previous laser photocoagulation had bettr results than unlasered eyes. Of patients without previous photocoagulation, 24% had 6-line failures at 12 months, compared to 8% of those with previous laser photocoagulation.

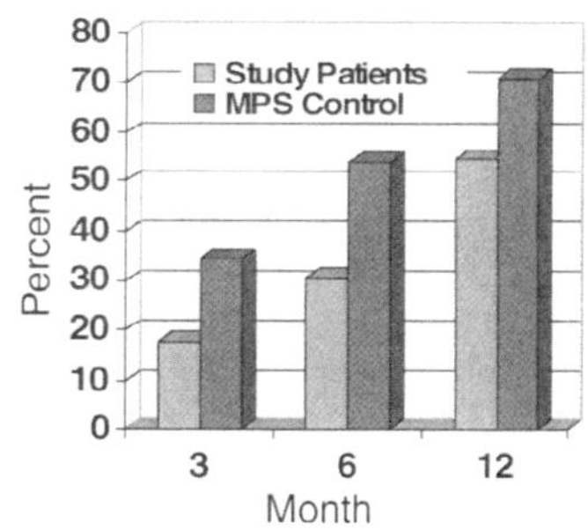

Fig. 13.3. Percent of patients showing 3-line visual loss

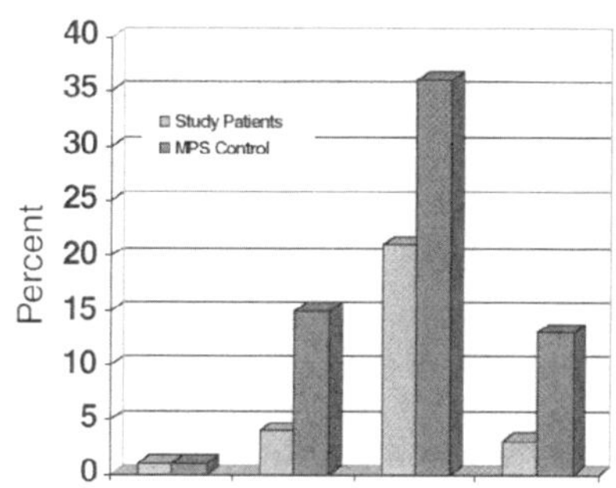

Fig. 13.4. Percent of patients showing 6-line visual loss according to age group

13.5 Discussion

Many studies have confirmed our experience that external beam irradiation has at the very least slowed the loss of visual acuity for some patients (Table 13.2) (Akmansu et al. 1998; Bergink et al. 1994, 1995; Berson et al. 1996; Brady et al. 1997; Donati et al. 1998; Finger et al. 1996; Freire et al. 1996; Hart et al. 1996; Hollick et al. 1996; Matsuhashi et al. 1996; Tholen et al. 1998; Valmaggia et al.1995, 1996). There are also other studies reporting no difference from the natural history of this progressive disease (Table 13.3) (Anders et al. 1998; D'Hollander et al. 1998; Harino et al. 1997; Krott et al. 1998; Pöstgens et al. 1997; Prettenhofer et al. 1998; Roesen et al. 1998; Spaide et al. 1998).

There is still no accepted standard protocol for radiotherapy. Several different fractionation schedules are used ranging from one fraction of 7.5 Gy (Char et al. 1999) to four fractions of 6 Gy (Bergink et al. 1994, 1995). Most investigators have utilized 14–16 Gy delivered in 1.8- to 2.0-Gy fractions. Some patients have been treated by plaque therapy (Finger et al. 1999; Jaakkola et al. 1999) and others with a proton beam (Yonemoto et al. 1999). The total dose

Table 13.2. Studies demonstrating a benefit of low dose radiotherapy for macular degeneration

Authors	N of treated patients	Dose	Authors' conclusion
THOLEN et al.	30	10 Gy 36 Gy	- 12 months - for occult CNV, there was no difference in incidence of severe visual loss for both 10 Gy and 36 Gy - 12 months - for classic CNV, there was a difference in severe visual loss for both 10 Gy and 36 Gy. 10 Gy postponed severe visual loss by a maximum of 18 months
DONATI et al.	46	4¥4 Gy	- VA maintained in 93% of eyes at 3 months - 17.5% demonstrated an increase in size of occult CNV, 75% demonstrated no change, and 6.5% demonstrated a decrease in si
CHAKRAVARTHY et al	9 10	5×3 Gy 5×2 Gy	- VA maintained or improved in 78% and 68% of treated patients at 6 and 12 months, respectively - Steady decline in VA in 6/7 control patients
BERGINK et al.	10 10 10 10	1×8 Gy 2×6 Gy 3×6 Gy 4×6 Gy	- Suggests a beneficial effect of radiotherapy at total dose of 12 or more
FINGER et al., BERSON et al.	75	12–15 Gy/ 1.75 to 1.8 Gy fraction	- 79% were within 2 lines of pretreatment VA - Stabilization of CNV in 92% at 3 months
FREIRE et al.	39 2	8×1.8 Gy 5×2 Gy	- 3 months - 65.8% no change in VA, 27% improvement subjectively
VALMAGGIA et al.	12 34	4×1.25 Gy 4×2 Gy	- VA loss better than natural history of ARMD
MATSUHASHI et al.	10	7×2 Gy	- Statistically significant difference between irradiated patients and control group when comparing changes on funduscopic exam and angiogram - No difference in VA between two groups
HART et al.	41	5×2 Gy 6×2 Gy 5×3 Gy 5×3 Gy	- Mean 12% decrease from baseline VA through 2-year follow-u irradiated eyes - Mean 50% decrease from baseline VA at 1 year and 75% decrease at 2 years in control group - No difference between dose groups
HOLLICK et al.	25	11–12.5 Gy in 5 fraction	- Visual acuity maintained or improved in 53% of eyes at 1 year
BRADY et al.	249 27 2	8×1.8 Gy 10×2 Gy 5×2 Gy	- At 2–3 months, 65.8% had no change in VA and 27% had improved VA
AKMANSU et al.	25	6×2 Gy	- VA stable or improved in 76% at 1month and in 80% at 3 months - Stabilization of CNV in 65%

required to control the disease process is unknown. THOLEN et al. (1998) reported an improvement in visual acuity at higher total doses (36 Gy) but with a 25% incidence of retinopathy. This high complication rate would be unusual unless large fractional doses were used. Overall, there have been no serious complications from low-dose radiotherapy reported in the literature.

Treatment of ARMD with low-dose radiotherapy will remain controversial until a large multi-institutional prospective randomized study is undertaken. There have, however, been two small, randomized, single-institution studies comparing low-dose radiotherapy to observation. BERGINK et al. (1998) randomized 74 patients with subfoveal CNV causing a drop in central vision to radiotherapy or observation.

Table 13.3. Studies demonstrating no benefit of low dose radiotherapy to macular degeneration

Authors	N of treated Patients	Dose	Authors' conclusion
Spaide et al.	91	5×2 Gy	- At 1 year, 49.4% of treated patients lost 3 or more lines of VA vs. 38.1% control patients
Krott et al.	73	8×2 Gy	- 7 months - significantly better VA in irradiated eyes - Long term VA - no significant difference
Anders et al.	76	6×2 Gy	- No significant difference between groups prior to therapy - No difference in VA after 12 months - Patients with LogMar 0.2 had more improvement with radiotherapy
D'Hollander et al.	104	10×2 Gy	VA not better than natural course of ARMD
Prettenhofer et al.	40	8×1.8 Gy	- 6 months - VA maintained in 42% and improved in 5% - 12 months - VA stable in 15% and worsened in 85% - No difference from natural course of ARMD
Roesen et al.	56	10×2 Gy	- 6 months - 15 patients with stable VA within 1 line on ETDRS and 27 with loss of more than 1 line - 12 months - four patients with stable VA within 1 line, 17 patients with loss of 2 lines or more - No significant benefit
Harino et al.	11 6	10 Gy 21 Gy	- VA no different from controls
Pöstgens et al.	100	4×0.5 Gy	- Mean visual acuity similar in irradiated and control groups at 1, 2, 5, and 10 years

The treatment group received four fractions of 6 Gy. Though the visual acuity in both groups declined, the radiotherapy group had significantly better (p=0.03) 3-line failure rates than the observation group (32% vs. 52.2%). In addition, there was significant improvement (p=0.002) in the incidence of severe visual loss (6 lines or more) in the radiotherapy group (8.8% vs. 40.9). No complications or side effects were noted. Char et al. (1999) randomized 27 patients with CNV to a single fraction of 7.5 Gy or observation. The visual loss was less in the irradiated group (p=0.046).

As noted previously, all of the published studies demonstrate that visual acuity declines progressively despite laser photocoagulation or radiotherapy. Radiotherapy may, however, slow the progression of the disease and arrest it in some patients. Our study demonstrates that patients with previous laser therapy fared better. The explanation is unknown, but this suggests that combined modality therapy may be better than single modality therapy. Our study was not randomized and does not have a long enough follow-up to assess the true benefit of low-dose irradiation. We await the results of large, randomized, prospective, controlled studies now in progress.

References

Akmansu M, Dirican B, Ozturk B, Egehan I et al (1998) External radiotherapy in macular degeneration: our technique, dosimetric calculation, and preliminary results. Int J Radiat Oncol Biol Phys 40:923–927

Alberti W (1986) Radiotherapy of choroidal hemangioma. Int J Radiat Oncol Biol Phys 12:122–123

Anders N, Stahl H, Dorn A et al (1998) Radiotherapy of exudative senile macular degeneration – a prospective controlled study. Ophthalmologe 95(11):760–764

Bergink GJ, Deutman AF, Van den Broek JE et al (1994) Radiation therapy for subfoveal choroidal neovascular membranes in age related macular degeneration: a pilot study. Graefes Arch Clin Exp Ophthalmol 232:591–598

Bergink GJ, Deutman AF, Van den Broek JE et al (1995) Radiation therapy for age-related subfoveal choroidal neovascular membranes. Doc Ophthalmol 90:67–74

Bergink GJ, Hoyng CB, van der Maazen RW, Vingerling JR et al (1998) A randomized controlled clinical trial on the efficacy of radiation therapy in the control of subfoveal choroidal neovascularization in age-related macular degeneration: radiation versus observation. Graefes Arch Clin Exp Ophthalmol 236(5):321–325

Berson AM, Finger PT, Sherr DL et al (1996) Radiotherapy for age-related macular degeneration: preliminary results of a potentially new treatment. Int J Radiat Oncol Biol Phys 36:861–865

Brady LW, Freire JE, Longton WA et al (1997) Radiation therapy for macular degeneration: technical considerations and preliminary results. Int J Radiat Oncol Bio Phys 39(4):945–948

Chakravarthy U, Biggart JH, Gardiner TA et al (1989a) Focal irradiation of perforating eye injuries with iodine-125 plaques. Curr Eye Res 8:1241–1250

Chakravarthy U, Gardiner TA, Archer DB et al (1989b) A light microscopic and autoradiographic study of irradiated ocular wounds. Curr Eye Res 8:337–347

Chakravarthy U, Houston RF, and Archer DB (1993) Treatment of age-related subfoveal choroidal neovascular membranes by teletherapy: a pilot study. B J Ophthal 77:265–273

Char DH, Irvine AI, Posner MD, Quivey J et al (1999) Randomized trial of radiation for age-related macular degeneration. Am J Ophthalmol 127(5):574–578

Colombo F, Benedetti A, Pozza F et al (1989) Linear accelerator radiosurgery of cerebral arteriovenous malformations. Neurosurgery 24:833

D'Hollander F, Stalmans P, Van Limbergen E, Leys A (1998) Retrospective study on the evolution of visual acuity after external beam radiotherapy (20 Gy, 2 Gy fractions) for subfoveal choroidal neovascular membranes in ARMD. Bull Soc Belge Ophthalmol 270:27–34

Donati G, Pournaras CJ, Soubrane D, Quaranta M et al (1998) Radiotherapy of occult neovascularization in senile macular degeneration: initial results of a pilot study. Klin Monatsbl Augenheilkd 212:321–323

Egbert PR, Donaldson SS, Kambiz M, Rosenthal AR (1978) Visual results and ocular complications following radiotherapy for retinoblastoma. Arch Ophthalmol 96:1826

Finger PT, Berson A, Sherr D et al (1996) Radiation therapy for subretinal neovascularization. Ophthalmology 103:878–889

Finger PT, Berson A, Ng T, Szechter A (1999) Ophthalmic plaque radiotherapy for age-related macular degeneration associated with subretinal neovascularization. Am J Ophthalmol 127(2):170–177

Freire J, Longton WA, Miyamoto CT, Brady LW et al (1996) External radiotherapy in macular degeneration: technique and preliminary subjective response. Int J Radiat Oncol Biol Phys 36:857–860

Gagnon JD, Ware CM, Moss WT, Stevens KR (1980) Radiation management of bilateral retinoblastoma: the need to preserve vision. Int J Radiat Oncol Biol Phys 6:669

Ganley JP, Roberts J (1983) Eye conditions and related need for medical care among persons 1–74 years of age: United States, 1971–72. Vital Health Stat 228:1–69

Harino S, Oshima Y, Tsujikawa K et al (1997) Treatment of age-related subfoveal choroidal neovascularization by low dose external radiation: a preliminary study. Nippon Ganka Gakkai Zasshi 101:341–348

Hart PM, Chakravarthy U, MacKenzie G, Archer DB, Houston RF (1996) Teletherapy for subfoveal choroidal neovascularization of age-related macular degeneration: results of follow up in a non-randomized study. Br J Ophthalmol 80:1046–1050

Hollick EJ, Goble RR, Knowles PJ, Ramsey MC et al (1996) Radiotherapy treatment of age-related subfoveal neovascular membranes in patients with good vision. Eye 10:609–616

Jaakkola A, Heikkonen J, Tarkkanen A, Immonen I (1999) Visual function after strontium-90 plaque irradiation in patients with age-related subfoveal choroidal neovascularization. Acta Ophthalmol Scand 77:57–61

Klein R, Klein BEF, Linton KLP (1992) Prevalence of age-related maculopathy: the Beaver Dam Eye Study. Ophthalmology 99:933–943

Krott R, Staar S, Muller RP et al (1998) External beam radiation in patients suffering from exudative age-related macular degeneration. A matched-pairs study and 1-year clinical follow up. Graefes Arch Clin Exp Ophthalmol 236(12):916–921

Leibowitz HM, Krueger DE, Maunder LR et al (1980a) The Framingham eye study monograph VI: macular degeneration. Surv Ophthalmol 24:428–457

Leibowitz HM, Krueger DE, Maunder LR et al (1980b) The Framingham eye study monograph: an ophthalmological and epidemiological study of cataract, glaucoma, diabetic retinopathy, macular degeneration, and visual acuity in a general population of 2631 adults, 1973–1975. Surv Ophthalmol 24 [Suppl]: 335–610

Macular Photocoagulation Study Group (1982a) Argon laser photocoagulation for senile macular degeneration: results of a randomized clinical trial. Arch Ophthalmol 100:912–918

Macular Photocoagulation Study Group (1982b) Laser photocoagulation of subfoveal neovascular lesions in age-related macular degeneration: updated findings from two clinical trials. Arch Ophthalmol 111:1200–1209

Macular Photocoagulation Study Group (1991a) Argon laser photocoagulation for neovascular maculopathy: five-year results from randomized clinical trial. Arch Ophthalmol 109:1109–1114

Macular Photocoagulation Study Group (1991b) Argon laser photocoagulation for neovascular maculopathy: three-year results from randomized clinical trial. Arch Ophthalmol 104:694–701

Macular Photocoagulation Study Group (1991c) Laser photocoagulation of subfoveal neovascular lesions in age related macular degeneration: results of a randomized clinical trial. Arch Ophthalmol 109:1220–1231

Macular Photocoagulation Study Group (1994a) Laser photocoagulation for juxtafoveal choroidal neovascularization: five-year results from randomized clinical. Arch Ophthalmol 112:500–509

Macular Photocoagulation Study Group (1994b) Visual outcome after laser photocoagulation for subfoveal choroidal neovascularization secondary to age-related macular degeneration: the influence of initial lesion size and initial visual acuity. Arch Ophthalmol 112:480–488

Matsuhashi H, Takahashi D, Noda Y et al (1996) Low dose radiation therapy for choroidal neovascularization in age-related macular degeneration. Nippon Ganka Gakkai Zasshi 100:803–809

Mitchell P, Smith W, Attebo K, Wang JJ (1995) Prevalence of age-related maculopathy in Australia: the Blue Mountains Eye Study. Ophthalmology 102:1450–1460

Parsons JT, Fitzgerald CR, Hood CI et al (1983) The effects of irradiation on the eye and optic nerve. Int J Radiat Oncol Biol Phys 9:609–622

Parsons JT, Mendenhall WM, Mancusco AA et al (1988) Malignant tumors of the nasal cavity and ethmoid and sphenoid sinuses. Int J Radiat Oncol Biol Phys 14:11

Petrovich Z, Astrahan M, Luxton G et al (1993) Primary malignant melanoma of the uvea: radioactive plaque therapy and other treatment modalities. In: Radiotherapy of intraocular and orbital tumors. Springer, Berlin Heidelberg New York, pp 31–41

Plowman PN, Harnett AN (1986) Radiotherapy in benign orbital disease. 1. Complicated ocular angiomas. Br J Ophthalmol 72:286–288

Plowman PN, Hungerford JL (1997) Radiotherapy for ocular angiomas. Br J Ophthalmol 81:258–259

Pöstgens H, Bodanowitz S, Kroll P (1997) Low dose radiation therapy for age-related macular degeneration. Graefes Arch Clin Exp Ophthalmol 235:656–661

Prettenhofer U, Haas A, Mayer R, Oechs A et al (1998) The photon therapy of subfoveal choroidal neovascularization in age-dependant macular degeneration – the results of a prospective study in 40 patients. Strahlenther Onkol 174:613–617

Roesen B, Scheider A, Kiraly A et al (1998) Choroid neovascularization in senile macular – 1-year follow-up after radiotherapy. Ophthalmologe 95:461–465

Schilling H, Sauerwein W, Lommatzsch A et al (1997) Long-term results after low dose ocular irradiation for choroidal haemangiomas. Br J Ophthalmol 81:267–273

Spaide RF, Guyer DR, McCormick B, Yannuzzi LA et al (1998) External beam radiation therapy for choroidal neovascularization. Ophthalmology 105:24–30

Steiner L, Lindquist C, Adler JR et al (1992) Clinical outcome of radiosurgery for cerebral arteriovenous malformations. J Neurosurg 77:1

Tholen AM, Meister A, Bernasconi PP, Messmer EP (1998) Radiotherapy for choroidal neovascularization in age-related macular degeneration – a pilot study using low versus high dose photon beam radiation. Ophthalmologe 95:691–698

Valmaggia C, Bischoff P, Ries G (1995) Low dosage radiotherapy of subfoveal neovascularization in age-related macular degeneration: preliminary results. Klin Monatsbl Augenheilkd 206:343–346

Valmaggia C, Bischoff P, Ries G (1996) Low dosage radiotherapy of subfoveal neovascularization in age-related macular degeneration: results after 6 weeks and 6 months. Klin Monatsbl Augenheilkd 208:315–317

Vingerling JR, Dielemans I, Hofman A et al (1995) The prevalence of age-related maculopathy in the Rotterdam Study. Ophthalmology 102:205–210

Yonemoto LT, Slater JD, Friedrichsen EJ (1996) Phase I/II study of proton beam irradiation for the treatment of subfoveal choroidal neovascularization in age-related macular degeneration: treatment techniques and preliminary results. Int J Radiat Oncol Biol Phys 36:867–871

14 Virtual Three-Dimensional CT Simulation of Radiotherapy for Exudative Age-Related Macular Degeneration

PETER NIEHOFF, N. KOVÁCS, and G. KOVÁCS

CONTENTS

14.1 Introduction

The irradiation of benign diseases demands exact planning and precise treatment delivery. When using radiotherapy for age-related macular degeneration (ARMD), the size and location of the globe, the smallness of the macular area to be treated, and the proximity of the lens as well as the opposite globe and other structures must all be taken into consideration (CHARLES and BROWN 1975). Conventional x-ray simulation cannot provide an exact presentation of the soft tissue structures of the eye (DINGES et al. 1998; KARLSSON et al. 1995; VINH HUNG et al. 1998). Virtual simulation captures more information in a format allowing multiplanar reconstruction and creation of digital radiographs all in one session. The patient is then free to leave and the radiation oncologist can design the treatment program when convenient (NIEHOFF et al. 1998). The lens, macula, and optic nerve can be outlined, a plan constructed, and verification achieved using multiplanar reconstruction and digital radiographs before delivering the first treatment (CONWAY and ROBINSON 1997; STEPHENSON and WILEY 1995).

P. NIEHOFF, MD
G. KOVÁCS, MD
Clinic for Radiation Therapy (Radio-oncology), University Hospital Kiel, Arnold Heller Strasse 9, 24105 Kiel, Germany
N. KOVÁCS, MD
Department of Ophthalmology and Orbital Centre, University Hospital Kiel, Arnold Heller Strasse 9, 24105 Kiel, Germany

14.2 Technical Background

Prerequisites for implementation of virtual simulation are computed tomographic (CT) scan with laser crosses, a virtual simulator, and a 3-D treatment planning program, as well as a network connection. A DICOM3 standard is recommended for secure data transfer. Optionally, it is possible to use a 3-D treatment planning system with the ability for multiplanar reconstruction if a virtual simulator is not available (Conway and Robinson 1997).

14.3 Preparation

14.3.1 Positioning

To secure repeatable and precise positioning, the head is fixed in the radiation position using a thermoplastic mask with the eye visible (THORTON et al. 1991; VERHEY et al. 1982; WILLNER et al. 1997) (Fig. 14.1). To avoid eye movements during CT imaging and later during the radiation course, we used the light fixation method (ETER et al. 1998) (Fig. 14.2).

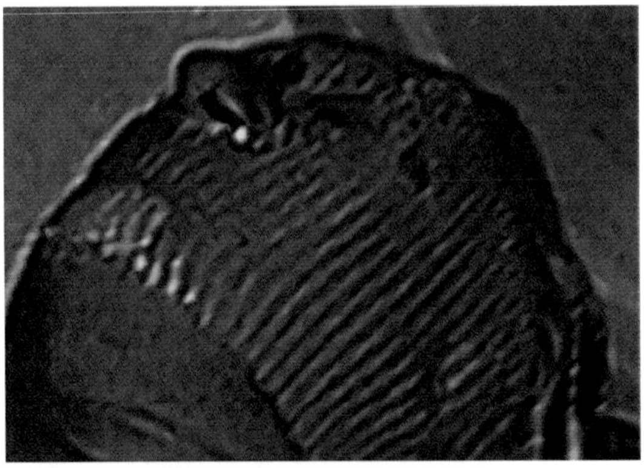

Fig. 14.1. Patient positioning

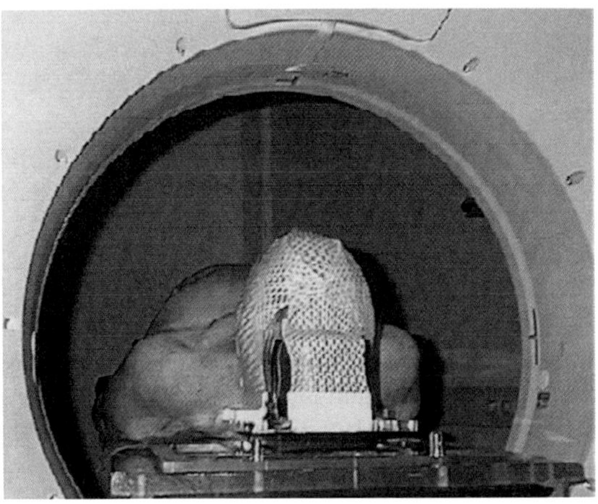

Fig. 14.2. Light fixation during CT

14.3.2
CT Acquisition

For virtual 3-D simulation and treatment planning, a CT database of the total skull was generated. We used a spiral CT (Picker 2000). The plane thickness was 2 mm in the orbital region and 5 mm outside the region of interest. To avoid setup errors on the virtual simulator and on the linear accelerator, laser crosses were marked on the mask with metal pearls. The CT database was then transferred onto the workstation of the virtual simulator.

14.4
Virtual Simulator

14.4.1
Isocenter Definition, Definition of Organs at Risk, and Target Volume

Further compilation of the CT database was carried out on the virtual simulator using the AqSim 3.4 and 4.0 programs (Picker).

The plane of stratification with the metal pearls was marked as the central beam and isocenter. If the metal pearls deviated from the laser crosses, a correction at the virtual simulator was carried out (Ragan et al. 1993). Evaluation of 17 patients showed a mean deviation of 3.44 mm on the *x*-axis and 0.66 mm on the *y*-axis. Table 14.1 shows the individual deviation of the metal pearls from the laser crosses.

The radiation-sensitive lenses were outlined as critical organs. Lenses could be clearly identified on the CT because eye movements were avoided by using the light-fixing method. In addition, the ipsilateral optic nerve was contoured. The macula is anatomically difficult to define on a CT image; the target volume was defined as a 4-mm area temporal to the optic disc over three planes (Fig. 14.3).

Table 14.1. Deviation of metal pearls from laser crosses

	Patient<?1>	Coordinates (mm)
	x	*y*
1	0.8	0.5
2	1.6	0
3	3.7	2
4	5.3	1
5	2.5	0
6	5.3	2
7	4.9	0
8	1.6	0
9	4.1	0
10	4.1	0
11	2.9	1
12	1.2	0
13	1.2	0
14	3	0
15	5.3	2
16	8.8	0
17	0	2
Mean	3.44	0.67
SD	2.15	0.84
Min	0	0
Max	8.8	2

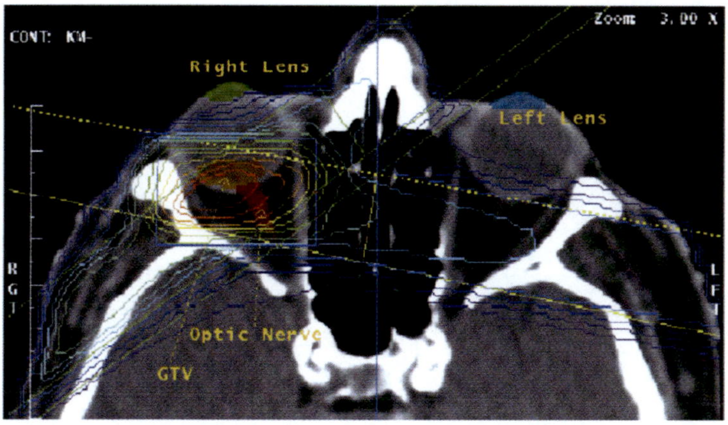

Fig. 14.3. Treatment plan

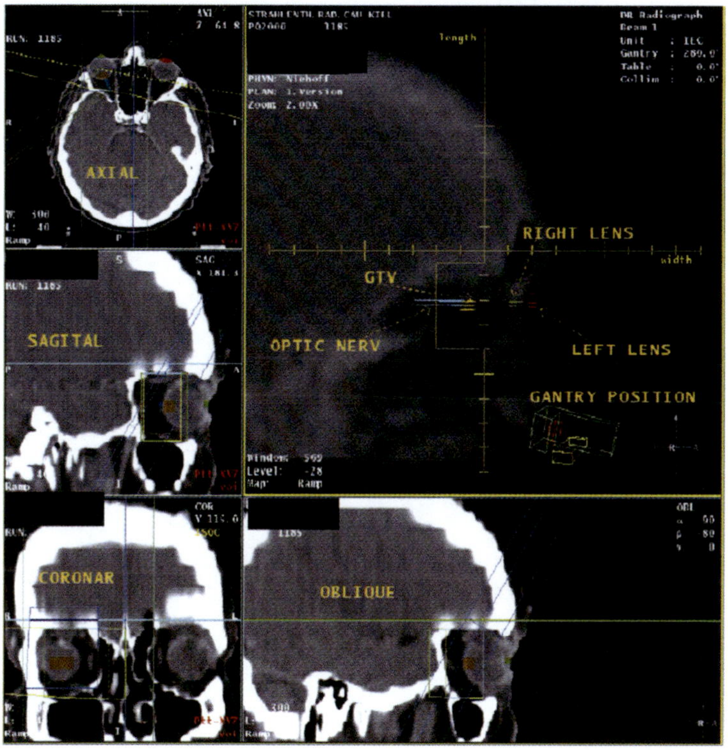

Fig. 14.4. Beam's eye view of treatment plan

14.4.2
Treatment Schedule

The total dose applied was 18 Gy using a daily fractionation of 2 Gy of 6-MV photons. (Bergink et al. 1995; Sasai et al. 1997) An asymmetrical noncoplanar treatment plan was calculated utilizing the treatment planning program Cadplan 3.0 (Varian) (Fig. 14.4).

Oriented on the Beekley spots, we chose an asymmetrical treatment plan to avoid possible displacements during the first adjustment at the Linac (Ragan et al. 1993). The noncoplanar technique allows an optimal dose distribution to the given target volume with maximum protection of critical organs while sparing the contralateral eye. We prefer a three-beam technique using two lateral tilted beams and one noncoplanar cranial beam.

14.4.3
Documentation and Verification

Documentation of the asymmetrical and noncoplanar treatment plan is technically impossible on a conventional x-ray simulator, and only the bony structures of the orbital region are presented. This provides only an approximate anatomical control (Karlsson et al. 1995). In contrast, using a virtual simulator it is possible to control and document the complete treatment plan and visualize soft tissue structures. Multiplanar reconstructions and digital radiographs offer the radiotherapist control of each beam's eye view image. The critical organs and target volume (soft tissue structures) are also presented.

Before the first treatment, field control images are performed using the double processing method. Field control images are compared with the hard copies from the virtual simulator. Treatment is started when correct positioning has been verified (VALICENTI et al. 1997) (Fig. 14.5).

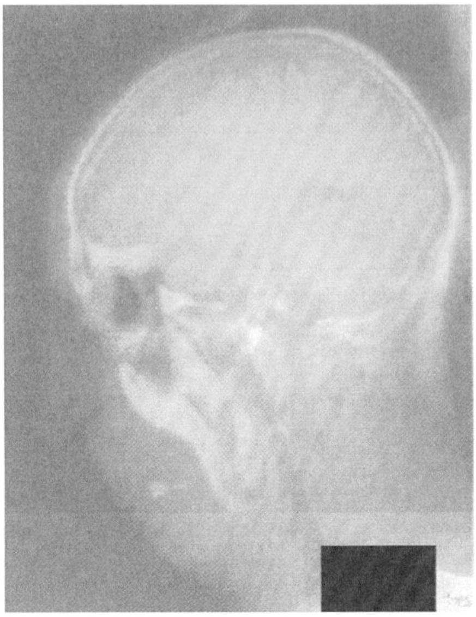

Fig. 14.5. Digital superimposition of MRI and field control image showing good alignment

14.5 Clinical Experience

14.5.1 Patients

We treated 47 eyes at Kiel University from March 1998 to December 1998. All patients were examined ophthalmologically with fluorescein angiography, and visual acuity was recorded. Pretreatment visual acuity was between 0.005 and 0.5. We included 25 eyes of 23 patients in our follow-up.

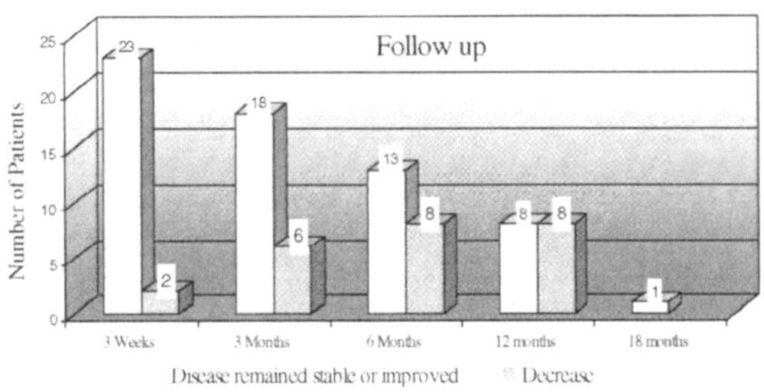

Fig. 14.6. Preliminary results

14.5.2 Results

The mean follow-up was 5.5 months (median 6 months). Follow-up investigations were performed after 3 weeks, 3 months, and 6 months. Three weeks after treatment, 92% of the patients had stable or improved visual acuity(2 lines or more). Six months after treatment, we observed stable or improved visual acuity in 13 of 21 eyes, and after 12 months 50% of the treated eyes were stable or improved (Fig. 14.6). No radiation-related side effects were observed.

14.6 Conclusions

Virtual 3-D CT simulation offers advantages for both the radiotherapist and the patient (MAH et al. 1998). It is a noninvasive, time-saving technique.

The patient profits in that he needs only one appointment for preparing and planning of radiotherapy. Documentation at the conventional simulator is no longer necessary. An advantage for the radiotherapist is the use of CT imaging itself: he can accomplish the complete simulation, planning, and documentation with one CT database on the screen. The variable image presentations with multiplanar reconstructions and digital radiographs allow better control of the treatment plan and dosimetry based on the certain identification of critical organs and the target volume (Valicenti et al. 1997)

In the observed cohort, 18-Gy fractionated external beam radiation led to stable visual acuity in at least 50% of the patients for 6 months.

References

Bergink GJ, Deutman AF, Van de Broek JE, Van Daal WA, Van de Maazen RM (1995) Doc Opthalmol 90(1):67–74

Charles MW, Brown N (1975) Dimensions of the human eye relevant to radiation protection. Phys Med Biol 2:202–218

Conway J, Robinson MH (1997) Br J Radiol70:106–118

Dinges S, Koswig S, Buchali A, Wurm R, Schlenger L, Böhmer D, Budach V (1998) Strahlenther Onkol 174 [Suppl 2]:28–30

Eter N, Schüller H, Spitznas M, Klein W, Schüttoff T (1998) Fixation monitoring during radiation therapy for subfoveal neovascularization Graefes Arch Clin Exp Ophthalmol 236(11):806–10

Karlsson U, Kirby T, Orrison W, Lionberger M (1995) Ocular globe topography in radiotherapy. Int J Radiat Oncol Biol Phys 33(3):705–712

Mah K, Danjoux CE, Manship S, Makhani N, Cardoso M, Sixel Ke (1998) Int J Radiat Oncol Biol Phys 41(5):997–1003

Niehoff P, Zimmermann JS, Schultze J, Kimmig B (1998) Virtuelle CT-Simulation von standard und individuellen Feldern mit AcQSim – Genauigkeitsprüfung mit dem konventionellen Simulator. Strahlenther Onkol 174:28

Ragan DP, He T, Mesina CF, Ratanatharathorn V (1993), Med Phys 20(2):379–380

Sasai K, Murata M, Takahshi M, Ogura Y, Ngata Y, Nishimura Y, Hiraoka M (1997) Radiation therapy for ocular choroidal neovascularization (phase I/II study): Preliminary report. Int J Radiat Oncol Biol Phys 39(1):173–178

Stephenson JA, Wiley AL Jr (1995) Current techniques in three-dimensional CT simulation and radiation treatment planning Oncology (Huntingt) 11:1225–1232, 1235–1240

Thorton AF Jr, Ten Haken RK, Gerhardsson A, Correll M (1991) Three-dimensional motion analysis of an improved head immobilization stem for simulation, CT, MRI, and PET imaging Radiother Oncol 20 (4):224–228

Valicenti RK, Waterman FM, Corn BW, Curran WJ Jr (1997) Int J Radiat Oncol Biol Phys 39(5):1131–1135

Verhey LJ, Goitein M, McNulty P, Munzenrider JE, Suit HD (1982) Precise positioning of patients for radiation therapy. Int J Radiat Oncol Biol Phys 8(2):289–294

Vinh Hung V, Verellen D, Van de Steene J, Nys F, Bijdekerke P, Linthout N, Classens CP, Storme G (1998) Int J Radiat Oncol Biol Phys 41(3):271–277

Willner J, Flentje M, Bartengeier K (1997) CT Simulation in stereotactic brain radiotherapy – analysis of isocenter reproducibility with mask fixation. Radiother Oncol 45(1):83–88

15 Radiation Therapy for Age-Related Macular Degeneration – a Wet Type Summary

LUTHER W. BRADY, JOHN E. LAHANIATIS, JORGE FREIRE, CURTIS T. MIYAMOTO, BIZHAN MICAILY, and THEODORE E. YAEGER

Age-related macular degeneration (ARMD) is the leading cause of legal blindness in persons over the age of 65, with most patients demonstrating the non-exudative or dry form (NATIONAL ADVISORY EYE COUNCIL 1998; KLEIN et al. 1992). However, approximately 90% of severe visual loss occurs secondarily to the exudative or wet type. It has been estimated that 5%–10% of all patients with age-related macular degeneration have the wet type.

The Macular Photocoagulation Study (MPS) demonstrated the benefit of laser photocoagulation over observation for the treatment of the classic extrafoveal or juxtafoveal choroidal neovascularization and for a subset of patients with subfoveal choroidal neovascularization (MPS GROUP 1982, 1991a, b, 1994a, b). However, severe visual loss often results with or without laser treatments (MPS Group 1982, 1991a, b, 1993, 1994a, b). It is well known that the majority of patients with choroidal neovascularization do not meet the MPS guidelines for laser therapy and therefore this disease process complicating ARMD often remains an untreatable blinding disorder.

As a consequence of these findings, alternative therapies for choroidal neovascularization are needed, and the list of experimental treatments is extensive. These treatments have included steroids, antioxidants, vitamins, and antibiotics, as well as other antiangiogenic therapies aimed at inhibiting choroidal neovascularization (D'AMATO et and ADAMIS 1995).

Radiation therapy has known antiangiogenic properties and been proposed as a modality for treatment of patients with severe visual loss in the exudative type of ARMD. The concept for this treatment modality originated in the observation and results of treatment of hemangiomas of the orbit and choroid with low-dose fractionated radiation therapy and the benefit that accrued as a consequence of that treatment program. However, even though the outlook for the use of radiation therapy in exudative ARMD is promising, most studies have been uncontrolled or nonrandomized in character, with relatively short periods of follow-up.

The radiation therapy techniques used in treating the wet type macular degeneration involved delivery of low dose fractionated radiation therapy with external beam radiation therapy technologies (BRADY et al. 1997, FREIRE et al. 1996; SAGERMAN et al. in this volume), or brachytherapy techniques (FINGER et al. 1996 and in this volume). The evolution of treatment with external beam radiation techniques has been directed toward precise localization of the treatment volume to include the macula and its immediate surrounding tissues while sparing other structures within the orbit. This can be determined by the utilization of three-dimensional reconstructed computed tomography and, with appropriate three-dimensional reconstructed treatment planning, the area can be treated with a high level of precision while sparing the lens, the opposite eye, and other vital structures in and around the orbit (FREIRE et al. 1996). Most of the reported patient series have used low-dose fractionated radiation therapy techniques (HART et al. 1995, HORINO et al. 1997, HOLLICK et al. 1996, MATSUHASKI et al. 1996, PÖSTGENS et al. 1997, SCHLEICHER et al. 1997, SPAIDE et al. 1998, STALMANS et al. 1997, VALMAGGIA et al. 1996). The major effort has been directed toward identifying the appropriate total radiation dose to be delivered through the area of the macula to maximize the potential benefit that might accrue from the treatment regimen. Over the years of investigation, the most frequently employed dose has been 20 Gy in ten fractions of 2 Gy each delivered in a 2-week period.

L.W. BRADY, MD
Professor of Clinical Oncology and Professor, Department of Radiation Oncology, Hahnemann University Hospital, Broad and Vine Streets, Mail Stop 200, Philadelphia, PA 19102, USA
J.E. LAHANIATIS, MD
C.T. MIYAMOTO, MD
B. MICAILY, MD
J. FREIRE, MD
Department of Radiation Oncology, Thomas Jefferson University, Philadelphia, PA 19107, USA
T.E. YAEGER, MD
Regional Oncology Center, Halifax Medical Center, Daytona Beach, FL 32115, USA

The brachytherapy technology proposed by Finger et al. (1996) has used sealed radioactive sources, primarily palladium-103 in the form of a plaque that can be placed over the area for treatment delivering radiation to a small field while sparing the normal surrounding ocular and nonocular tissues. The advantages are related to the limitation of normal tissue radiation dosage and the specific localization characteristics of the plaque in directing the treatment to the macula. Disadvantages of the brachytherapy include the need for surgical invasion in order to suture the plaque in the appropriate position for the appropriate time.

Other radiation therapy techniques have been developed using the cyclotron generating beams of protons, or charged nuclei that can be directed toward the area delivering the energy at the maximum point utilizing the Bragg peak (Yonemoto et al. 1996). This method allows for the delivery of relatively high doses of radiation at the depth of the treatment area while sparing overlying normal tissue. Other technologies relative to radiation therapy involve stereotactic radiosurgery or stereotactic radiotherapy, where radiation can be delivered to a small volume by a stereotactically localized target of the macula (Arndt 1993). This can be done by x-rays or by gamma rays from the gamma knife. The most commonly used approach in the treatment of ARMD of the wet type is external beam radiation therapy employing photons.

All patients accepted in the treatment program for macular degeneration should have a thorough ophthalmologic examination to confirm the diagnosis and to develop baseline values against which future studies can be compared. The patients accepted for radiation therapy are those who have the wet type of ARMD.

With the development of highly specific, precisely defined radiation therapy technologies, the treatment program can be carried out without the risk of major toxicities to the structures in and around the orbit. Three-dimensional reconstructed treatment techniques should be utilized for identification of the area to be treated in the patient, who is immobilized by a prefabricated head restraint or custom-molded face mask in order to insure accuracy and reproducibility of positioning. Simulation is carried out with the patient in this immobilized position, allowing for reproducibility of positioning and treatment on a day-to-day basis (Freire et al. 1996).

The rationale for radiation therapy is based on the limited number of patients who meet the criteria for the application of laser photocoagulation, even though this remains the only proven therapy for choroidal neovascularization complicating ARMD. The MPS did demonstrate that laser treatment was beneficial in decreasing the risk of severe visual acuity loss in patients with classic, well-defined extrafoveal and juxtafoveal choroidal neovascularization (MPS Group 1982, 1994, 1991). Despite this benefit, however, at least one half of the treated eyes suffered severe visual loss usually associated with recurrence or persistence of the disease process. Therefore, there is a major and significant need for adjunctive therapies to decrease the rate of recurrence and perhaps to treat the disease effectively without major loss of vision or complications relative to the treatment program. Radiation therapy has been proposed as one of these alternative treatment regimens for exudative ARMD because of the known radiosensitivity of vascular endothelial cells. The capillary endothelium has long been recognized as radiosensitive, and therefore the basic biologic consideration for its use is appropriate and proper. The radiation dosage being utilized in the treatment of choroidal vascular neovascularization is lower than that which would cause toxicities to the cornea, conjunctiva, lacrimal system, retina, or optic nerve, and, because the lens is scrupulously excluded from the treatment field, even the potential for radiation cataract exists.

The radiation dosage chosen employs standard fractionation of external beam therapy in daily fractions of 2 Gy each for a total dose of 20 Gy over a 2-week period. When fraction sizes greater than 2.5 Gy are used, there is a predisposition to toxicity, especially if the total dose exceeds 35 Gy–45 Gy by conventional fractionation or less when alternate fractionation schemes are used.

The data that have been presented indicate the absence of significant side effects related to treatment and the potential for benefit that accrues as a consequence of the treatment program. A summary of the data would indicate those reports that indicate favorable responses (Becker et al. 1999; Bergink et al. 1994, 1995; Berson et al. 1996; Chakravarthy et al. 1993; Finger et al. 1996; Freire et al. 1996; Gibbs et al. 1999; Gruschow et al. 1999; Imgart et al. 1999; Proceedings of the meeting on age-related macular degeneration 1999; Roeper et al. 1999; Sagerman et al. in this volume; StaAr et al. 1999; Valmaggia et al. 1995), those with no change (Breyer et al 1999; Gelisken et al. 1999; Prottenhofer et al. 1998), and those with no significant effect noted (Augsburger et al.; Chakravarthy et al.; Vareilles et al. 1999; Weinberger et al. 1999).

At the present time, more than 2000 patients worldwide have been treated with radiation therapy and a significant number have been reported in peer review publications. However, it remains uncertain whether radiation therapy is beneficial. Fine et al. (personal communication) have embarked upon the development of a randomized control trial to evaluate the benefits from radiation therapy in the treatment of the choroidal neovascularization process with the randomization between photodynamic therapy with laser photocoagulation and radiation therapy delivering 20 Gy in five fractions of 4 Gy each. Criticism has been leveled at this scheme because of a significant risk of radiation retinopathy and other changes in the normal structures of the eye being irradiated. However, there is a need to proceed within an appropriately designed and properly conceived project to evaluate the benefit that might be accrued as a consequence of the treatment program. The most helpful publication by Bergink et al., where 74 patients with classic, mixed, or occult subfoveal choroidal neovascularization were randomized to observation versus external beam radiation therapy, revealed that at 1 year 52.2% of the observation group versus 32% of the radiation group had lost 3 or more lines of visual acuity (p=0.08). Six or more lines of visual acuity loss was observed in 40.9% of the observation group versus 8.8% of the radiation group (p=0.002) of Bergink et al. (1998). A greater beneficial treatment effect was found for mixed or occult choroidal neovascularization than for the classic type. This publication indicated that visual acuity preservation was significantly better for the radiation group at 1-year follow-up. Other randomized clinical trials are ongoing in the United States and United Kingdom, including those by Marcus et al. (Marcus et al. 1996, 1997a, b), Shiels et al. (1997), and Chakravarthy et al. (personal communication).

In summary, radiation therapy has demonstrated positive beneficial effects in the treatment of choroidal neovascularization and, therefore, emerges as a promising treatment of this disease process. However, additional randomized control trials will be needed to assess the short-term, intermediate, and long-term benefit as a consequence of this treatment program. With the appropriate choice of radiation dosage, toxicities can be considerably reduced to an essentially minor dimension compared to the benefit that would accrue from treatment. Evaluation in this disease process is made more difficult by the vagaries in the progression and stability of the disease. The optimum dose for treatment is probably 20 Gy in ten fractions of 2 Gy delivered over a 2-week period, but other data indicate that 30–35 Gy in fractions of 2–2.5 Gy each appear to be relatively safe while possessing the potential to inhibit choroidal neovascularization. The reported studies have demonstrated no significant short-term side effects but a large measure of positive benefit. Clearly, radiation therapy is a promising, readily available treatment method for exudative ARMD.

References

Akmansu M et al (1998) External radiotherapy in macular degeneration: our technique, dosimetric calculation, and preliminary results. Int J Radiation Oncology Biol Phys 40:923–927

Arndt J (1993) Focused gamma radiation: the gamma knife. In: Phillips MH (ed) Physical aspects of stereotactic radiosurgery. Plenum, New York

Augsburger J et al z

Becker et al (1999) Proceedings of the meeting on age-related macular degeneration: new aspects of treatment. Hamburg

Bergink GJ et al (1994) Radiation therapy for subfoveal choroidal neovascular membranes in age-related macular degeneration: a pilot study. Graefes Arch Clin Exp Ophthalmol 232:591–598

Bergink GJ et al (1995) Radiation therapy for age-related subfoveal choroidal neovascular membranes. Doc Ophthalmol 90:67–74

Bergink GJ et al (1998) A randomized controlled clinical trial on the efficacy of radiation therapy in the control of subfoveal choroidal neovascularization in age-related macular degeneration: radiation versus observation. Graefes Arch Clin Exp Ophthalmol 236:321-325

Berson AM et al (1996) Radiotherapy for age-related macular degeneration: preliminary results of a potentially new treatment. Int J Radiat Oncol Biol Phys 36:861–865

Brady LW et al (1997) Radiation therapy for macular degeneration: Technical considerations and preliminary results. Int J Radiation Oncology Biol Phys 39:945–948

Breyer et al (1999) Proceedings of the meeting on age-related macular degeneration: new aspects of treatment. Hamburg

Chakravarthy U, Houston RF, Archer DB (1993) Treatment of age-related subfoveal neovascular membranes by teletherapy: a pilot study. Br J Ophthalmol 77:265–273

D'Amato R, Adamis A (1995) Angiogenesis inhibition in age-related macular degeneration. Ophthalmology 102:1261–1262

Finger PT et al (1996) Radiation therapy for subretinal neovascularization. Ophthalmology 103:878–889

Freire JE et al (1996) External radiotherapy in macular degeneration: technique and preliminary subjective response. Int J Radiat Oncol Biol Phys 36:857–860

Gelisken et al (1999) Proceedings of the meeting on age-related macular degeneration: new aspects of treatment. Hamburg

Gibbs et al (1999) Proceedings of the meeting on age-related macular degeneration: new aspects of treatment. Hamburg

Gruschow et al (1999) Proceedings of the meeting on age-related macular degeneration: new aspects of treatment. Hamburg

Harino S et al (1997) Treatment of age-related subfoveal choroidal neovascularization by low-dose external radiation: a preliminary study. Nipppon Ganka Gakkai Zasshi 101:341–348

Hart PM, Archer DB, Chakravarthy U (1995) Asymmetry of disciform scarring in bilateral disease when one eye is treated with radiotherapy. Br J Ophthalmol 79:562–568

Hart PM et al (1996) Teletherapy for subfoveal choroidal neovascularization of age-related macular degeneration: results of follow-up in a non-randomized study, Br J Ophthalmol 80:1046–1050

Hollick EJ et al (1996) Radiotherapy treatment of age-related subfoveal neovascular membranes in patients with good vision. Eye 10:609–616

Imgart et al (1999) Proceedings of the meeting on age-related macular degeneration: new aspects of treatment. Hamburg

Klein R, Klein BEF, Linton KLP (1992) Prevalence of age-related maculopathy: the Beaver Dam Eye Study. Ophthalmology 99:933–943

Macular Photocoagulation Study Group (1982) Argon laser photocoagulation for senile macular degeneration: results of a randomized clinical trial. Arch Ophthalmol 100:912–918

Macular Photocoagulation Study Group (1991a) Argon laser photocoagulation for neovascular maculopathy after five years: results from randomized clinical trials. Arch Ophthalmol 109:1109–1114

Macular Photocoagulation Study Group (1991b) Laser photocoagulation of subfoveal neovascular lesions in age-related macular degeneration. Arch Ophthalmol 109:1220-1231

Macular Photocoagulation Study Group (1993) Laser photocoagulation of subfoveal neovascular lesions in age-related macular degeneration: updated findings from two clinical trials. Arch Ophthalmol 111:1200–1209

Macular Photocoagulation Study Group (1994a) Laser photocoagulation for juxtafoveal choroidal neovascularization: five-year results from randomized clinical trials. Arch Ophthalmol 112:500–509

Macular Photocoagulation Study Group (1994b) Visual outcome after laser photocoagulation for subfoveal choroidal neovascularization secondary to age-related macular degeneration: the influence of initial lesion size and initial visual acuity. Arch Ophthalmol 112:480–488

Marcus D et al (1996) The Radiation of Age-Related Macular Degeneration (ROARMD) Study. Invest Ophthalmol Vis Sci 37 [Suppl]:1016

Marcus D et al (1997a) External beam irradiation of recurrent choroidal neovascular membranes in age-related macular degeneration. Invest Ophthalmol Vis Sci 38 [Suppl]: 4476

Marcus D et al (1997b) The Radiation of Age-Related Macular Degeneration (ROARMD) Study: a multicenter trial. Paper presented at the International Symposium on Radiation Therapy for Macular Degeneration. New York

Matsuhashi H et al (1996) Low-dose radiation therapy for choroidal neovascularization in age-related macular degeneration. Nippon Ganka Gakkai Zasshi 100:803–809

National Advisory Eye Council (1998) Vision research, a national plan: 1994–1998, Pub No. NIH 93-3186. National Institutes of Health, Bethesda

Pöstgens H et al (1997) Low-dose radiation therapy for age-related macular degeneration. Graefes Arch Clin Exp Ophthalmol 235:656–661

Proceedings of the meeting on age-related macular degeneration (1999) New aspects of treatment. Hamburg

Prottenhofer U, Haas A, Mayer R, Oechs A et al (1998) The photon therapy of subfoveal choroidal neovascularization in age-dependent macular degeneration – the results of a prospective study in 40 patients. Strahlentherapie und Onkologie 174(12):613–617

Roeper B et al (1999) Proceedings of the meeting on age-related macular degeneration: new aspects of treatment. Hamburg

Schleicher et al (1997) Radiotherapy of macular degeneration. experience with two fractionation schemes. Front Radiat Ther Oncol 30:253–258

Shiels C et al (1997) Extra-macular sparing technique for radiation treatment of age-related macular degeneration. Paper presented at the International Symposium on Radiation Therapy for Macular Degeneration. New York

Spaide RF et al (1998) External beam radiation therapy for choroidal neovascularization. Ophthalmology 105:24–30

Staar S et al (1999) Proceedings of the meeting on age-related macular degeneration: new aspects of treatment. Hamburg

Stalmans P et al (1997) External beam radiotherapy (20 Gy, 2 Gy fractions) fails to control the growth of choroidal neovascularization in age-related macular degeneration: a review of 111 cases. Retina 17:481–492

Valmaggia C, Bischoff P, Ries G (1995) Low dosage radiotherapy of subfoveal neovascularization in age-related macular degeneration: preliminary results. Klin Monatsbl Augenheilkd 206:343–346

Valmaggia C, Bischoff P, Ries G (1996) Low dosage radiotherapy of subfoveal neovascularization in age-related macular degeneration: results after 6 weeks and 6 months. Klin Monatsbl Augenheilkd 208:315–317

Vareilles et al (1999) Proceedings of the meeting on age-related macular degeneration: new aspects of treatment. Hamburg

Weinberger et al (1999) Proceedings of the meeting on age-related macular degeneration: new aspects of treatment. Hamburg

Yonemoto LT, Slater JD, and Friedrichsen EJ (1996) Phase I/II study of proton beam irradiation for the treatment of subfoveal choroidal neovascularization in age-related macular degeneration: treatment techniques and preliminary results. Int J Radiat Oncol Biol Phys 36:867–871

16 External Beam Radiotherapy in Age-Related Macular Degeneration – an Ineffective Treatment Approach?

SUSANNE STAAR, R. KROTT, M. KOCHER, R.P. MUELLER, and K. HEIMANN

CONTENTS

16.1 Introduction

Age-related macular degeneration (ARMD) is the leading cause of progressive and irreversible loss of vision in the elderly population, affecting approximately one in three people over the age of 65. It is currently incurable and is characterized by progressive degeneration of the sensory retina, supporting retinal pigment epithelium (RPE), and choriocapillaris, which constitutes the blood supply to the outer retina (BRESSLER et al 1990; CHERASKIN 1992; SOUBRANE et al. 1990; STEVENS et al. 1997; VINGERLING et al. 1995). Historically, ARMD was first reported as „senile" macular degeneration in 1885 by Otto Haab (HAAB 1885). In 1967, Gass clarified the understanding of ARMD, indicating that drusen, senile macular degeneration, and senile disciform macular degeneration represent a single disease entity in different phases (GASS 1967). In early stages of this disease, clinical examination reveals multiple yellow spots or drusen, which are lipid-rich deposits beneath the basement membrane of the RPE. Later in the course there may be a progressive atrophy of the choriocapillaris, RPE, and retina (STEVENS et al. 1997). The progressive loss of central vision results from either an exudative process involving subretinal neovascularization or this atrophic process involving the retinal epithelium and choriocapillaris in the macula. The majority of ARMD (80%) is of the atrophic or „dry" form. The most severe „wet" form is characterized by serous or hemorrhagic detachments of the retina and choroidal neovascularization (CNV). It is observed in about 20% of patients with ARMD (LEIBOWITZ et al. 1980). The wet form of ARMD generally progresses to destructive disciform scarring of the macula and fibrovascular scars involving the choroid and sensory retinal lesions. These patients develop progressive blindness, and visual acuity (VA) better than 20/200 in this phase is rare. Control of the natural course of ARMD, especially the wet neovascular form, is difficult (AVERTY et al. 1996).

Radiation therapy may induce two reactions. First, radiation may stop the inflammatory process from producing cytokines and angioproliferating substances and second, the proliferating vascularity may be occluded. Radiobiologically, the very low total and fractional doses (<1 Gy) needed for inflammatory diseases stand in contrast to the need for relatively high single doses to induce occlusion of pathological vascularization. These two possible effects may be achieved with irradiation to the eye. If regression occurs, vision may be stabilized or even improved.

S. STAAR, MD
Department of Radiation Oncology, University of Cologne, Josef-Stelzmann-Strasse 9, 50933 Cologne, Germany
R. KROTT, MD
Department of Ophthalmology, University of Cologne, Josef-Stelzmann-Strasse 9, 50933 Cologne, Germany
M. KOCHER, MD
R.-P. MUELLER, MD
Department of Radiation Oncology, University of Cologne, Josef-Stelzmann-Strasse 9, 50933 Cologne, Germany
K. HEIMANN, MD
Department of Ophthalmology, University of Cologne, Josef-Stelzmann-Strasse 9, 50933 Cologne, Germany

16.2 Materials and Methods

16.2.1 Patient Selection Criteria and Pretreatment Procedures

From January 1996 to October 1997, a total of 287 elderly patients with the classical type of wet ARMD were treated with external beam radiation therapy. All patients enrolled in this study did not meet the criteria of small, well-defined subfoveal neovascularization (Fig. 16.1) and were unsuitable for laser coagulation according to the criteria of the Macular Photocoagulation Study (MPS) group (Macular Photocoagulation Study Group 1990, 1991, 1993).

Before radiation treatment, all patients had complete eye examination with notation of vision according to standard, unmasked, Early Treatment Diabetic Retinopathy Study (ETDRS) refraction, pupillary, ocular motor, and slit lamp examinations as well as measurements of intraocular pressure using the Goldmann tonometer. Ophthalmoscopy was performed with direct, indirect, and contact lens techniques as needed. Only patients with clinical signs of wet ARMD including CNV and retinal pigment epithelial changes were included. The best corrected VA was not worse than 20/320 on the ETDRS chart. The CNV lesions had to be subfoveal. For all patients, the basal dimensions and extent of the subretinal neovascular membranes were determined by red-free fundus photography and digital fluorescein angiography. The lesion size was calculated as relative size compared to the optic nerve head of the same eye. Within 1 week after angiography, a detailed discussion was held and informed consent obtained from all patients. Treatment was initiated within another 10–14 days. Patients had to be able to return for all study visits at 3-month intervals for a minimum of 1-year follow-up.

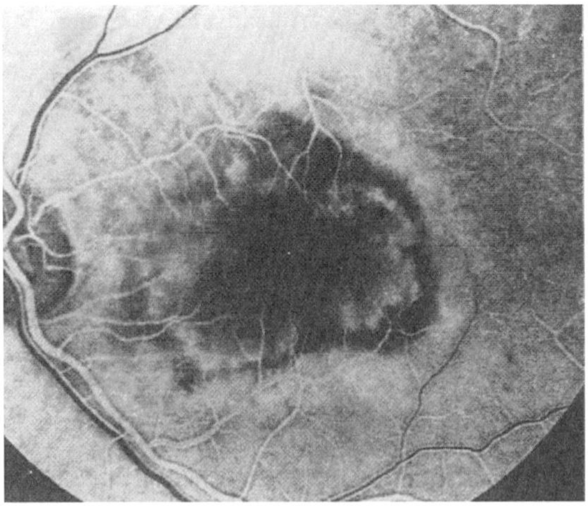

Fig. 16.1. Fluorescein angiogram with typical hyperfluorescence of CNV in ARMD

16.2.2 Patients' Characteristics

This first analysis is restricted to a group of 73 out of 287 patients with a minimum follow-up of 11 months. The median follow-up for this cohort is 13.3 months, with a range from 11.1 to 16.9 months. There were 50 women and 23 men with a median age of 74.3 years (range 52.2–88.8). Risk factors included hypertension with medical treatment in 32%, diabetes in 6%, and myopia in 5%. About two thirds of the patients (65%) were smokers (Table 16.1). All these patients had typical signs of the classical type of wet ARMD with blood, exudates, subfoveal membranes, and retinal pigment epithelial and neurosensory detachments. Classic subretinal neovascular lesions were characterized by well-demarcated areas of hyperfluorescence discerned in the early phases of fluorescein angiogram which progressed during the later phases. The fluorescein angiograms were graded at baseline for location and size of neovascularization. Only patients with subfoveal neovascularization were eligible for this study. Despite low-vision aids, no additional therapy had been allowed. Eighteen patients qualified for radiation therapy but refused treatment. The follow-up of these patients was compared to a matched pairs analysis unpaired *t*-test

Table 16.1. Patient characteristics

Total number of patients	287
Treatment period	1/1996–10/1997
Patients	
with minimum follow-up of 11 months	73
Male	23
Female	50
Male:Female	1:3
Median age	74 years
Range of age	52.2–88.8 years
Smoking (>20 years)	65%
Hypertension (with daily medical treatment)	32%
Diabetes (beginning >45 years of age)	6%
Myopia	5%

of 18 irradiated patients. The main characteristics, patient age and gender, VA, refraction, and size of subretinal neovascularization were equal in both groups.

16.2.3 Radiation Therapy

All patients were treated in the Department of Radiation Oncology, University of Cologne. Patients were supine and immobilized with a thermoplastic head mask, with the head in normoextension. Computed tomography was performed for treatment planning and followed by simulation.

Irradiation was administered with 5-MeV or 6-MeV photons (Linac SL 25, Elekta, Stockholm, Sweden). Field size was 3×3 cm in source skin distance (SSD) technique. Patients were treated with a lateral oblique field angled posteriorly 3°–5° to spare the lens and contralateral eye as much as possible (Fig. 16.2). For three patients with cardiac pacemakers, radiotherapy was applied with a cobalt-60 unit with a half beam block technique. All patients received single daily fractions of 2 Gy five times per week to a total reference dose of 16 Gy according to ICRU 50.

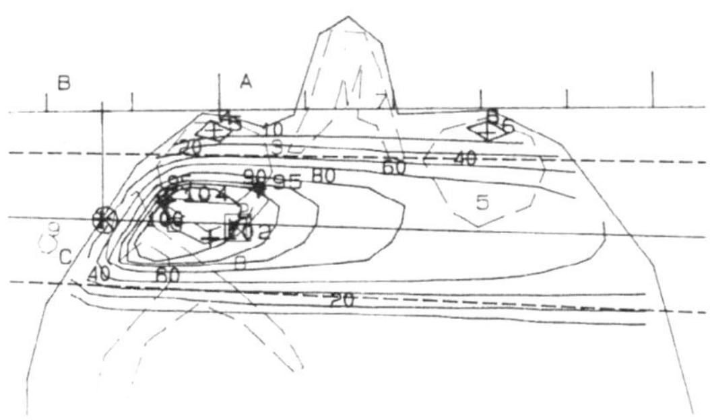

Fig. 16.2. Dose distribution for a lateral oblique (275°) 6-MV photon beam. Total dose was 16 Gy in 2-Gy daily fractions

16.2.4 Follow-Up

Patients were asked to return for the first follow-up 2 months after irradiation (3 months after diagnosis of wet ARMD). Further follow-up examinations were scheduled for 6, 9, and 12 months after radiotherapy. The patients had ETDRS VA measurements with protocol refraction, slit lamp biomicroscopy, ophthalmoscopy, and fundus photography. At the 3- and 12-month follow-up, the patients had repeat fluorescein angiography. Additionally, all patients were evaluated at each follow-up specifically for possible radiation side effects.

16.3 Results

External beam radiotherapy was applied to 287 patient eyes suffering from CNV due to ARMD. This first analysis includes 73 patients with a minimum follow-up of 11 months and a median follow-up of 13.3 months. Initial median VA was 20/80 on the ETDRS scale. After radiotherapy, the VA dropped by 1 line or more in 46 patients (63%), improved by 1 line or more in 17 (23.3%), and was stabilized in ten (13.7%) during the first year of follow-up.

In all, about two thirds of treated patients had no objective measurable benefit from radiotherapy. Subjectively, half of the patients reported somewhat better or clearer vision after irradiation. The analyysis of median VA using the ETDRS scale shows a continuous decrease in vision from 20/80 before radiotherapy to 20/400 at the end of the first year of follow-up (Fig. 16.3). The ophthalmic examination showed a growth of the choroidal neovascularization in 71/73 eyes (97.3%); only one eye improved and one remained stable. For a matched pairs analysis and comparative calculation, the ETDRS VA of all patients was transferred into the logarithmic minimum angle of resolution (log MAR) scale (Table 16.2). This notation for VA is the incorporation of the visual angle notation into the 0.1 log unit chart size progression. In the matched pairs analysis of 18 irradiated versus 18 nontreated patients, at the beginning there was an equal distribution of gender (thirteen women, five men), refraction, VA, and membrane size. (p=0.94). For the untreated group, there was a

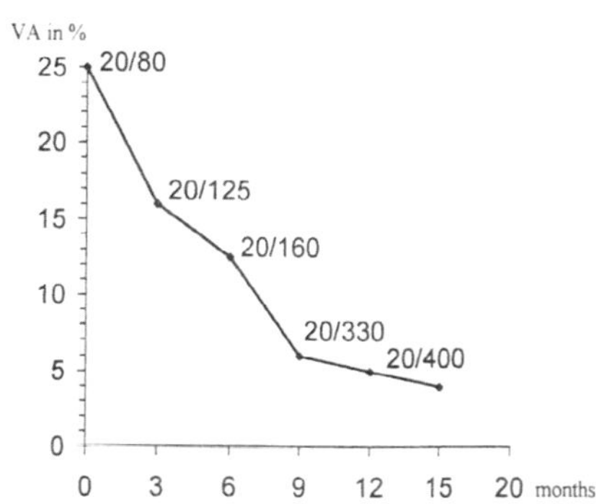

Fig. 16.3. Development of median visual acuity (VA) according to ETDRS (73 patients)

Table 16.2. Log MAR compared with ETDRS chart

Log MAR	ETDRS
0.0	20/20
0.1	20/25
0.2	20/32
0.3	20/40
0.4	20/50
0.5	20/63
0.6	20/80
0.7	20/100
0.8	20/125
0.9	20/160
1.0	20/200
1.1	20/250
1.2	20/330
1.3	20/400
1.4	20/500
1.5	20/660
1.6	20/800
1.7	20/1000
1.8	Hand movements at 20 cm

Log MAR, visual acuity using the logarithmic minimal angle of resolution; ETDRS, Early Treatment Diabetic Retinopathy Study refraction.

decrease in VA in 16/18 patients (89%) during 1-year follow-up. One patient had stable vision and another showed slight improvement. In the matched group of patients with radiotherapy, VA was unchanged after 1 year for two, but 16/18 patients (89%) had a decrease in VA. With a drop to 20/160 during the first 7 months, VA decreased more slowly for irradiated patients, compared to 20/250 for the control group (p=0.035). After 13 months, the median VA was 20/330 on the ETDRS scale (1.2 log MAR) for the treatment group and 20/400 (1.3 log MAR) for controls (Fig. 16.4). The difference is not statistically significant (p=0.243). The growth pattern of choroidal neovascularization in irradiated eyes at the final follow-up evaluation was fairly similar to the changes in untreated fellow eyes for most patients. The size of subretinal membranes doubled during 1 year in both groups (Fig. 16.5). None of the patients developed complications such as keratitis, retinopathy, or cataract. Ophthalmoscopy and fluorescein angiography did not show occlusion of choroidal new vessels as a result of radiotherapy at any time in the follow-up periods (Fig. 16.6).

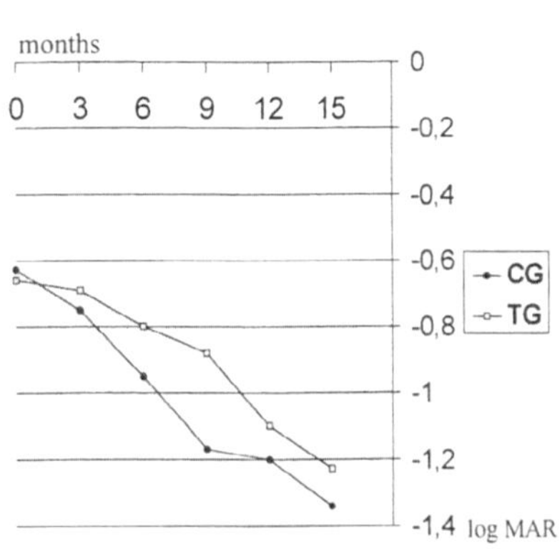

Fig. 16.4. Follow-up of visual acuity. Matched pairs analysis of the treatment group (*TG*) versus control group (*CG*)

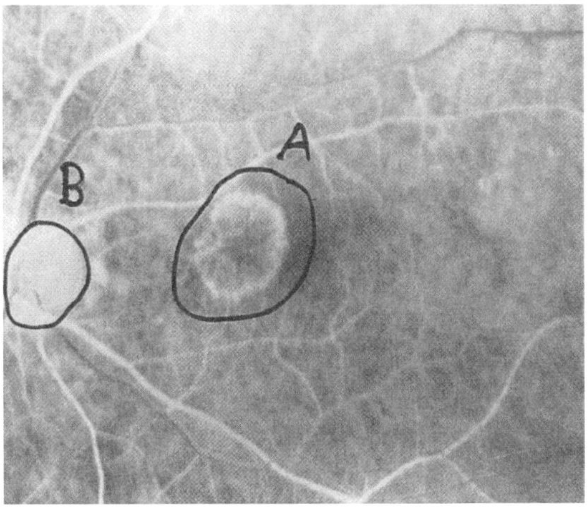

Fig. 16.5. Measurement of the relative size of CNV (*A*) in relation to the optic nerve head (*B*)

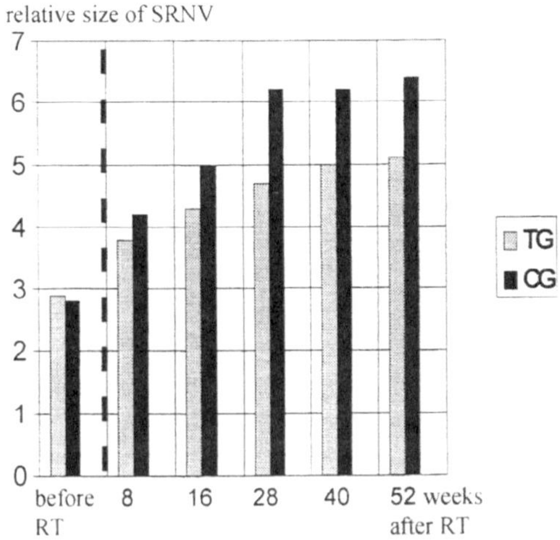

Fig. 16.6. Growth of subretinal neovascularization. Matched pairs analysis of the treatment group (*TG*) versus control group (*CG*)

16.4 Discussion

Subfoveal choroidal neovascularization in patients with ARMD is associated with a poor visual prognosis. Unfortunately, only a minority of patients with well-defined lesions that do not extend under the center of the fovea are suitable for laser photocoagulation. When the CNV is present within the foveal zone, VA will be 20/200 or worse in approximately 70% of the affected eyes within 18 months (BRESSLER et al. 1988). The treatment of CNV with external beam radiotherapy is based on the hypothesis that ionizing radiation may prevent the proliferation of endothelial cells necessary for neovascularization and may induce the obliteration of aberrant vessels (ARCHER 1993). Previous experimental and clinical studies have demonstrated that low-dose ionizing radiation may selectively damage proliferating new vessels and induce secondary vessel obliteration while sparing the retina and optic nerve (PARSONS et al. 1994). Chakravarthy et al. published one of the first reports suggesting a possible beneficial therapeutic effect of radiotherapy in wet ARMD by maintaining central VA and inducing regression of the CNV size with total doses of 10 Gy in 2-Gy fractions or 15 Gy in 3-Gy fractions. Visual acuity stabilized or improved in 63% of 19 irradiated patients at 12 months. There was a significant regression of CNV in 77% of the 19 patients 1 year after radiation treatment (CHAKRAVARTHY et al. 1993).

The current analysis was initiated to examine the VA changes in patients treated with external beam irradiation for subfoveal choroidal neovascularization due to ARMD. The change in VA of a group of untreated patients refusing radiation therapy was compared by matched pairs analysis to that of an irradiated group of patients with similar characteristics. The analysis revealed that patients treated with radiation therapy had only small, short-term benefit, losing VA somewhat more slowly than patients without any treatment. In all patients, there was a continuous, significant decrease in VA during 1-year follow-up. Measurements of the size of subretinal vascularizations showed an ongoing CNV process which was not stopped by radiation treatment.

The data from the current study suggest that 16 Gy in eight fractions of 2-Gy external beam photon therapy is not very beneficial in treating CNV due to ARMD. These results are in contrast to other published studies reporting significant efficacy of radiotherapy in subretinal neovascularization (BERGINK et al. 1995; BERSON et al. 1996; FINGER et al. 1996; HARINO et al. 1997; HART et al. 1996; HOLLICK et al. 1996; VALMAGGIA et al 1996). In these studies, patients treated with radiotherapy for CNV experienced less VA loss than untreated patients. The design of our study differed from these studies in important ways. The current study measured vision using the ETDRS scale with standardized refraction. A number of baseline covariates were assessed, such as size of CNV in fluorescein angiogram, and analyzed during several follow-ups. This study compared the change in VA after external beam radiotherapy (EBRT) to that of a nontreated control group with the same baseline characteristics.

Although the VA could not be stabilized by the 16-Gy EBRT, there might be a greater benefit with alternate doses and fractionation schedules. The total dose of 16 Gy in our study was selected primarily because similar doses have been used in past studies reporting a beneficial effect from EBRT with total doses varying between 5 Gy and 24 Gy. Valmaggia and colleagues (VALMAGGIA et al. 1996) saw no difference in response between doses of 5 Gy and 8 Gy. The Belfast group found similar results with doses of 10 Gy, 12 Gy, and 15 Gy (CHAKRAVARTHY et al. 1993). The study of Harino and coworkers (HARINO et al 1997) showed no difference in response to doses between 10 Gy and 21 Gy. Bergink and colleagues (BERGINK et al. 1995) treated four groups of patients consisting of ten patients each with doses of 8 Gy, 12 Gy, 18 Gy, and 24 Gy. They found a response with possibly favorable results for patients receiving higher doses of radiotherapy. However, these groups of patients were not matched for baseline characteristics and had varying types and extent of CNV. The follow-up was shorter for patients with total doses of 18 Gy and 24 Gy. The exact biologic force behind the initiation and development of CNV in ARMD is unknown. Choroidal neovascularization lesions removed surgically were much larger than expected by ophthalmic examination including fluorescein angiography (LOPEZ et al. 1991; RUBIN et al 1996).

Studies on the effects of radiation on vascular endothelial cells showed radiation induced morphologic responses as well as DNA breaks, decreased cell replication, and reduced prostaglandin synthesis and production (LOPEZ et al. 1991; HOSOI et al. 1993; MOOTERI et al. 1996; RUBIN et al. 1996). Radiation also results in increased cell permeability and adhesion (WATERS et al. 1996) and may induce vascular endothelial cell apoptosis (EISSNER et al. 1995) at doses comparable to or less than those used in our current study. Comparable to the results of our study, other investigations in the last 2 years also did not find EBRT effective in CNV with doses of 20 Gy in ten fractions (STALMANS et al. 1997) or 10 Gy in five fractions (SPAIDE et al. 1998). Stalmans and colleagues (STALMANS et al. 1997) analyzed the results of 20-Gy EBRT in patients with classic or mixed classic and occult CNV. They found a continuous increase in size and rapid growth of CNV during follow-up of 12–30 months. Spaide and coworkers (SPAIDE et al. 1998) applied 10 Gy in five fractions. Ninety-one patients were included in this trial. The mean baseline VA was 20/80 before radiotherapy and 20/200 after 1-year follow-up. At 1 year, 49.1% of patients with radiotherapy and 38.1% of a control group had lost 3 or more lines of VA (p=0.16). The authors concluded that EBRT of 10 Gy was not effective in CNV and patients should not be treated with this dose scheme.

Recognition of the presence of occult CNV seems to be important in the management of ARMD. A recent study by the MPS group (MACULAR PHOTOCOAGULATION STUDY GROUP 1996) showed that juxtafoveal lesions with classic CNV but no occult CNV benefit from laser treatment. For radiotherapy, there might be a greater benefit for patients with occult CNV (SPAIDE et al. 1998).

In general, testing VA is often difficult in these patients with poor vision. For this reason, the results of our study are also based on the objective determination of growth of CNV on control angiograms. In our experience, VA often remains relatively spared in a proportion of patients with definitive growth of CNV. This observation may explain the differences in study outcomes based on vision.

There are no good animal models for subretinal neovascularization, and there is still no exact way to know the best dose of radiation needed to treat human CNV. The final answer to the question of whether external beam therapy is beneficial in patients with CNV due to ARMD has to come from a randomized trial including patients with well-balanced characteristics of their medical history and CNV lesions as well as a minimum median follow-up of 1 year. We await the results of a randomized double-blinded multicenter German trial of 16-Gy EBRT versus „placebo“ radiotherapy in patients with the classical form of wet ARMD.

References

Archer DB (1993) Doyne Lecture. Responses of retinal and choroidal vessels to ionizing radiation. Eye 7:1–13

Averty RL, Fekrat S, Hawkins BS et al (1996) Natural history of subretinal hemorrhage in age-related macular degeneration. Retina 16:183–189

Bergink GJ, Deutman AF, Van den Broek JE et al (1995) Radiation therapy for age-related subfoveal choroidal neovascularization membranes. A pilot study. Doc Ophthalmol 90:67–74

Berson AM, Finger PT, Sherr DL et al (1996) Radiotherapy for age-related macular degeneration: Preliminary results of a potentially new treatment. Int J Radiat Oncol Biol Phys 36:861–865

Bressler NM, Bressler SB, Fine SL (1988) Age-related macular degeneration. Surv Ophthalmol 32:375–412

Bressler SB, Maguire MG, Bressler NM et al (1990) Relationship of drusen and abnormalities of the retinal pigment epithelium to the prognosis of neovascular macular degeneration. Arch Ophthalmol 108:1442–1447

Chakravarthy U, Houston RF, Archer DB (1993) Treatment of age-related subfoveal neovascular membranes by teletherapy: A pilot study. Br J Ophthalmol 77:265–273

Cheraskin E (1992) Macular degeneration: How big is the problem? J Natl Med Assoc 84:873–876

Eissner G, Kohlhuber F, Grell M et al (1995) Critical involvement of transmembrane necrosis factor-alpha endothelial programmed cell death mediated by ionizing radiation and bacterial endotoxin. Blood 86:4181–4193

Finger PT, Berson A, Sherr DL et al (1996) Radiation therapy for subretinal neo-vascularization. Ophthalmology 103:878–889

Gass JDM (1967) Pathogenesis of disciform detachment of the neuroepithelium (parts I and III). Am J Ophthalmol 63:573–711

Haab O (1885) Erkrankungen der Macula lutea. Zentralblatt Augenheilkd 9:384–391

Harino S, Oshima Y, Tsujikawa K et al (1997) Treatment of age-related subfoveal choroidal neovascularization by low-dose external radiation: A preliminary study. Nippon Ganka Gakkai Zasshi 101:341–348

Hart PM, Chakravarthy U, MacKenzie G et al (1996) Teletherapy for subfoveal choroidal neovascularization of age-related macular degeneration: Results of follow-up in a non-randomized study. Br J Ophthalmol 80:1046–1050

Hollick EJ, Goble RR, Knowles PJ et al (1996) Radiotherapy treatment of age-related subfoveal neovascular membranes in patients with good vision. Eye 10:609–616

Hosoi Y, Yamamoto M, Ono T et al (1993) Prostacyclin production in cultured endothelial cells is highly sensitive to low doses of ionizing. Int J Radiat Biol Phys 63:631–638

Leibowitz H, Krueger D, Maunder L et al (1980) The Framingham Eye Study monograph: An ophthalmological and epidemiological study of cataract, glaucoma, diabetic retinopathy, macular degeneration, and visual acuity in a general population of 2631 adults. Surv Ophthalmol 24:335–610

Lopez PF, Grossniklaus HE, Lambert HM et al (1991) Pathologic features of surgically excised subretinal neovascular membranes in age-related macular degeneration. Am J Ophthalmol 112:647–656

Macular Photocoagulation Study Group (1990) Krypton laser photocoagulation for neovascular lesions of age-related macular degeneration. Results of a randomized clinical trial. Arch Ophthalmol 108:816–824

Macular Photocoagulation Study Group (1991) Laser photocoagulation of subfoveal neovascular lesions in age-related macular degeneration. Results of a randomized clinical trial. Arch Ophthalmol 109:1220–1231

Macular Photocoagulation Study Group (1993) Laser photocoagulation of subfoveal neovascular lesions of age-related macular degeneration. Updated findings from two clinical trials. Arch Ophthalmol 111:1200–1209

Macular Photocoagulation Study Group (1996) Occult choroidal neovascularization. Arch Ophthalmol. 114:400–412

Mooteri SN, Podolski JL, Drab EA et al (1996) WR - 1065 and radioprotection of vascular endothelial cells. II. Morphology. Radiat Res 145:217–224

Parsons JT, Bova FJ, Fitzgerald CR et al (1994) Radiation retinopathy after external beam irradiation: Analysis of time-dose factors. Int J Radiat Oncol Biol Phys 30:765–773

Rubin DB, Drab EA, Kang HJ et al (1996) WR - 1065 and radioprotection of vascular endothelial cells. 1. Cell proliferation, DNA synthesis and damage. Radiat Res 145:210–216

Soubrane G, Coscas G, Francais C et al (1990) Occult subretinal new vessels in age-related macular degeneration. Ophthalmology 97:649–657

Spaide RF, Guyer DR, McCormick B et al (1998) External beam radiation therapy for choroidal neovascularization. Ophthalmology 105:24–30

Stalmans P, Leys A, Van Limbergen E (1997) External beam radiotherapy (20 Gy, 2-Gy fractions) fails to control the growth of choroidal neovascularization in age-related macular degeneration: A review of 111 cases. Retina 17:481–492

Stevens TS, Bressler NM, Maguire MG et al (1997) Occult choroidal neovascularization in age-related macular degeneration. A natural history study. Arch Ophthalmol 115:345–350

Valmaggia C, Bischoff P, Ries G et al (1996) Niedrig-dosierte Radiotherapie der subfoveolären Neovaskularisationen bei altersabhängiger Makuladegeneration. Klin Monatsbl Augenheilkd 208:315–317

Vingerling JR, Dielemans I, Hofman A et al (1995) The prevalence of age-related maculopathy in the Rotterdam Study. Ophthalmology 102:205–210

Waters CM, Taylor JM, Molteni A et al (1996) Dose-response effects of radiation on the permeability of endothelial cells in culture. Radiat Res 146:321–328

Clinical Studies of Age-Related Macular Degeneration (ARMD)

17 Results of a Prospective, Randomized, Double-Blind Multicenter Trial on Radiation Therapy of Age-Related Macular Degeneration (RAD Study)

CAREN BELLMANN, KRISTINA UNNEBRINK, J. DEBUS, RITA ENGENHART-CABILLIC, M. WANNENMACHER, and FRANK G. HOLZ FOR THE RAD-STUDY GROUP*

CONTENTS

17.1 Background

Age-related macular degeneration (ARMD) is the leading cause of legal blindness in Western nations for persons beyond 50 years of age (BRESSLER et al. 1988, KLEIN et al. 1992; LEIBOWITZ et al. 1980; WORMALD 1995). The most frequent cause of severe visual loss associated with ARMD is the growth of neovascular membranes from the choriocapillaris into the subretinal space. This usually results in irreversible degeneration of the overlying neurosensory retina. Laser treatment has been shown to be beneficial in patients presenting with well-defined choroidal neovascularization (CNV) (MACULAR PHOTOCOAGULATION STUDY GROUP 1986, 1991, 1994). However, about 50% of patients will develop recurrences during the subsequent clinical course. In addition, laser photocoagulation of initially subfoveal membranes is associated with irreversible destruction of foveal neurosensory retina (MACULAR PHOTOCOAGULATION STUDY GROUP 1991). Furthermore, the majority of patients with exudative ARMD have neovascular membranes that cannot be clearly delineated using angiographic examination (FREUND et al. 1993). The visual results from treating these occult CNV are disappointing (SOUBRANE et al. 1990). Therefore, the visual prognosis is disappointing for most patients and new, effective, and safe forms of treatment are needed.

Recently, alternate therapeutic approaches for subfoveal CNV have been developed. These include surgical removal, which is currently being evaluated in randomized clinical studies (submacular surgery trials). However, unavoidable concurrent removal of retinal pigment epithelial cells in the macular area has been shown to limit functional outcome. Experience with macular rotation and transplantation of retinal or iris pigment epithelial cells is still limited to a few pilot studies and needs further evaluation (ALGVERE et al. 1994; ECKARDT et al. 1999; MACHEMER and STEINHORST 1993; NINOMIYA et al. 1996; REZAI et al. 1997; THOMAS et al. 1992; SCHEIDER et al. 1999). Pharmacological treatment using anti-angiogenic drugs (interferon alfa-2a) have either failed to show a therapeutic effect (PHARMACOLOGICAL THERAPY FOR MACULAR PHOTOCOAGULATION STUDY GROUP 1997; THOMAS and IBANEZ 1993) or are still under investigation (thalidomide, integrin antagonists, etc.) (CHALLA et al. 1998; D'AMATO et al. 1994), whereby potential side effects may limit their use in elderly patients (CIULLA et al. 1998). Favorable effects of photodynamic therapy in the presence of subfoveal CNV in ARMD have been noted, indicating

C. BELLMANN, MD
Department of Ophthalmology, University Hospital Heidelberg, Im Neuenheimer Feld 400, 69120 Heidelberg, Germany
K. UNNEBRINK, MD
Department of Biostatistics, University Hospital Heidelberg, Im Neuenheimer Feld 400, 69120 Heidelberg, Germany
J. DEBUS, MD
R. ENGENHART-CABILLIC, MD
M. WANNENMACHER
Department of Radiotherapy, University Hospital Heidelberg, Im Neuenheimer Feld 400, 69120 Heidelberg, Germany
F. G. HOLZ, MD
Department of Ophthalmology, University Hospital Heidelberg, Im Neuenheimer Feld 400, 69120 Heidelberg, Germany

that treated patients have better visual outcome than untreated patients (Schmidt-Erfurth 1999). When compared with these treatment modalities, theoretical advantages of radiotherapy include absence of iatrogenic mechanical or laser damage or systemic side effects. In addition, patients with occult neovascular membranes are treatable.

The scientific rationale for using radiotherapy in a benign disease characterized by neovascular growth is based on experimental and clinical evidence indicating that proliferating endothelial cells are susceptible to radiation (Archambeau et al. 1998; De Gowin et al. 1974; Hosoi et al. 1993; Johnson et al. 1982; Mooteri et al. 1996; Raicu et al. 1993; Rosander and Zackrisson 1995; Rubin et al. 1996; Verheij et al. 1994; Waters et al. 1996). Benign intracerebral arteriovenous malformations as well as choroidal hemangiomas have been shown to regress using ionizing beams (Engenhart et al. 1994; Schilling et al. 1997; Scott et al. 1991). These observations led to several pilot studies that used radiotherapy in the treatment of CNV.

The first report on radiation therapy for exudative ARMD dates back to 1973 (Sautter and Utermann 1973). A recent pilot study showed a favorable outcome after percutaneous teletherapy with total doses of 10–15 Gy (Chakravarthy et al. 1993). Other studies have been performed since then, the majority of which appear to confirm a beneficial therapeutic effect (Akmansu et al. 1998; Bergink et al. 1994, 1995, 1998; Berson et al. 1996; Chakravarthy et al. 1993, 1997, 1998; Hart et al. 1995, 1996, 1997; Hollick et al. 1996; Finger et al. 1996, 1998; Freire et al. 1996; Jaakkola et al 1998, 1999; Krott et al. 1998; Moyers et al. 1999; Schittkowski et al. 1998; Valmaggia et al. 1997), while others did not (Augsburger 1998; Holz et al. 1997; Roesen et al. 1998; Spaide et al. 1998; Stalmans et al. 1997).

The conflicting data from these studies and the variable outcome in the natural course of CNV prompted us to undertake this large-scale randomized, prospective, double-masked, clinical multicenter trial to test the efficacy of external beam irradiation in patients with subfoveal CNV secondary to ARMD (Radiation Therapy for Age-related Macular Degeneration [RAD] Study Group 1999).

17.2 Patients and Methods

17.2.1 Patient Selection, Inclusion, and Exclusion Criteria

Consecutive patients from nine ophthalmologic and radiotherapeutic tertiary referral centers in Germany were enrolled in this study. Participating centers were: Benjamin Franklin University Hospital, Free University of Berlin, University of Münster and St. Franziskus Hospital Münster, and the universities of Erlangen-Nürnberg, Freiburg, Hannover, Heidelberg, Munich, Regensburg, and Würzburg. Informed consent was obtained from each patient prior to recruitment. Patients had to be 50 years of age or older and be able to return for all study visits in the 1-year follow-up period. They had to have clinical signs of exudative ARMD with subfoveal involvement in the study eye. The CNV lesions had to be equal to or less than six disc areas in size and classified as either occult or classic – classic CNV included mixed CNV with both classic and occult components. Duration of symptoms in the study eye had to be equal to or less than 6 months. The fellow eye had to have clinical signs of exudative or nonexudative ARMD, including drusen and characteristic changes of the retinal pigment epithelium. For measurement of visual acuity, the modified Early Treatment of Diabetic Retinopathy Study (ETDRS) protocol and ETDRS charts were used (Ferris et al. 1982). The best corrected visual acuity in the study eye had to be 20/320 or better (Snellen equivalent), measured within 2 weeks before start of treatment.

Patients with additional eye diseases that could compromise visual acuity in the study eye or with sub-, intra-, or prefoveal hemorrhage, previous macular laser photocoagulation, photodynamic therapy, or treatment with antiangiogenic drugs were excluded from this trial.

17.2.2 Method of Radiation Therapy and Sham Treatment

Radiation treatment was applied with a single lateral port covering the entire posterior pole using 4 MV–6 MV photons or 15–16 MeV electrons. The anterior beam edge was placed at the bony canthus, and the field size measured 2.5×2.5 cm to 4.0×4.0 cm. To minimize radiation-induced side effects, the treatment table was angled 20° and the beam 15° posteriorly. The dose was computer-calculated to the reference point at the posterior pole. A total macular dose of 16 Gy was administered at 2 Gy per treatment; the eight fractions were given over a 10-day period since treatment was not performed on weekends.

Patients in the placebo group were likewise planned and placed in the linear accelerator for eight fractions, but with eight doses of 0 Gy. Machine noise during irradiation was simulated and the technicians were instructed not to inform patients about the mode of treatment. The sham treatment method was spread out over the same time course as the radiation treatment.

Randomization was performed by telephone by the Biostatistics and Data Center, Heidelberg, Germany. To ensure blinding of patients and ophthalmologists, only the respective radiation therapy departments were informed by letter about treatment allocation.

17.2.3 Evaluations and Patient Follow-up

Baseline examinations performed within 2 weeks before initiating radiation therapy included visual acuity, routine slit lamp biomicroscopy, ophthalmoscopy, and swinging flashlight testing. They were repeated at each follow-up examination 3, 6, and 12 months after irradiation. Fluorescein angiography and fundus photography were performed in a standardized manner on every patient at baseline and 6 and 12 months. The fluorescein angiograms were graded at baseline for location and type of CNV. All angiograms were read by reviewers in the Heidelberg University Department of Ophthalmology and blinded to treatment assignments.

17.2.4 Statistical Analysis

Statistical analysis was performed by the Institute of Biostatistics, University of Heidelberg. The main endpoint was the number of lines of vision lost at 12 months. The study was planned with a sufficient number of patients to detect a difference between mean loss in treatment and control groups of 1.5 lines with a power of 90%. Analysis was done according to the principle of intention-to-treat, i.e., every patient in the treatment group allocated at randomization was analyzed. For analysis of continuous parameters, a Mann-Whitney U-Test was performed and, for discrete parameters, Fisher's exact test.

17.3 Results

17.3.1 Recruitment and Randomization

A total of 205 patients were recruited between February 1996 and October 1997. One hundred one patients were randomly allocated to treatment with 8×2 Gy and 104 to 8×0-Gy placebo treatment (control group).

17.3.2 Demographic Data

The proportions of men and women in the two groups were not significantly different (p=0.57). The patients randomly allocated to the treatment group were younger than those allocated to sham treatment (treatment group 72.2±6.8 years, control group 74.9±6.0 years, p=0.003) (Table 17.1). Smoking habits were very similar (control group 53% nonsmokers, 35% former smokers, 13% current smokers; treatment group 51% nonsmokers, 32% former smokers, 17% current smokers; p=0.68). The two groups were similar at baseline with regard to history of hypertension. When the status of fellow eyes was compared, there was no statistically significant difference observed with respect to atrophic versus neovascular ARMD.

Table 17.1. Demographic data

Age	n	Mean±SD	Q1	Median	Q3	Min	Max	p
Total	205	73.6±6.6	69	74	78	54	88	0.003
Control	104	74.9±6.0	71	75	79	61	88	
Treatment	101	72.2±6.8	68	72	77	54	87	

SD, Standard deviation; Q1, first quartile; Q3, third quartile

Table 17.2. Change in visual acuity: lines of vision lost at 1-year follow-up

	n	Mean±SD	Q1	Median	Q3	Min	Max	p
All patients								
Control	95	3.7±3.8	1	3	6	-3	13	0.528
Treatment	88	3.5±4.7	0	3	6	-8	14	
Occult CNV								
Control	59	3.4±3.8	1	2	5	-3	13	0.804
Treatment	55	3.4±4.9	0	2	6	-8	14	
Classic and mixed classic and occult CNV								
Control	36	4.3±3.9	1	4	8	-3	13	0.465
Treatment	33	3.7±4.4	0	4	6	-3	14	

SD, standard deviation; Q1 first quartile; Q3, third quartile.

Table 17.3. Percentage losing 3 lines of vision at 1-year follow-up

	n	%	p
All patients			
Control	5	52.6	0.88
Treatment	8	51.1	
Occult CNV			
Control	9	49.2	0.85
Treatment	5	47.3	
Classic and mixed classic and occult CNV			
Control	6	58.3	1.00
Treatment	3	57.6	

17.3.3 Efficacy Evaluation

One hundred eighty-three patients (89.3%) completed the 1-year follow-up and thus provided data about the main endpoint of the trial (Fig. 17.1).

Mean reduction in visual acuity was 3.5±4.7 lines in the 8×2 Gy treatment group and 3.7±3.8 lines in the 8×0 Gy control group after 1 year; this difference was not statistically significant (p=0.53, Mann-Whitney U-test) (Table 17.2). At 1 year, 51.1% of treated patients and 52.6% of controls had lost three or more lines (p=0.88) (Table 17.3). Thus, in this randomized double-blind study, radiation therapy at a dose of eight fractions of 2 Gy provided no benefit in treating subfoveal CNV secondary to ARMD.

17.3.4 Subgroup Analysis

The fluorescein angiogram reading center at the Department of Ophthalmology, University of Heidelberg, classified 83 patients (41 randomized to the treatment group, 42 to the control group) as having classic or mixed classic and occult CNV and 122 patients (treatment group 60, control group 62) as having occult CNV. Visual acuity in the patients with classic or mixed classic and occult CNV dropped by 3.7±4.4 lines in the treatment group (n=33) vs. 4.3±3.9 lines in the control group (n=36, p=0.47). In the occult CNV group, visual acuity dropped by 3.4±4.9 lines in the treatment group (n=55) vs. 3.3±3.8 lines in the control group (n=59, p=0.80).

17.3.5 Safety Analysis

Four patients (treatment group three, control group one) died before the 1-year follow-up visit. These deaths (due to cancer, myocardial infarction, pulmonary embolism) were unrelated to radiation treatment and not unexpected in this age group. Phosphenes during treatment were noted by one patient (1%) in the control group and two (2.1%) in the treatment group (p=0.612). Neither radiation retinopathy nor radiation optic neuropathy was noted in any of the patients surveyed. Cataract formation during the review period was detected in 12 (16.0%) control patients vs. seven (10.3%) in the treatment group (p=0.218). Complaints of dry eye symptoms were recorded in 38 (45.2%) control and 30 (40.0%) treated patients (p=0.525)

17.4 Discussion

In this study, visual acuity changes were compared between patients treated with radiotherapy and those receiving sham treatment. External randomization was performed to ensure blinding of both patients and ophthalmologists. Only the radiation therapists were informed of the treatment allocation. The dose regimen of 16 Gy of 6-MV photons in eight fractions applied in this trial did not preserve visual acuity. The mean reduction in visual acuity was 3.5±4.7 lines in the 8×2-Gy treatment group and 3.7±3.8 lines in the 8×0-Gy control group. At 1 year, 51.1% of treated patients and 52.6% of controls lost three or more lines. Since there was no difference in development of lens opacities in either group during the review period, changes in visual acuity were assumed to have resulted from the macular disease process.

The dose regimen applied herein was based on clinical experience from previously reported pilot studies, the results of which were interpreted to indicate a therapeutic effect (BERGINK et al. 1994, 1995, 1998; BERSON et al. 1996; CHAKRAVARTY et al. 1993, 1997, 1998; HART et al. 1995, 1997; HOLLICK et al. 1996; FINGER et al. 1996, 1998; FREIRE et al. 1996; KROTT et al. 1998; SCHITTKOWSKI et al. 1998; VALMAGGIA et al. 1997). Since there is no appropriate animal model for choroidal neovascular membranes, there are no experimental data which would allow accurate determination of an effective dose. Dose regimens applied in former studies range broadly from 5 Gy to 24 Gy. Chakravarthy and coworkers found a beneficial effect with both 10 Gy and 15 Gy, with no difference in response (CHAKRAVARTHY et al. 1993). Likewise, a subsequent report by the Belfast Group showed no difference between 10, 12, and 15 Gy (HART et al. 1996). Bergink and coworkers applied four different total dosages including 8, 12, 18, and 24 Gy and concluded from their data that higher doses may have a more favorable effect on the dose-response relationship (CHAKRAVARTHY 1997). Valmaggia et al. interpreted their observations to mean that both 5 Gy and 8 Gy of fractionated radiotherapy would have a beneficial effect (VALMAGGIA et al. 1997).

To our knowledge, the study reported here is the first that includes a randomized control group with sham treatment, the rationale being to minimize bias in determination of the main outcome parameter, i.e., visual acuity, and thus enhance the internal validity of our study. Furthermore, only one delivery method was used, allowing accurate interindividual comparison.

In this study, no adverse events from radiation therapy were noted during the review period of 12 months. Neither radiation retinopathy nor optic neuropathy was noted in any of the patients surveyed. However, with the dose regimen applied, these side effects are unlikely to occur, according to data from the literature on radiobiological effects on these tissues (BROWN et al. 1982; MERIAM et al. 1972; PARSONS et al. 1994). However, elderly patients with possible vascular compromise, especially in the retinal and optic nerve circulation, might be more susceptible to radiation damage (PARSONS et al. 1994).

Findings on the efficacy of radiation therapy for neovascular ARMD have been controversial to date. While the majority of studies found a beneficial effect (CHAKRAVARTHY et al. 1993, 1997, 1998; AKMANSU et al. 1998; BERGINK et al. 1994, 1995, 1998; BERSON et al. 1996;, HART et al. 1995, 1996, 1997; HOLLICK et al. 1996; FINGER et al. 1996, 1998; FREIRE et al. 1996; MOYERS et al. 1999; JAAKKOLA et al. 1998, 1999; KROTT et al. 1998; SCHITTKOWSKI et al. 1998; VALMAGGIA et al. 1997), some authors concluded that there was no difference or even a worse outcome than with the natural history (AUGSBURGER 1998; HOLZ et al. 1997; ROESEN et al. 1998; SPAIDE et al. 1998; STALMANS et al. 1997). In the study of CHAKRAVARTHY et al. (1993), 19 patients were treated with 10–15 Gy vs. seven who declined treatment and served as controls. There were significant differences in visual acuity and membrane size between the two groups during the review period. However, as the study was not randomized, these groups were probably prone to selection bias, e.g., the patients in the control group may have had particular reasons for declining treatment. None of these had been thought suitable for laser treatment before, but five of the treated patients had received previous treatment with laser. The authors concluded that prospective randomized trials are necessary to achieve reliable results (CHAKRAVARTHY et al. 1993).

The same group reported a retrospective analysis of 11 patients with bilateral ARMD (HART et al. 1995). They compared outcome in eyes receiving radiation therapy with that of untreated fellow eyes and concluded that the results after treatment were significantly better at the end of each individual's observation time. However, in each case the eye which received radiotherapy was the second eye to be involved, and the disciform response in the fellow eye had probably evolved much farther. They argue that the mean follow-up time of 28 months in treated eyes was long enough for the disciform response to have ceased evolving. However, five of the 11 treated eyes had review periods of less than 24 months, whereas the duration of disciform disease in all fellow eyes was more than 32 months, with a mean of 64.5 months (HART et al. 1996).

BRADY et al. (1997) and STALMANS et al. (1997) published uncontrolled trials, i.e., without compariison with untreated patients. BRADY et al. (1997) reported on the subjective visual acuity after 2–3 weeks and 2–3 months of 278 patients treated with radiation therapy and conclude that many patients will have improved or stable vision after treatment with low-dose irradiation. Besides the lack of a control group, it is difficult to draw conclusions from the presented data because of the short-term review period. STALMANS et al. (1997) observed 111 patients for a longer period of time (at least 1 year) and had to conclude that „radiotherapy failed to control growth of CNV and was ineffective in stabilizing vision."

SPAIDE et al. (1997) compared 91 patients treated with radiation therapy (5×2 Gy) with 119 historical controls. They concluded that external beam radiation was not effective in the treatment of CNV secondary to AMD, although general comparisons with historical controls tend to overemphasize differences between treatments (SPAIDE et al. 1998; SACKS et al. 1982).

The only randomized, controlled trial under discussion reported so far is the study by BERGINK et al. (1998). Thirty-six patients treated with 4×6 Gy and 32 untreated patients were compared with regard to loss of visual acuity and size of the neovascular membrane. The authors state that the sample size was calculated for the „proportion of patients losing more than 1 or more Snellen lines of vision and ending up with visual acuities of <0.1." The main difference between the trial reported by BERGINK et al. (1998) and our study is the blinding of patients and ophthalmologists for treatment assignment. We introduced the described sham treatment to avoid the *possibility* that patients' and examiners' commitment to measurement of visual acuity might be influenced by the knowledge of whether they received radiation therapy. It is interesting to note that, with the objective endpoint reported by BERGINK et al. (1998), the two groups showed no difference at all in size of the neovascular membrane (p=0.5).

Several reasons may be considered why radiation treatment as applied here is not effective for neovascular ARMD. The underlying etiology of the disease is not affected by this mode of therapy. Degenerative changes in the outer retina associated with ARMD include focal and diffuse deposition of debris in Bruch's membrane, various aging changes of the retinal pigment epithelium, and alterations at the level of the choriocapillaris and neurosensory retina (BIRD 1996; HOLZ et al. 1994a, b; PAULEIKHOFF et al. 1990; YOUNG 1987). Therefore, the angiogenic stimulus resulting from these changes would be expected to persist even if radiation therapy temporarily affects proliferating cells. Experience from photodynamic therapy has shown that closure of a neovascular net may be achieved after a single treatment session, but vascular channels have been shown to reopen, and therefore repeated treatments were necessary (SCHMIDT-ERFURTH et al. 1999). Repetition of radiotherapy, however, is limited because of potentially severe radiation-associated side effects, including optic atrophy and radiation retinopathy (BROWN et al. 1982a, b; MERIAM et al. 1972; PARSONS et al. 1994; FAJARDO and BERTHRAM 1988; THÖLEN et al. 1998).

An alternative explanation for why radiation therapy was ineffective in this study may be that the total dose and/or doses of the individual fractions were too low. It might be argued that higher doses could give different results. Bergink and coworkers' report might serve to support this view. However, with the advent of photodynamic therapy (PDT), applying higher radiation doses with a potentially higher risk of adverse effects seems even more questionable. In addition, the data presented in this double-blind, randomized study do not even show a trend toward better functional outcome in treated patients. Therefore, it appears unlikely that higher doses would make a profound difference and that another large-scale trial is warranted.

17.5 Conclusion

In this randomized study, radiation therapy at a dose of 16 Gy in eight fractions of 2 Gy provided no benefit as a treatment for subfoveal CNV secondary to ARMD with regard to visual acuity at 1-year follow-up. We therefore conclude that radiotherapy at this dose regimen should not be applied in these patients. From the data presented, it cannot be ruled out that alternate doses or radiation fractionation schemes might have a beneficial effect on the course of the disease.

* The RAD-Study Group

Steering committee: Frank G. Holz, MD; Rita Engenhart-Cabillic, MD; Kristina Unnebrink, PhD; Maria Pritsch, PhD
Biostatistis and data centre: Kristina Unnebrink, PhD; Jutta Schmitt; Maria Pritsch, PhD
Data and Safety Monitoring Board: Rolf Holle, PhD; Rolf-Peter Müller, MD; Thomas J. Wolfensberger, MD
Photography/Fluorescein Angiography Reading Center: Frank G. Holz, MD; Caren Bellmann, MD; Florian Schütt, MD; Stephanie Staudt, MD

Clinical centers

Freie Universität Berlin, University Hospital Benjamin Franklin
Department of Ophthalmology: Michael Foerster, MD; Miriam Gross-Jendroska, MD; Simone Potthöfer, MD; Norbert Bornfeld, MD; Markus Kleineidam, MD; Tim Behme, MD
Department of Radiation Therapy: Thomas Wiegel, MD; Wolfgang Hinkelbein, MD
University of Erlangen-Nürnberg
Department of Ophthalmology: Ulrich Schönherr, MD; Thomas Amann, MD; Christian Y. Mardin; Gottfried O.H. Naumann
Department of Radiation Therapy: Ulrike Schuchardt, MD; Ludwig Keilholz, MD; Rolf Sauer, MD
University of Freiburg
Department of Ophthalmology: Lutz L. Hansen, MD; Mechthild Scheuerbrandt, MD; Peter Jahnknecht, MD; Günter Schlunck, MD
Department of Radiation Therapy: Karl Henne, MD; Hermann Frommhold, MD
University of Hannover
Department of Ophthalmology: Rolf Winter, MD; Ulrich Steinhorst, MD; Mayk Steiner, MD; Heink de Groot, MD
Department of Radiation Therapy: Frank Placke, MD; Dirk Rades, MD; Johann Hinrich Karstens, MD
University of Heidelberg
Department of Ophthalmology: Frank G. Holz, MD; Caren Bellmann, MD; Florian Schütt, MD; Donate Taufenbach, MD; Hans E. Völcker, MD
Department of Radiation Oncology: Rita Engenhart-Cabillic, MD; Jürgen Debus, MD; Martin Fuss, MD; Michael Wannenmacher, MD
University of München
Ludwig-Maximilians-University, Department of Ophthalmology: Andreas Scheider, MD; Michael W. Ulbig, MD; Bernhard Roesen, MD
Technische Universität, Department of Radiation Oncology: Hans J. Feldmann, MD; Anca-Ligia Grosu, MD; Michael Molls, MD
Münster
St. Franziskus-Hospital, Department of Ophthalmology: Daniel Pauleikhoff, MD; Martin Radermacher, MD; Georg Spital, MD; Christian Müller, MD; Lisette Hobin
University of Münster, Department of Radiation Therapy: Ulrich Schäfer, MD; Dorothea Riesenbeck, MD; Normann Willich, MD
University of Regensburg
Department of Ophthalmology: Peter Gabel, MD; Arne Bunse, MD; Sonja Ottmann, MD
Department of Radiation Therapy: Michael Allgäuer, MD; Irene Rube, MD; Manfred Herbst, MD
Department of Radiation Therapy (Klinikum Passau): Anton Atzinger, MD
University of Würzburg
Department of Ophthalmology: Wolfgang F. Schrader, MD; Peter Fischer, MD
Department of Radiation Therapy: Michael Flentje, MD; Anja Herrmann, MD

References

Akmansu M, Dirican B, Öztürk B et al (1998) External radiotherapy in macular degeneration: our technique, dosimetric calculation, and preliminary results. Int J Radiat Oncol Biol Phys 40:923–927

Algvere PV, Berglin L, Gouras P, Sheng Y (1994) Transplantation of fetal retinal pigment epithelium in age-related macular degeneration with subfoveal neovascularization. Graefes Arch Clin Exp Ophthalmol 232:707–716

Archambeau JO, Mao XW, Yonemoto LT et al (1998) What is the role of radiation in the treatment of subfoveal membranes: review of radiobiologic, pathologic, and other considerations to initiate a multimodality discussion. Int J Radiat Oncol Biol Phys 40:1125–1136

Augsburger JJ (1998) External beam radiation therapy is not effective in the treatment of age-related macular degeneration. Arch Ophthalmol 116:1509–1511

Bergink GJ, Deutman AF, Van den Broek JECM et al (1995) Radiation therapy for age-related subfoveal choroidal neovascular membranes. A pilot study. Doc Ophthalmol 90:67–74

Bergink GJ, Deutman AF, van den Broek JFCM, Daal et al (1994) Radiation therapy for subfoveal choroidal neovascular membranes in age-related macular degeneration. A pilot study. Graefes Arch Clin Exp Ophthalmol 232:591–598

Bergink GJ, Hoyng CB, van der Maazen RWM et al (1998) A randomized controlled clinical trial on the efficacy of radiation therapy in the control of subfoveal choroidal neovascularization in age-related macular degeneration: radiation versus observation. Graefes Arch Clin Exp Ophthalmol 236:321–325

Berson AM, Finger PT, Sherr DL et al (1996) Radiotherapy for age-related macular degeneration: preliminary results of a potentially new treatment. Int J Radiat Oncol Biol Phys 36:861–865

Bird AC (1996) Age-related macular disease. Br J Ophthalmol 80:2–3

Brady LW, Freire JE, Longton WA et al (1997) Radiation therapy for macular degeneration: Technical consideration and preliminary results. Int J Radiat Oncol Biol Phys 39:945–948

Bressler NM, Bressler SB, Fine SL (1988) Age-related macular degeneration. Surv Ophthalmol 32:375–413

Brown GC, Shields JA, Sanborn G et al (1982a) Radiation optic neuropathy. Ophthalmology 89:1489–1493

Brown GC, Shields JA, Sanborn G et al (1982b) Radiation retinopathy. Ophthalmology 89:1494–1501

Chakravarthy U (1997) Radiation therapy for age-related macular degeneration [letter]. JAMA 278:288

Chakravarthy U, Houston RF, Archer DB (1993) Treatment of age-related subfoveal neovascular membranes by teletherapy: A pilot study. Br J Ophthalmol 77:265–273

Chakravarthy U, Hart P, Finger P (1998) External beam radiation therapy for CNV. Ophthalmology 105:1790–1792

Challa JK, Gillies MC, Penfold PL et al (1998) Exudative degeneration and intravitreal triamcinolone: 18-month follow-up. Aust N Z J Ophthalmol 26:277–281
Ciulla TA, Danis RP, Harris A (1998) Age-related macular degeneration: Review of experimental treatments. Surv Ophthalmol 43:134–146
D'Amato RJ, Loughan MS, Flynn E, Folkman J (1994) Thalidomide is an inhibitor of angiogenesis. Proc Natl Acad Sci USA 91:4082–4085
De Gowin RL, Lewis LJ, Hoak JC et al (1974) Radiosensitivity of human endothelial cells in culture. J Lab Clin Med 84:42–48
Eckardt C, Eckardt U, Conrad HG (1999) Macular rotation with and without counter-rotation of the globe in patients with age-related macular degeneration. Graefes Arch Clin Exp Ophthalmol 237:313–325
Engenhart R, Wowra B, Debus J et al (1994) The role of high-dose, single-fraction irradiation in small and large intracranial arteriovenous malformations Int J Radiat Oncol Biol Phys 30:521–529
Fajardo LF, Berthrong M (1988) Vascular lesions following radiation. Pathol Annu 23:297–330
Ferris FL III, Kassoff A, Bresnick GH, Bailey I (1982) New visual acuity charts for clinical research. Am J Ophthalmol 94:91–96
Finger PT, Berson A, Sherr D et al (1996) Radiation therapy for subretinal neovascularization. Ophthalmology 103:878–889
Finger PT, Chakravarthy U, Augsburger JJ (1998) Radiotherapy and the treatment of age-related macular degeneration. External beam radiation therapy is effective in the treatment of age-related macular degeneration. Arch Ophthalmol 116:1507–1511
Freire J, Longton WA, Miyamoto CT et al (1996) External radiotherapy in macular degeneration: Technique and preliminary subjective response. Int J Radiat Oncol Biol Phys 36:857–860
Freund KB, Yannuzzi, LA, Sorenson JA (1993) Age-related macular degeneration and choroidal neovascularization. Am J Ophthalmol 115:786–791
Hart PM, Archer DB, Chakravarthy U (1995) Asymmetry of disciform scarring in bilateral disease when one eye is treated with radiotherapy. Br J Ophthalmol 79:562–568
Hart PM, Chakravarthy U, MacKenzie G et al (1996) Teletherapy for subfoveal choroidal neovascularisation of age-related macular degeneration: Results of follow-up in a nonrandomised study. Br J Ophthalmol 80:1046–1050
Hart PM, Archer DB, Chakravarthy U (1997) Teletherapy in the management of patients with age-related macular degeneration complicated by subfoveal neovascularisation: An overview. Front Radiat Ther Oncol 30:229–237
Hollick EJ, Goble RR, Knowles PJ et al (1996) Radiotherapy treatment of age-related subfoveal neovascular membranes in patients with good vision. Eye 10:609–616
Holz FG, Sheraidah G, Pauleikhoff D, Bird AC (1994a) Analysis of lipid deposits extracted from human macular and peripheral Bruch's membrane. Arch Ophthalmol 112:402–406
Holz FG, Wolfensberger TJ, Piguet B et al (1994b) Bilateral macular drusen in age-related macular degeneration: Prognosis and risk factors. Ophthalmology 101:1522–1528
Holz FG, Engenhart R, Bellmann C et al (1997) Stereotactic radiation therapy for subfoveal choroidal neovascularization secondary to age-related macular degeneration. Front Radiat Ther Oncol 30:238–246
Hosoi Y, Yamamoto M, Ono T, Sakamoto K (1993) Prostacyclin production in cultured endothelial cells is highly sensitive to low doses of ionizing radiation. Int J Radiat Biol 63:631–638
Husain D, Miller JW, Michaud N et al (1996) Intravenous infusion of liposomal benzoporphyrin derivative for photodynamic therapy of experimental choroidal neovascularization. Arch Ophthalmol 114:978–985
Jaakkola A, Heikkonen J, Tommila P et al (1998) Strontium plaque irradiation of subfoveal neovascular membranes in age-related macular degeneration. Graefes Arch Clin Exp Ophthalmol 236:24–30
Jaakkola A, Heikkonen J, Tarkkanen A, Immonen I (1999) Visual function after strontium-90 plaque irradiation in patients with age-related subfoveal choroidal neovascularization. Acta Ophthalmol Scand 77:57–61
Johnson LK, Longenecker JP, Fajardo LF (1982) Differential radiation response of cultured endothelial cells and smooth myocytes. Anal Quant Cytol 4:188–198
Klein R, Klein BEK, Linton KLP (1992) Prevalence of age-related maculopathy. The Beaver Dam Eye Study. Ophthalmology 99:933–943
Kliman G, Puliafito CA, Stern D et al (1994) Phthalocyanine photodynamic therapy: New strategy for closure of choroidal neovascularization. Lasers Surg Med 15:2–10
Krott R, Staar S, Müller RP et al (1998) External beam radiation in patients suffering from exudative age-related macular degeneration. A matched-pairs study and 1-year clinical follow-up. Graefes Arch Clin Exp Ophthalmol 236:916–921
Leibowitz HM, Krueger DE, Maunder LR et al (1980) The Framingham Eye Study monograph: An ophthalmological and epidemiological study of cataract, glaucoma, diabetic retinopathy, macular degeneration, and visual acuity in a general population of 2631 adults, 1973–1975. Surv Ophthalmol 24 [Suppl]:335–610
Lin SC, Lin CP, Feld JR et al (1994) The photodynamic occlusion of choroidal vessels using benzoporphyrin derivative. Curr Eye Res 13:513–522
Machemer R, Steinhorst UH (1993) Retinal separation, retinotomy, and macular relocation: II. A surgical approach for age-related macular degeneration? Graefes Arch Clin Exp Ophthalmol 231:635–641
Macular Photocoagulation Study Group. (1986) Argon laser photocoagulation for neovascular maculopathy Three-year results from randomized clinical trials. Arch Ophthalmol 104: 694–701
Macular Photocoagulation Study Group (1991) Laser photocoagulation of subfoveal neovascular lesions in age-related macular degeneration. Results of a randomized clinical trial. Arch Ophthalmol 109:1220–1231
Macular Photocoagulation Study Group (1994) Laser photocoagulation for juxtafoveal choroidal neovascularization. Five-year results from randomized clinical trials. Arch Ophthalmol 112:500–509
Meriam GR Jr, Szechter A, Focht EF (1972) The effects of ionizing radiation on the eye. Front Radiat Ther Oncol 6:346–385
Miller JW, Walsh AW, Kramer M et al (1995) Photodynamic

therapy of experimental choroidal neovascularization using lipoprotein-delivered benzoporphyrin. Arch Ophthalmol 113:810–818

Mooteri SN, Podolski JL, Drab EA et al (1996) WR-1065 and radioprotection of vascular endothelial cells. II. Morphology. Radiat Res 145:217–224

Moyers MF, Galindo RA, Yonemoto LT et al (1999) Treatment of macular degeneration with proton beams. Med Phys 26:777–782

Ninomiya Y, Lewis JM, Hasegawa T, Tana Y (1996) Retinotomy and foveal translocation for surgical management of subfoveal choroidal neovascular membranes. Am J Ophthalmol 122:613–621

Parsons JT, Bova FJ, Fitzgerald CR et al (1994) Radiation retinopathy after external beam irradiation: Analysis of time-dose factors. Int J Radiat Oncol Biol Phys 30:765–773

Pauleikhoff D, Harper CA, Marshall J, Bird AC (1990) Aging changes in Bruch's membrane. A histochemical and morphologic study. Ophthalmology 97:171–178

Peyman GA, Moshfeghi DM, Moshfeghi A et al (1997) Photodynamic therapy for choriocapillaris using tin ethyl etiopurpurin (SnET2). Ophthalmic Surg Lasers 28:409–417

Pharmacological Therapy for Macular Degeneration Study Group (1997) Interferon-2a is ineffective for patients with choroidal neovascularization secondary to age-related macular degeneration. Results of a prospective randomized placebo-controlled clinical trial. Arch Ophthalmol 115:865–872

Radiation Therapy for Age-Related Macular Degeneration Study Group (1999) A prospective, randomized, double-masked trial on radiation therapy for neovascular age-related macular degeneration (RAD Study). Ophthalmology 106:2239–2247

Raicu M, Vral A, Thierens H, De Ridder L (1993) Radiation damage to endothelial cells in vitro, as judged by the micronucleus assay. Mutagenesis 8:335–339

Rezai KA, Kohen L, Wiedemann P, Heimann K (1997) Iris pigment epithelium transplantation. Graefes Arch Clin Exp Ophthalmol;235:558–562

Roesen B, Scheider A, Kiraly A et al (1998) Choroidale Neovaskularisation bei altersbezogener Makuladegeneration. Einjahresergebnisse nach Strahlentherapie. Ophthalmologe 95:461–465

Rosander K, Zackrisson B (1995) DNA damage in human endothelial cells after irradiation in anoxia. Acta Oncol 34:111–116

Rubin DB, Drab EA, Kang HJ et al (1996) WR-1065 and radioprotection of vascular endothelial cells. I. Cell proliferation, DNA synthesis, and damage. Radiat Res 145:210–216

Sacks H, Chalmers TC, Smith H Jr (1982) Randomized versus historical controls for clinical trials. Am J Med 72:233–240

Sautter H, Utermann D (1973) Gesichtspunkte zur medikamentösen Behandlung der degenerativen „senilen" Maculaaffektionen. Ber Dtsch Ophthalmol Ges 197:573–585

Scheider A, Gündisch O, Kampik A (1999) Surgical extraction of subfoveal choroidal new vessels and submacular haemorrhage in age-related macular degeneration: Results of a prospective study. Graefes Arch Clin Exp Ophthalmol 237:10–15

Schilling H, Sauerwein W, Lommatzsch A et al (1997) Long-term results after low dose ocular irradiation for choroidal haemangiomas. Br J Ophthalmol 81:267–273

Schittkowski MP, Schneider H, Ziegler PG et al (1998) Niedrig dosierte, fraktionierte, perkutane Teletherapie bei subfovealen choroidalen Neovaskularisationen. Ophthalmologe 95:466–472

Schmidt-Erfurth U, Miller JW, Sickenberg M et al (1999) Photodynamic therapy with Verteporfin for choroidal neovascularization caused by age-related macular degeneration. Arch Ophthalmol 117:1177–1187

Scott TA, Augsburger JJ, Brady LW et al (1991) Low dose ocular irradiation for diffuse choroidal hemangiomas associated with bullous nonrhegmatogenous retinal detachment. Retina 11:389–393

Soubrane G, Coscas G, Francais C, Koenig F (1990) Occult subretinal new vessels in age-related macular degeneration. Natural history and early laser treatment. Ophthalmology 97:649–657

Spaide RF, Guyer DR, McCormick B et al (1998) External beam radiation therapy for choroidal neovascularization. Ophthalmology 105:24–30

Stalmans P, Leys A, Van Limbergen E (1997) External beam radiotherapy (20 Gy, 2 Gy fractions) fails to control the growth of choroidal neovascularization in age-related macular degneration: A review of 111 cases. Retina 17:481–492

Thölen AM, Meister A, Bernasconi PP, Messmer EP (1998) Radiotherapie von subretinalen Neovaskularisationsmembranen bei altersabhängiger Makuladegeneration (AMD). Niedrig- versus hochdosierte Photonenbestrahlung. Ophthalmologe 95:691–698

Thomas MA, Ibanez HE (1993) Interferon alfa-2 in the treatment of subfoveal choroidal neovascularization. Am J Ophthalmol 115:563–568

Thomas MA, Grand MG, Williams DF et al (1992) Surgical management of subfoveal choroidal neovascularization. Ophthalmology 99:952–968

Valmaggia C, Bischoff P, Ries G et al (1997) Low dose radiation for subfoveal choroidal neovascularization in age-related macular degeneration. A pilot study: Radiotherapy for age-related macular degeneration. Doc Ophthalmol 93:317–326

Verheij M, Koomen GC, van Mourik JA, Dewit L (1994) Radiation reduces cyclooxygenase activity in cultured human endothelial cells at low doses. Prostaglandins 48:351–366

Waters CM, Taylor JM, Moltenio A, Ward WF (1996) Dose-response effects of radiation on the permeability of endothelial cells in culture. Radiat Res 146:321–328

Wormald R (1995) Assessing the prevalence of eye disease in the community. Eye 9:674–676

Young RW (1987) Pathophysiology of age-related macular degeneration. Surv Ophthalmol 31:291–306

18 External Beam Radiotherapy as a Treatment for Choroidal Neovascularisation in Age-Related Macular Degeneration

USHA CHAKRAVARTHY

CONTENTS

18.1 Introduction

Radiotherapy for choroidal neovascularisation (CNV) in age-related macular degeneration (AMD) has been proposed as a treatment modality which merits investigation on the basis of a number of uncontrolled pilot studies which have suggested that low doses of ionising radiation can stabilise vision and induce regression of subfoveal CNV. Our initial pilot study used two fractionation regimes in patients with angiographic diagnosis of classic subfoveal CNV. Nineteen patients were assigned to receive either 10 Gy (2 Gy in five fractions) or 15 Gy (3 Gy in five fractions) of 6-MV photons from a linear accelerator. Seven patients who declined treatment were followed up as controls. With a mean follow-up of 12 months, visual acuity was unchanged in 63% of the treated group. By contrast, visual acuity showed steady deterioration in six out of seven patients, who were concurrently followed and represented a nonrandomised control group (CHAKRAVARTHY et al. 1993).

U. CHAKRAVARTHY, MD
Professor of Vision Science, Consultant Ophthalmologist, Queen's University of Belfast, Royal Victoria Hospital, Belfast BT12 6BA, Northern Ireland

In patients receiving 10 Gy of radiation to the macula of the affected eye, the rate of regression of the neovascular membrane was slower than that observed in those who received 15 Gy, although final visual acuity was similar between groups. This lack of difference could have represented a lack of power to detect a difference owing to the small size of the pilot study or the absence of any real difference between the two doses of radiotherapy. As 3-Gy fractions are known to be associated with a higher risk of optic neuropathy (HARRIS and LEVENE 1976), we initiated a different fractionation schedule consisting of 12 Gy delivered in six fractions of 2 Gy. The nominal standard dose (NSD) was calculated and did not exceed 850 rets when treatment was carried out to specified fractionation schedules and the total dose was 10 Gy, 12 Gy, or 15 Gy. Our follow-up data on 45 patients and 13 controls for periods of up to 60 months confirmed that radiotherapy was associated with better acuity in treated eyes (HART et al. 1996). No retinal vessel or optic nerve damage ascribable to radiotherapy was found in this series. This is in accordance with previously published findings where detrimental changes due to radiation were not shown to occur with NSD values below than 1500 rets (HARRIS and LEVENE 1976). On the basis of these findings, we concluded that a multicentre randomised controlled clinical trial was warranted to confirm or refute a role for external beam radiotherapy (EBRT) in the management of subfoveal CNV of AMD. This was commenced in the United Kingdom in December 1995. Patients were required to be over 60 and have no diabetes, severe hypertension, or life-threatening malignancy. The inclusion criteria also stipulated a fluorescein angiographic diagnosis of classic subfoveal CNV in an eye with acuity equal to or better than 20/200 and unsuitable for laser photocoagulation by Macular Photocoagulation Study Group (MPS)-defined criteria (MACULAR PHOTOCOAGULATION STUDY GROUP 1991). The dose of radiotherapy used was 12 Gy, as the NSD for a daily fractionation regime with fraction sizes of 2 Gy is 621 rets, giving a wider margin of safety than 15 Gy, which could potentially have an NSD in excess of 850 rets.

18.2 Experimental Studies Supporting a Role for Radiotherapy in Choroidal Neovascularisation in Age-Related Macular Degeneration

Radiation therapy was proposed as an alternative treatment for CNV in AMD because of the known radiosensitivity of vascular endothelial cells. The radiosensitivity of capillary endothelium has long been recognised by in vivo studies (Johnson et al. 1982; Law 1981; Rheinhold et al. 1973). Furthermore, proliferating endothelial cells in neovascular tissue are even more radiosensitive, as cells suffer more extensive DNA damage when they are replicating than when they are quiescent. On histopathological examination, capillaries within irradiated tissue demonstrate characteristic features which include swelling of the endothelium, increased permeability, necrosis, and destruction of segments of the blood vessel (Law 1981). In tissue culture, cells derived from large-vessel endothelium suffer growth inhibition when exposed to a single dose of 8.7 Gy (Johnson et al. 1982). Retinal endothelial cells are even more radiosensitive, as a single radiation dose of approximately 5 Gy is sufficient to arrest division in 99% of cultured retinal endothelial cells (Chakravarthy et al. 1989a). Thus, the potential exists for radiotherapy to inhibit neovascular growth and induce regression by the induction of programmed cell death in the component cells and also by the modification of the growth factor profile within the neovascular complex.

Support for a possible role for radiation therapy in AMD comes from studies conducted in our laboratories which demonstrated that the neovascular component of healing ocular wounds is significantly reduced by continuous focal exposure to gamma rays at doses exceeding 9.5 Gy (Chakravarthy et al. 1989a, b). These experiments demonstrated that the adjacent normal choroid and retina were not adversely affected, thus emphasising the radioresistance of the neural retina. Choroidal neovascular lesions contain inflammatory cells believed to be involved in (a) the pathogenesis of CNV, (b) the release of enzymatic products, and (c) remodelling of the lesion. The inflammatory response may recruit additional macrophages that induce neovascularisation through production of cytokines and angiogenic growth factors (Grossniklaus et al. 1992). Low doses of radiation inhibit the inflammatory process and the formation of scar tissue. These additional effects of radiation may further compromise expansion of the CNV and cause involution of the vascular complex.

18.3 Clinical Studies Supporting a Role for Radiotherapy in CNV in AMD

Stereotactic radiosurgery using a single high dose induces obliteration and regression of arteriovenous malformations of the central nervous system (Flickinger et al. 1996). In practice, however, the treatment of ocular vascular abnormalities by irradiation usually involves fewer fractions and lower doses than those used for cerebral vascular malformations. Radiation therapy has also been used to inhibit benign vascular ocular and nonocular tumors (Plowman et al. 1988; Scott 1991). Choroidal haemangiomata respond to external beam irradiation (EBRT) at doses of 12 Gy–40 Gy in standard fractions of less than 2 Gy, and radiation-induced complications are not usually observed after such treatment (Plowman et al. 1988; Scott 1991). Also, proton beam irradiation and plaque brachytherapy to a total dose of 50 Gy are generally considered effective but relatively safe treatment modalities for the management of choroidal haemangiomata. Thus, the accrued evidence suggests that relatively low doses of ionising radiation applied in standard fractions can induce regression of vascular tumours and supports its application as a potential treatment modality in CNV in AMD.

Nevertheless, an important consideration when contemplating the irradiation of ocular structures is the development of sight-threatening complications, of which the most pertinent are radiation retinopathy and optic neuropathy. Factors which influence their development are the total dose delivered, daily fraction size, pre-existing microangiopathy or diabetes, previous or concurrent chemotherapy, and radiation field topography (Harris and Levene 1976; Chan and Shukovsky 1976; Aristizibal et al. 1977). Sight-threatening radiation retinopathy is characterised by delayed onset of a slowly progressive occlusive vasculopathy that may lead to capillary nonperfusion, retinal vessel incompetence, neovascularisation, macular oedema, and visual loss (Archer et al. 1991). The dose at which retinopathy develops is variable and differs, depending on whether treatment is delivered by brachytherapy or teletherapy. Present scientific knowledge suggests that brachytherapy at doses in excess of 150 Gy or teletherapy in excess of 50 Gy to ocular structures could result in serious postradiation complications (Archer et al. 1991). The risk of significant injury to the retina and optic nerve with the treatment regimes used in the pilot studies of CNV to date is therefore considered low.

18.4 Summary of Phase I Studies of External Beam Radiotherapy for CNV of AMD

A number of reports are now available on the use of low dose EBRT in exudative or wet AMD (Bergink et al. 1994, 1995; Berson et al. 1996; Brady et al. 1997; Finger et al. 1996; Freire et al. 1996; Postgens et al. 1997; Prettenhoffer et al. 1998; Sasai et al. 1997; Spaide et al. 1998; Stalmans et al. 1998; Yonemoto et al. 1996). All these studies were phase I/II trials. While the majority of them appear to suggest that visual acuity is stabilised and risk of severe visual loss reduced in treated patients, some have found no beneficial effect. The results of all these phase I/II trials, whether identifying a benefit or lack of benefit, need to be interpreted with caution. Firstly, none of them included randomised, prospective controls, and follow-up times were short. Although visual loss is usually rapid in individuals with subfoveal classic CNV, in a significant number of patients vision may be maintained over a protracted and variable period of time (Macular Photocoagulation Study Group 1994). Therefore, the relatively short follow-up time in the studies using EBRT may have caused overestimation of the treatment benefit. Secondly, a number of these studies included patients with occult CNV only. In the absence of a classic CNV component, natural history studies of exudative AMD have shown an even more variable outcome in terms of the protracted nature of visual loss (Bressler et al. 1988). Thus, the studies reporting a beneficial effect when patients with only occult disease are treated with EBRT may have erroneously attributed maintenance of vision to treatment when in reality it may simply have reflected the slow natural history of the disease process. These pitfalls may have been avoided by the recruitment of a concurrent control group.

Several studies using EBRT have shown no treatment benefit (Postgens et al. 1997; Spaide et al. 1998; Stalmans et al. 1998). These studies are similarly flawed, as they lack adequate control groups and follow-up is short. Their results do not provide sufficient reason to reject EBRT as a potential treatment modality.

A wide variety of doses and fractionation schedules were used in the phase I studies (Bergink et al. 1994, 1995; Berson et al. 1996; Brady et al. 1997; Finger et al. 1996; Freire et al. 1996; Postgens et al. 1997; Prettenhoffer et al. 1998; Sasai et al. 1997; Spaide et al. 1998; Stalmans et al. 1998; Yonemoto et al. 1996). A few studies have used relatively large fraction sizes and in extreme cases the entire dose may have been given as one fraction (Yonemoto et al. 1996). Such nonstandard fractionation regimes cause difficulties when attempting to evaluate the biological effectiveness of the dose. In two studies which attempted a dose escalation approach, a tendency toward better outcome was noted with higher doses in terms of regression of CNV and better vision (Hart et al. 1996; Bergink et al. 1994). As individual phase I studies are often too small to evaluate, we decided to pool the data from a number of treating centres in an attempt to model the effect of radiotherapy on the natural history of CNV. We created a database with data acquired from the literature or obtained directly from investigators (nine centres) who used EBRT to treat CNV in AMD. Analysis of the pooled data showed that baseline acuity and prior use of laser photocoagulation were associated with poor visual outcome. After correcting for confounding factors, the biologically effective dose (BED), which allows for fractionation schedules, was found to be a weak predictor of visual outcome, with those studies using higher doses reporting better outcome. In clinical oncological practice when seeking to minimise normal tissue effects, it is standard clinical practice to keep fraction sizes lower than 2 Gy. On the other hand, where radiotherapy is used to treat benign disease (e.g. acoustic neuroma, haemangiomas, etc), larger fraction sizes are often required. It could be argued therefore that CNV composed of what may be described as granulation tissue from a low grade inflammatory process responds better to higher fractions of radiation, which is in accordance with the findings from analysis of the pooled data.

18.5 Randomised Clinical Trials of Radiotherapy in the Treatment of CNV of AMD

At present there appear to be at least six ongoing randomised clinical trials involving EBRT in exudative AMD. The known details of these studies are given in Table 18.1.

Table 18.1. Overview of ongoing randomised clinical trials (RCT) involving external beam radiotherapy (EBRT) in exudative AMD. The ROARMD and RAD studies include sham treatment groups and are double-blinded. The other phase III trials are single-blinded, with refractionist and angiogram readers blinded to patient treatment status

Study name	Location	Design	Dose	Patients (n)	Results
Nijmegen Study	Rotterdam	Two armed single-centre RCT, observation versus EBRT, classic, occult, or mixed CNV, planned size 72 patients	24 Gy (6×4 Gy)	74	53% of controls and 32% of treated group lost 3 or more lines (p=0.03)
SFRADS	Belfast London Southampton UK	Two-armed multicentre RCT, observation versus EBRT, subfoveal classic +/- occult CNV, planned size 240 patients	12 Gy (6×2 Gy)	204	
ROARMD	Georgia, USA	Two-armed single centre study, observation versus EBRT, subfoveal classic CNV, planned size 60, two armed study of laser alone or laser+EBRT in extrafoveal CNV, planned size 60	14 Gy (7×2 Gy)	78 6	Awaited, numbers enrolled are too few, results not expected for some time
NYS	New York Study	Two-armed single centre study, observation versus EBRT, subfoveal classic, occult, or mixed CNV, planned size not known, XRT is given if there is 3-line loss of vision in controls	18 (9×2 Gy)	70	Awaited
RAD study	German Study	Two-armed multicentre study, observation versus EBRT, subfoveal classic, occult, or mixed, planned size 200	16 (8×2 Gy)	200	No difference in visual outcome between treatment and control groups at 1 year

The most compelling evidence for a beneficial effect comes from a study of EBRT in patients with classic, occult, or mixed type CNV which included randomised concurrent controls (Bergink et al. 1998). This study showed that after a follow-up of 12 months, 52.2% of patients randomised to observation lost three or more lines of vision versus only 32% of patients randomised to EBRT. When a drop of 6 lines or more in visual acuity was used as the criterion for evaluation, 41% of control patients and 8% of treated patients were found to have suffered such a loss (p<0.01). However, a multicentre randomised double-masked clinical trial (RAD study) of 200 patients with exudative AMD with 16 Gy of radiotherapy given in eight 2-Gy fractions failed to reveal any benefit after 1 year of follow-up (Holz et al. 1999). Reasons for this may include (a) a true inability of radiation to induce neovascular regression within the context of a CNV, (b) inadequacy of dose, and (c) the preponderance of subjects with occult CNV only, which is less likely to respond to therapies aimed at inducing neovascular regression. Other studies which recruited subjects with classic CNV only and used different dose and fractionation regimes will be reporting their findings shortly, and the role for radiotherapy in the management of this disease will become clearer.

18.6 Potential Benefits

It is highly unlikely that radiotherapy will result in improved vision in individuals with CNV of AMD, and the accrued evidence suggests that at best it may be associated with a slowing of visual loss. Even if the number of patients who experience severe loss of vision could be halved (the MPS reported 45% of patients with subfoveal CNV suffer a quadrupling of the visual angle by 36 months in the affected eye) (Macular Photocoagulation Study Group 1994), the benefits to maintaining vision-related quality of life could be highly significant.

In summary, there is evidence from both phase I/II and phase III clinical trials to suggest that radiotherapy could be beneficial in CNV in AMD (CHAKRAVARTHY and FINGER 1998). However, it is crucial to remember that phase I type studies have no further role in evaluating EBRT in CNV in AMD. Any future studies must be designed and executed as part of multicentre randomised controlled clinical trials.

References

Archer DB, Amoaku, WMK, Gardiner TA (1991) Radiation retinopathy, clinical, histopathological, ultrastructural, and experimental correlations. Eye 5:239-251

Aristizibal S, Caldwell WL, Avila J (1977) The relationship of time dose fractionation factors to complications in the treatment of pituitary tumours by irradiation. Int J Radiat Oncol Biol Phys 2:667-673

Bergink G et al (1998) A randomised controlled clinical trial on the efficacy of radiation therapy in the control of subfoveal choroidal neovascularization in age-related macular degeneration: Radiation versus observation. Graefes Arch Clin Exp Opthalmol 236:321-325

Bergink GJ, Deutman AF, VandenBroek JFCM et al (1994) Radiation therapy for sub-foveal choroidal neovascular membranes in age-related macular degeneration. Graefes Arch Clin Exp Opthalmol 232:591-598

Bergink GJ, Deutman AF, VandenBroek JE et al (1995) Radiation therapy for age-related subfoveal choroidal neovascular membranes. A pilot study. Docum Ophthalmol 90:67-74

Berson A, Finger PT, Sherr DL, Emery R, Alfieri A, Bosworth JL (1996) Radiotherapy for age-related macular degeneration: Preliminary results of a potentially new treatment. Int J Radiat Oncol Biol Phys 36:861-865

Brady LW, Freire JE, Longton WA et al (1997) Radiation therapy for macular degeneration: technical considerations and preliminary results. Int J Radiat Oncol Biol Phys 39:945-948

Bressler NM, Frost LA, Bressler SB, Murphy RP, Fine SL (1988) Natural course of poorly defined choroidal neovascularization associated with macular degeneration. Arch Ophthalmol 106:1537-1542

Chakravarthy U, Finger PT (1998) Radiation therapy is effective in age-related macular degeneration. Arch Ophthalmol 106:137-1542

Chakravarthy U, McQuaid M (1989) Radiosensitivity of retinal capillary endothelial cells and pericytes. Thirtieth meeting of the Association for Eye Research, Montpellier, p 89

Chakravarthy U, Biggart JH, Gardiner TA, Archer DB, Maguire CJF (1989a) Focal irradiation of perforating eye injuries with iodine-125 plaques. Curr Eye Res 8:1241-1250

Chakravarthy U, Gardiner TA, Archer DB, Maguire CJF (1989b) A light microscopic and autoradiographic study of irradiated ocular wounds. Curr Eye Res 8:337-347

Chakravarthy U, Houston RF, Archer DB (1993) Treatment of age-related sub-foveal neovascular membranes by teletherapy: A pilot study. Brit J Ophthalmol 77:265-273

Chan RC, Shukovsky LJ (1976) Effects of irradiation on the eye. Radiology 120:673-675

Finger PT, Berson A, Sherr D, Riley R, Balkin RA, Bosworth JL (1996) Radiation therapy for subretinal neovascularization. Ophthalmology 10:878-889

Flickinger JC, Pollock BE, Kondziolka D, Lunsford LD (1996) A dose response analysis of arteriovenous malformations after radiosurgery. Int J Radiol Oncol Biol Phys 1:873-879

Freire J, Longton WA, Miyamoto CT et al (1996) External radiotherapy in macular degeneration: technique and preliminary subjective response. Int J Radiat Oncol Biol Phys 36:857-860

Grossniklaus HE, Martinez JA, Brown VB, Lambert HM, Sternberg P, Capone A, Aaberg T, Lopez PF (1992) Immunohistochemical and histochemical properties of surgically excised subretinal neovascular membranes in age-related macular degeneration. Am J Ophthalmol 114:464-472

Harris JR, Levene MB (1976) Visual complications following irradiation for pituitary adenomas and craniopharyngiomas. Radiology 120:167-171

Hart PM, Chakravarthy U, Mackenzie G, Archer DB, Houston RF (1996) Teletherapy for sub-foveal choroidal neovascularization of age-related macular degeneration: results of follow-up in a nonrandomized study. Brit J Ophthalmol 80:1046-1050

Holz FG, EngerhartCabillic R, Unnebrink K et al (1999) A prospective randomized double-masked trial of radiotherapy for wet age-related macular degeneration (RAD study). Ophthalmology 106:2239-2247

Johnson K, Longenecker JP, Fajardo LF (1982) Differential radiation responses of cultured endothelial cells and smooth myocytes. Anal Quant Cytol 4:188-198

Law M (1981) Radiation-induced vascular injury and its relation to late effects in normal tissues. In: Lett, JAH (ed) Advances in radiation biology. Vol. 9. New York Academic Press, New York, pp 37-73

Macular Photocoagulation Study Group (1991) Laser photocoagulation of subfoveal neovascular lesions in age-related macular degeneration. Arch Ophthalmol 109:1220-1231

Macular Photocoagulation Study Group (1994) Visual outcome after laser photocoagulation for subfoveal choroidal neovascularization secondary to age-related macular degeneration. Arch Ophthalmol 112:480-488

Plowman PN, Harnett AN (1988) Radiotherapy in benign orbital disease. I. Complicated ocular angiomas. Br J Ophthalmol 72:286-288

Postgens H, Bodanowitz S, Kroll P (1997) Low-dose radiation therapy for age-related macular degeneration. Graefes Arch Clin Exp Opthalmol 235:656-661

Prettenhoffer U, Hass A, Mayer R, Ochhs A, Pakisch B, Stranzl H, Willfurth P, Hack A (1998) Photontherapie der subfovealen choroidalen Neovaskularisation bei altersabhangiger Makuladegeneration. Ergebnisse einer prospektiven Studie an 40 Patienten. Strahlenther Onkol 174:613.7

Rheinhold HW, Buisman GH (1973) Radiosensitivity of capillary endothelium. Brit J Radiol 46:54-57

Sasai K, Murata R, Mandai M, et al (1997) Radiation therapy for ocular chooidal neovascularization (phase I/II study): Preliminary report. Int J Radiat Oncol Biol Phys 39:173-178

Scott TA (1991) Low dose irradiation for diffuse choroidal

hemangioma associated with bullous nonrhegmatogenous retinal detachment. Retina 11:389–393

Spaide RF, Guyer DR, McCormick B et al (1998) External beam radiotherapy for choroidal neovascularisation. Ophthalmology 105:24–30

Stalmans P, Leys A et al (1998) External beam radiotherapy fails to control the growth of chroidal neovascularisation in age-related macular degeneration. A review of 111 cases. Retina 17:481–492

Yonemoto LT, Slater JD, Friedrichsen EJ et al (1996) Phase I/II study of proton beam irradiation for the treatment of subfoveal choroidal neovascularization in age-related macular degeneration: Treatment techniques and preliminary results. Int J Radiat Oncol Biol Phys 36:867–871

19 Long-Term Results of High Doses of External Radiotherapy for Age-Related Macular Degeneration with Subfoveal Neovascularization

MARTINE MAUGET-FAŸSSE, RÉGIS COQUARD, JEAN-PIERRE GERARD, and PHILIPPE MARTIN

CONTENTS

19.1 Introduction

Age-related macular degeneration (ARMD) is the leading cause of visual loss among patients over 65 in industrialized countries. In it, the most severe visual loss results from onset of choroidal neovascularization (CNV) (BRESSLER et al. 1988). Fluorescein angiography (FA) data reveal three CNV subgroups according to Macular Photocoagulation Study (MPS) guidelines (MACULAR PHOTOCOAGULATION STUDY GROUP 1996): classic without occult CNV, occult without classic CNV, and mixed (classic CNV associated with occult CNV). All types of CNV can be associated with pigment epithelium detachment (PED). Recently, indocyanine green angiography (ICG) has contributed to better recognition of clinical forms of CNV.

M. MAUGET-FAŸSSE, MD
Ophthalmologiste, Attachée des Hôpitaux de Lyon, Centre d'Imagerie et de Laser, 14 Rue Rabelais, Lyon, France
R. COQUARD, MD
Clinique St-Jean, 69003 Lyon, France
J.-P. GERARD, MD
Professor, Service de Radiothérapie, CENTRE HOSPITALIER LYON-Sud, Lyon, France
P. MARTIN, MD
Clinique St-Jean, 69003 Lyon, France

The natural course of CNV has a poor prognosis. BRESSLER et al. (1982) reported only 31% of 58 patients with stable visual acuity (VA) after an average follow-up period of 21 months. SOUBRANE et al. (1990) found after 3 years' observation that only 38% of 82 patients had stable VA.

Several trials have proven that laser photocoagulation (LP) of the extra- or subfoveal neovascular membrane is better than no treatment. (MACULAR PHOTOCOAGULATION STUDY GROUP 1990, 1991a, b, 1994). Indeed, LP of extrafoveal isolated classic CNV has been proven effective, but recurrences are frequent (more than 50% after 1 year) and only 10–15% of CNV cases meet the criteria for laser treatment according to MPS guidelines.

Laser photocoagulation of subfoveal CNV, either occult or classic, leads to the iatrogenic destruction of central fixation, producing immediate severe visual loss with an irreversible central scotoma. Most patients will not accept this, particularly those who still have vision of better than 20/125 with central fixation.

Even in the long term, the difference between the natural course of subfoveal or perifoveal photocoagulation is not clinically evident (SORENSON 1994). Recurrence is possible, and patients must receive good follow-up to retain maximum peripheral vision and good contrast sensitivity.

The application of new therapies to stop the angiogenesis process which is one characteristic of these lesions (D'AMATO 1995) is justified by the severity of the functional prognosis and by the number of restrictions on the use of laser therapy for large exudative lesions with retrofoveal CNV.

In 1999, QLT (QLT Phototherapeutics Inc., Vancouver, Canada) and Ciba-Vision (Ciba-Vision Inc., Duluth, Georgia, USA and Bülach, Switzerland) announced that photodynamic therapy (PDT) with verteporfin has been considered effective in exudative ARMD, particularly in mixed CNV with 50% or more classic CNV in the neovascular lesion. The study is still ongoing to determine how long is the interval before neovascularization relapses, how many times retreatment will be necessary, and if verteporfin is also effective in occult CNV.

For patients whose CNV is untreatable according to MPS guidelines and because this severe visual disease is typically bilateral, radiotherapy has been proposed as a new alternative treatment.

Numerous clinical pilot studies (BERGINK et al. 1994, 1998; CHAKRAVARTHY et al. 1993; CHAR et al. 1999; CHURCHILL et al. 1998; DONATI et al. 1999; FINGER et al. 1996, 1999; HART et al. 1996; HOLLICK et al. 1996; JAAKKOLA et al. 1998; RAD STUDY GROUP 1999; SPAIDE et al. 1998; STAAR et al. 1999; STALMANS et al. 1997; VALMAGGIA et al. 1995; and many others...) have described the effects of radiotherapy on CNV evolution and visual function employing different doses and techniques, and the results have been controversial.

BERGINK et al. (1998) reported a randomized study of 75 patients with occult, classic, and mixed types of CNV submitted to observation or radiation therapy. Twenty-four Gy of 6-MV photons were given in four fractions over a 3-week period. At 1-year follow-up, 30% of treated patients and 52% of the controls had lost 3 or more lines of VA. Conversely, STALMANS et al. (1997) concluded that radiation therapy (20 Gy, 2-Gy fractions) failed to control CNV of ARMD in a study including 111 patients. These results are difficult to compare due to differences in follow-up, dose-levels, and CNV type inclusion.

19.2 Materials and Methods

We conducted two studies of radiotherapy starting in 1994.

19.2.1 First Prospective Study

In the first prospective study (MAUGET-FAŸSSE et al. 1999), 212 patients (231 eyes) with age-related macular degeneration complicated with subfoveal CNV not eligible for laser therapy were treated with high doses of external radiotherapy.

Two teams treated them with two radiotherapy methods:

1. The lateral beam technique (72 eyes) using a 6-MV photon beam with hemicircular collimation. Twenty Gy in five fractions were delivered over 5 consecutive days (Fig. 19.1).
2. The lateral arc therapy technique, using a 25-MV photon minibeam with a cylindrical collimator dedicated to stereotactic radiosurgery. Twenty Gy (80 eyes) or 16 Gy (79 eyes) in five or four fractions were given over 5 or 4 consecutive days. This technique spares the fellow eye (159 eyes) (Fig. 19.2).

Patients included were 55 years or older diagnosed with active subfoveal CNV in at least one eye having evolving clinical symptoms with recent metamorphopsia or recent (within less than 6 months) decrease of VA. Both FA and ICG angiography demonstrated that CNV lesions were not amenable to laser therapy according to the MPS criteria.

Patients were excluded from the study if diagnosed with other causes of CNV (myopic eye), occlusive retinal vascular disease (diabetes mellitus, branch or central vein occlusion, uncontrolled systemic hypertension), evolutive glaucoma, previous radiotherapy for ocular or cerebral malignancies, CNV previously treated with laser photocoagulation, fibroglial and atrophic scars, or ongoing chemotherapy.

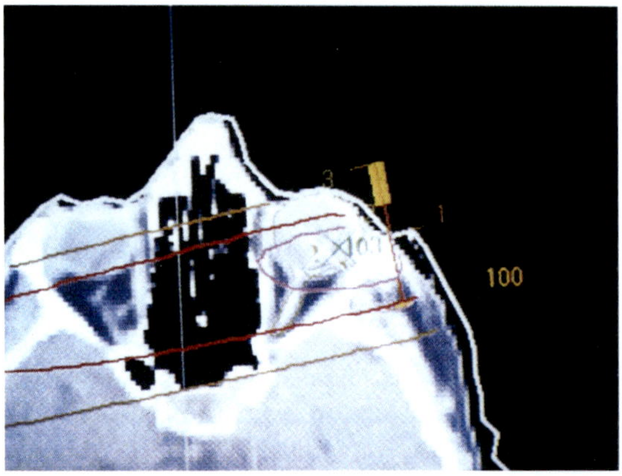

Fig. 19.1. The lateral beam technique: dosimetry

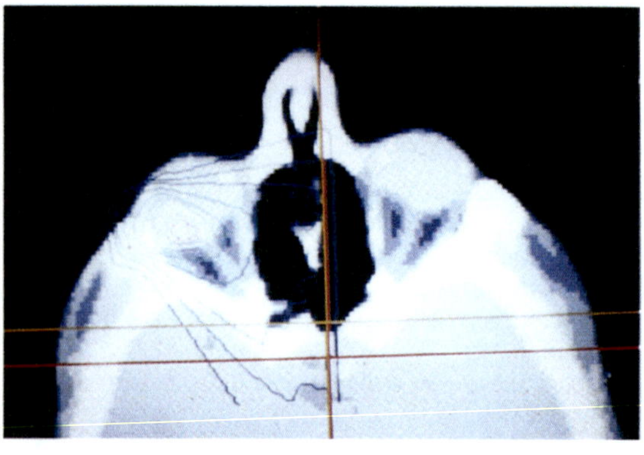

Fig. 19.2. The lateral arc technique: dosimetry

CNV was associated with PED in 36% of the eyes and classified as one of the following:

1. Occult CNV without classic 71.4% (165/231 eyes)
2. Mixed classic CNV associated with occult 26% (60/231 eyes)
3. Classic CNV without occult 2.6% (6/231 eyes)

At inclusion, 144 female (67.9%) and 68 male (32%) patients with a mean age of 77 years (range 56–95) were enrolled. One hundred sixteen right eyes (50.2%) and 115 left eyes (49.8%) were treated. In 145 patients (62.8%), fellow eyes were already affected by exudative ARMD. Complete functional and anatomical evaluation was done at baseline and 6, 12, 18, and 24 months after radiotherapy. At the scheduled follow-up visits at 6, 12, 18, and 24 months, data were available in 231, 154, 94, and 55 eyes, respectively.

The best VA was tested with the Early Treatment Diabetic Retinopathy Study (ETDRS) chart and a change of 2 lines was considered significant, with mean VA calculated using logarithmic minimum angle of resolution (log MAR) scores. Contrast sensitivity was measured with the Mentor or Pelli-Robson tests and CNV area was measured in both FA and ICG late-phase images with Tocpon Imagenet software (Topcon Corporation Japan). Digital FA and ICG were realized with a Topcon Imagenet Digital Imaging System (Topcon Corporation Japan).

Laser photocoagulation was applied when an increase of over 20% in CNV area was noted with VA less than 20/200 or when choroidal telangiectasia was diagnosed by ICG angiography.

Statistical analysis was performed using the Statistical Package for Social Science (SPSS) program.

19.2.2 A Second Prospective Study

A second prospective study analyzed retinal and choroidal side effects of radiotherapy given for ARMD. In it, we attempted to focus on risk factors, frequency, intensity, and treatment of the complications of radiotherapy. This analysis covered 270 patients (Mauget-Faÿsse et al. 2000).

Nineteen patients in this study had diabetes without diabetic retinopathy at inclusion. The doses were as follows: 15 Gy or less (four eyes), 16 Gy in four fractions (113 eyes), 18 Gy in five fractions (35 eyes), 20 Gy in five fractions (123 eyes), 24 Gy in six fractions (two eyes), 28.8 Gy in eight fractions (17 eyes), and more than 28.8 Gy (one eye). Patients had regular follow-up visits over a mean period of 15 months.

19.3 Results

19.3.1 Functional Results

19.3.1.1 Metamorphopsia

The number of patients complaining of metamorphopsia was statistically lower at 6 and 12 months after radiotherapy (p=0.1) and similar at 18 and 24 months, compared to the baseline values (paired comparison).

19.3.1.2 Visual Acuity

Thirty-one percent of patients had improved VA at 18 months and 32.7% at 24 months, 33% were stable at 18 months and 27% at 24 months, and 36% had VA loss at 18 months vs. 40% at 24 months. The relative frequencies of improvement and deterioration of VA were similar at 6, 12, 18, and 24 months. There were no statistical differences between the three types of CNV. Twenty-four months after treatment, the mean VA was worse in the PED group (p=0.03).

19.3.1.3 Contrast Sensitivity

Contrast sensitivity was assessed in 44 consecutive patients. Twenty-two of them (50%) and nine of 24 (37.5%) showed improved contrast sensitivity at 6 and 12 months.

19.3.2 Anatomical Results

Paired comparisons of CNV areas in FA and ICG angiography showed no significant change between inclusion and each follow-up visit. However, 12 and 18 months after treatment, 47% of the patients showed a CNV size reduction of 10% or more in both FA and ICG. No difference was found between occult and mixed CNV.

No statistical difference between the two radiotherapy groups was noted during the course of the study.

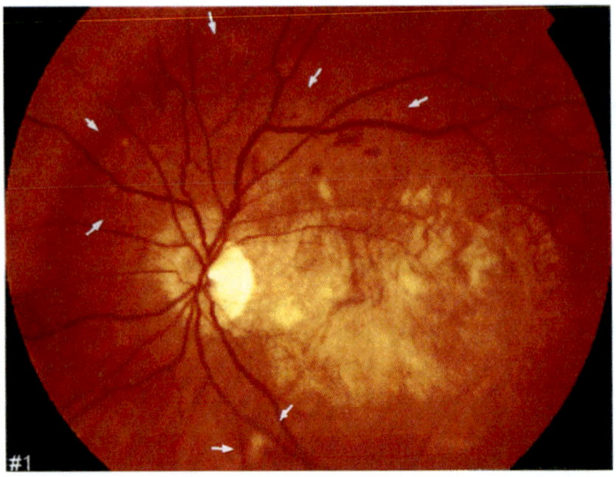

Fig. 19.3. Radiation retinopathy (*arrows*) 2 years after radiotherapy in a patient who received 20 Gy in 4-Gy fractions

19.3.3 Complications

Radiation retinopathy was noted in 15 eyes (5.1%) (Fig. 19.3). No radiation retinopathy was observed within 6 months after radiation. Most of them showed no functional impact and retinopathy remained limited. In five cases (three diabetic patients), radiation retinopathy was very severe, with extensive zones of ischemia leading to loss of vision. Panphotocoagulation was required to avoid neovascular glaucoma. This complication was clearly related to the radiation dose.

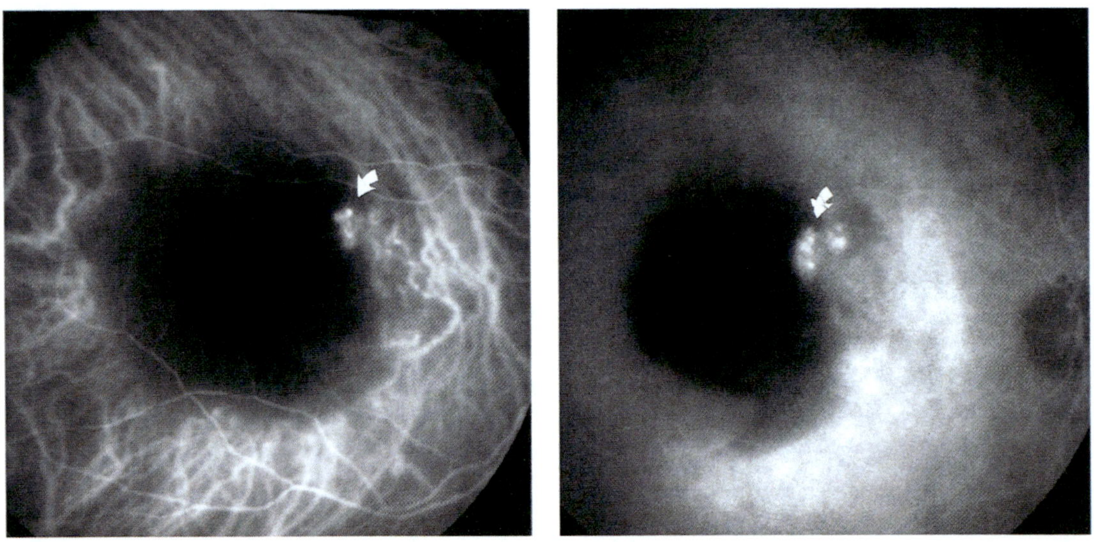
a b

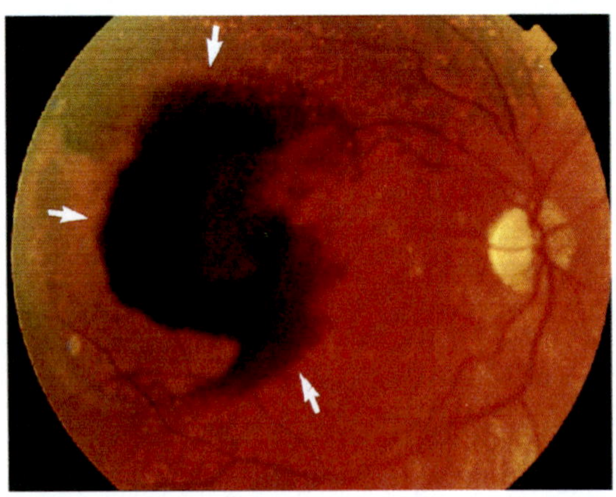
c

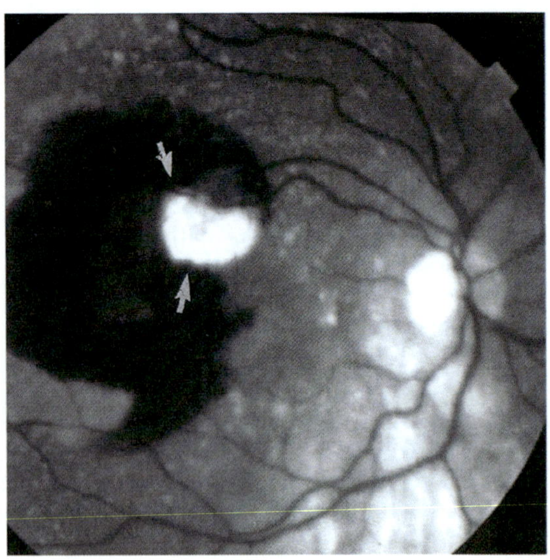
d

Fig. 19.4a–d. Choroidal telangiectasia (radiation-associated choroidal neovasculopathy) 18 months after radiotherapy in a patient who received 24 Gy in 4-Gy fractions. It is detected best on ICG angiography (*arrows*) (**a** 3mn38, **b** 16mn31) and associated with hemorrhage (**c** *arrows*). **d** red free photograph taken immediately after laser treatment, showing photocoagulation spots (*arrows*) of the choroidal telangiectasia

Bilateral neovascular glaucoma was seen in one patient (0.3%) and ischemic optic neuropathy in five eyes (1.7%).

Choroidal telangiectasia, also called radiation-associated choroidal neovasculopathy (Spaide et al. 1999) occurred in 19 eyes (6.4%) (Fig. 19.4). This was always associated with exudates and/or hemorrhages. Choroidal telangiectasia was seen earlier in patients treated with higher doses. It is imaged best by ICG angiography and easily missed by FA. The evolution of patients with choroidal telangiectasia was fair when treated with laser. On the contrary, those who were not treated underwent severe vision loss due to exudation, hemorrhage, and serous detachment of the retina. Choroidal telangiectasia occurred more frequently in patients with retinal pigmentary detachment (13/19, 68%) and with large neovascular surface (optic nerve area size >8) (9/19, 47%).

Venous occlusion was diagnosed in two eyes (0.75%).

Edematous retinopathy with major exudation (ORME) was seen in 31 eyes (10.5%) (Fig. 15.5). When not associated with choroidal telangiectasia, they recovered spontaneously.

Choroidal hematoma was observed in eight eyes (2.7%).

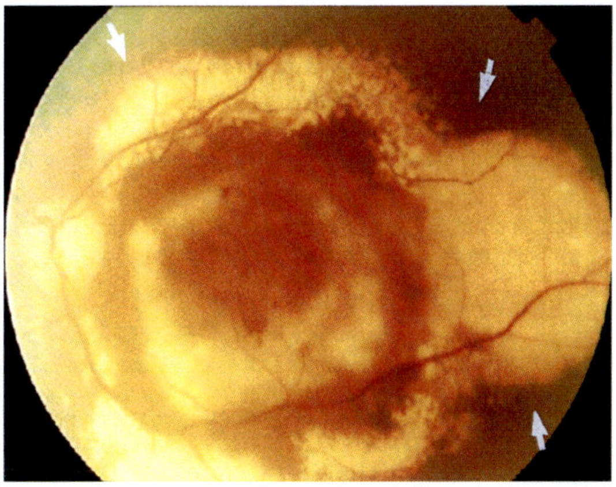

Fig. 19.5. Edematous retinopathy with major exudation 12 months after radiotherapy in a patient who received 20 Gy in 4-Gy fractions. *Arrows* show major accumulation of exudates around the neovascular lesion

19.4 Discussion and Conclusion

From our experience, radiotherapy for ARMD should not be done in diabetic patients. The high incidence of complications may be related to hypofractionation, and ICG angiography should be considered essential in the follow-up of patients treated with radiotherapy.

In comparison with the natural course of subfoveal CNV, the results of our first prospective study suggest that radiotherapy could stabilize visual and anatomical outcome in selected cases up to 24 months after irradiation.

Radiotherapy in ARMD requires careful follow-up, and ICG angiographies are essential (1) to detect the evolution of the CNV area and ascertain whether CNV has been stabilized by radiation therapy and (2) to detect and treat the potential choroidal telangiectasic complications. The occurrence of choroidal telangiectasia must be systematically checked. If present, it must be treated with laser. The prognosis is very poor if it is left untreated (Spaide et al. 1999).

So far, there have been few reports about choroidal and retinal complications of radiotherapy with doses lower than 40 Gy. The side effects that we observed were unexpected. The high dose per fraction used in this study may be responsible for these adverse events. At present, we recommend reducing the dose per session to 2-Gy fractions.

We need further indications from randomized clinical trials to identify predictive factors as an indication for radiotherapy for the exudative form of ARMD.

References

Bergink GJ, Deutman AF, Van den Broek JFCM, Van Daal WAJ, Van der Maazen RWM (1994) Radiation therapy for subfoveal choroidal neovascular membranes in age-related macular degeneration. Graefes Arch Clin Exp Ophthalmol 232:591–598

Bergink GJ, Hoyng CB, Van der Maazen RWM et al (1998) A randomized controlled clinical trial on the efficacy of radiation therapy in the control of subfoveal choroidal neovascularization in age-related macular degeneration: Radiation versus observation. Graefes Arch Clin Exp Ophthalmol 236:321–325

Bressler SB, Bressler NM, Fine SL et al (1982) Natural course of choroidal neovascular zone in senile macular generation. Am J Ophthalmol 93:157–163

Bressler NM, Bressler SB, Fine SL (1988) Age-related macular degeneration. Surv Ophthalmol 32:375–412

Chakravarthy U, Houston RF, Archer DB (1993) Treatment of age-related subfoveal neovascular membranes by teletherapy: A pilot study. Br J Ophthalmol 77:265–273

Char DH, Irvine AI, Posner MD (1999) Randomized trial of radiation for age-related macular degeneration. Am J Ophthalmol 127(5):574–578

Churchill AJ, Franks WA, Ash DV (1998) An alternative and more cost effective method of delivery of radiotherapy in age-related macular degeneration. Br J Ophtalmol 82:373–375
D'Amato RJ, Adamis AP (1995) Angiogenesis inhibition in age-related macular degeneration. [Editorial]. Ophthalmology 102:1261–1262
Donati G, Soubrane D, Quaranta M (1999) Radiotherapy for isolated occult subfoveal neovascularisation in age-related macular degeneration: A pilot study. Br J Ophthalmol 83(6):646–651
Finger PT, Berson A, Sherr D, Riley R, Belkin RA, Bosworth JL (1996) Radiation therapy for sub-retinal neovascularization. Ophthalmology 103:878–889
Finger PT, Berson A, Ng T, Szechter A (1999) Ophthalmic plaque radiotherapy for age-related macular degeneration associated with subretinal neovascularization. Am J Ophthalmol 127(2):170–177
Hart PM, Chakravarthy U, MacKenzie G, Archer DB, Houston RF (1996) Teletherapy for subfoveal choroidal neovascularization of age-related macular degeneration: Results of follow-up in a non-randomized study. Br J Ophthalmol 80:1046–1050
Hollick EJ, Goble RR, Knowles PJ, Ramsey MC, Deutsch G, Casswell AG (1996) Radiotherapy treatment of age-related subfoveal neovascular membranes in patients with good vision. Eye 10:609–616
Jaakkola A, Heikko J, Tommila P, Laatikanen L, Immomen I (1998) Strontium plaque irradiation of subfoveal neovascular membranes in age-related macular degeneration. Graefes Arch Clin Exp Ophthalmol 236:24–30
Macular Photocoagulation Study Group (1990) Krypton laser photocoagulation for neovascular lesion of age-related macular degeneration: Results of a randomized clinical trial. Arch Ophtalmol 108:816–824
Macular Photocoagulation Study Group (1991a) Argon laser photocoagulation for neovascular maculopathy. Five years' results from randomized clinical trials. Arch Ophthalmol 109:1109–1114
Macular Photocoagulation Study Group (1991b) Subfoveal neovascular lesions in age-related macular degeneration: Guidelines for evaluation and treatment in the macular photocoagulation study. Arch Ophtalmol 109:1242–1257
Macular Photocoagulation Study Group (1994) Visual outcome after laser photocoagulation for subfoveal choroidal neovascularization secondary to age-related macular degeneration. Arch Ophthalmol 112:480–488
Macular Photocoagulation Study Group (1996) Occult choroidal neovascularization. Influence on visual outcome in patients with age-related macular degeneration. Arch Ophthalmol 114:400–412
Mauget-Faÿsse M, Chiquet C, Milea D, Romestaing P, Gérard JP, Martin P, Koenig F (1999) Long-term results of radiotherapy for subfoveal choroidal neovascularisation in age-related macular degeneration Br J Ophthalmol 83(8):923–928
Mauget-Faÿsse M, Coquard R, Français-Maury C, Milea D, Chiquet C, Martin Ph, Romestaing P, Romanet JP, Gérard JP (2000) Radiothérapie dans la dégénérescence maculaire liée à l'age: Facteurs de risque de survenue des complications, prévention et traitement des effets secondaires. A propos d'une étude de 295 yeux traités. J Fr Ophtalmol 23(2)127–136
RAD Study Group (1999) A prospective, randomized, double-masked trial in radiation therapy for neovascular age-related macular degeneration (RAD Study); radiation therapy for age-related macular degeneration. Ophthalmology 106(12):2239–2247
Sorenson JA, Yannuzzi LA, Slakter JS, Guyer DR, Ho AC, Orlock DA (1994) A pilot study of digital indocyanine green videoangiography for recurrent occult choroidal neovascularization in age-related macular degeneration. Arch Ophthalmol 112:473–479
Soubrane G, Coscas G, Français C, Koenig F (1990) Occult subretinal new vessels in age-related macular degeneration. Natural history and early laser treatment. Ophthalmology 97:649–657
Spaide RK, Guyer DR, McCormick B, Yannuzzi LA, Burke K, Mendelsohn M, Haas A, Slakter JS, Sorenson JA, Fisher YL, Abramson D (1998) External beam radiotherapy for choroidal neovascularization. Ophthalmology 105:24–30
Spaide R, Leys A, Herrmann-Delemazure B (1999) Radiation-associated choroidal neovasculopathy. Ophthalmology 106(12):2254–2260
Staar S, Krott R, Mueller RP (1999) External beam radiotherapy for subretinal neovascularization in age-related macular degeneration: Is this treatment efficient? Int J Radiat Oncol Biol Phys 45(2):467–473
Stalmans P, Leys A, Van Limbergen E (1997) External beam radiotherapy (20 gy, 2-Gy fractions) fails to control the growth of choroidal neovascularization in age-related macular degeneration: A review of 111 cases. Retina 17:481–492
Valmaggia C, Bischoff P, Ries G (1995) Low dose radiation on the subfoveal neovascular membranes in age-related macular degeneration. Klin Monatsbl Augenheilkd 206(5):343–346

20 Low-Dose Radiotherapy for Age-Related Macular Degeneration with Subfoveal Choroidal Neovascularization: Update of Results of the St. Gallen Prospective Randomized Study

CHRISTOPHE VALMAGGIA, GERHARD RIES, PETER COSSMANN, PETER BISCHOFF, and HUGO NIEDERBERGER

CONTENTS

20.1 Introduction

Based on long-term experience in our hospital with low dose radiotherapy of age-related macular degeneration (AMD), we performed a prospective randomized study between November 1994 and February 1999. The aim of this double-blind study was to evaluate the extent of subfoveal choroidal neovascularization (CNV) and analyze the level of visual acuity after treatment with different radiation doses.

20.2 Methods

The patients were informed in detail about their disease, the available therapeutic possibilities, and the study protocol of our investigation. Informed consent was obtained. The study was approved by the ethical committee of the Kantonsspital St. Gallen. All patients were over 50 years of age and complained of rapidly worsening visual acuity, central scotoma, or metamorphopsia.

The presumed clinical diagnosis was confirmed in each case by two experts from the Department of Ophthalmology after examination using simultaneous fluorescein and indocyanine green angiography (BISCHOFF et al. 1995). The subfoveal CNV in AMD was classified as either classic or occult as defined by the Macular Photocoagulation Study Group (MPS) (MACULAR PHOTOCOAGULATION STUDY GROUP 1991). Eyes with foveal hemorrhage were not included in our study due to a possible spontaneous resolution which would positively falsify results in visual acuity. Eyes with severe hemorrhage or serous pigment epithelial detachment impeding the correct measurement of CNV were excluded.

The patients were stratified into four different subgroups according to CNV type and size and duration of symptoms:

1. Subgroup A: patients with classic CNV of less than two times papillar size (3.54 mm^2) and a history of less than 3 months
2. Subgroup B: patients with classic CNV of less than two times papillar and a history of more than 3 months
3. Subgroup C: patients with classic CNV of more than two times papillar size and a history of more than 3 months
4. Subgroup D: patients with occult CNV

This stratification provides a homogeneous distribution of the patients in the three different groups considered, which received total doses of 1 Gy, 8 Gy, or 16 Gy, respectively. Patients were randomized according to this stratification and treated in our Department of Radiation Oncology. Collaborators in the Department of Ophthalmology and the patients were not aware of the applied radiation dose. On the other hand, the colleagues in the Department of Radiation Oncology were informed only about the eye being treated and the stratification code.

C. VALMAGGIA, MD
Department of Ophthalmology, Kantonsspital, 9007 St. Gallen, Switzerland
G. RIES, MD
Professor, Department of Radiation Oncology, Kantonsspital, 9007 St. Gallen, Switzerland
P. COSSMANN
Department of Medical Physics Radiation, Inselspital, 3010 Bern, Switzerland
P. BISCHOFF, MD
H. NIEDERBERGER
Department of Ophthalmology, Kantonsspital, 9007 St. Gallen, Switzerland

Radiotherapy was administered with a 6-MV linear accelerator (Clinac 600, Varian Assoc., Palo Alto, Calif., USA). Patients were fixed in a shell in supine position. Treatment consisted of a single lateral field (3×4 cm^2). This field was placed 1.5 cm posteriorly to the cornea in such a way that the anterior margin did not extend beyond the outer bony canthus. The dose of 1 Gy (4×0.25 Gy), 8 Gy (4×2 Gy), or 16 Gy (4×4 Gy) was applied at the posterior pole of the afflicted eye on four consecutive days. We chose the group with a dose of 1 Gy as controls because no significant effect could be obtained on CNV with such a low total radiation dose (FELTEN 1968). The dose of 8 Gy was expected to have an anti-inflammatory effect leading to lesion of the macrophages and consecutive diminished release of cytokines and growth factors (REINHOLD et al. 1988; BICKNELL and HARRIS 1991; HAIMOVITZ-FRIEDMANN et al. 1991). The dose of 16 Gy should entail an additional antiangiogenic effect with lesion of the endothelial cells of the vessels of CNV and consecutive obliteration (LIPOWSKY et al. 1988; ALLEN et al. 1981). To spare the lenses, a half-blocked beam technique was used. With this technique, the macula of the opposite eye received approximately 70% of the prescribed dose, e.g., about 0.7 Gy, 5.6 Gy, and 11.2 Gy respectively. We deliberately used such a field arrangement to get a prophylactic effect on the nonafflicted eye. The lenses received approximately 15% of the total dose, e.g., about 0.15 Gy, 1.2 Gy, and 2.4 Gy respectively.

At the time of treatment as well as after 6, 12, and 18 months, we assessed the best corrected distance visual acuity with a letter chart at 1 m to 5 m and the best corrected magnification need with text of different sizes at 25 cm (Fritz Buser, SZB, Olten, Switzerland). For both parameters, vision was considered stable if it remained within one line of baseline. At each examination, we performed simultaneous fluorescein and indocyanine green angiography in order to document the CNV size. Videotapes of the angiography were reviewed by two experts from the Department of Ophthalmology. The pictures were digitized with a special software program (Sigma Scan, Image Measurement Software, Version 4.0, SPSS Inc., Chicago, Ill., USA) to measure accurately the CNV size in mm^2.

The chi-square and crosstable tests were used for statistical purposes. According to our earlier experience, we expected about 30% more stabilization of visual acuity in the 8-Gy and 16-Gy groups than in the 1-Gy group. Each group had to include at least 50 patients for a significance level of 0.05 and a power of 0.80.

20.3 Results

As of June 1999, 144 patients had been examined at 6 months, 112 at 12 months, and 91 at 18 months following treatment. Women comprised 57% of the collective and men comprised 43%. The mean age was 75 years. Subfoveal CNV was diagnosed as classic in 57% of cases and as occult in 43%. After starting our investigation, nine patients had to abandon the study due to severe illness and eight patients died. Follow-up was unsuccessful in 17 due to loss of interest. Controls are still planned for 36 patients who have not yet completed follow-up.

After 6, 12, and 18 months, distance visual acuity had worsened by two lines or more as follows: 1-Gy group 44.2%, 61.1%, and 50% respectively; 8-Gy group 23.4%, 30.8%, and 35.3%; 16-Gy group 26%, 35.1%, and 51.7%. A decrease in distance visual acuity of two lines or more was observed significantly

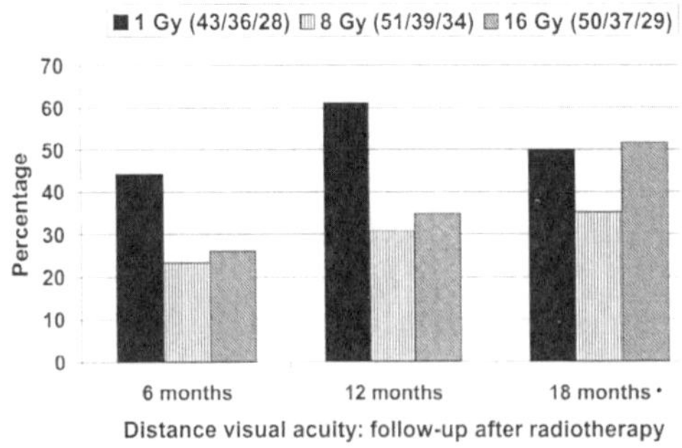

Fig. 20.1. Percentage of eyes with decrease in distance visual acuity of two or more lines from baseline after 6, 12, and 18 months in the 1-Gy control group (*solid line*) and the 8-Gy (*dotted line*) and 16-Gy (*broken line*) treatment groups

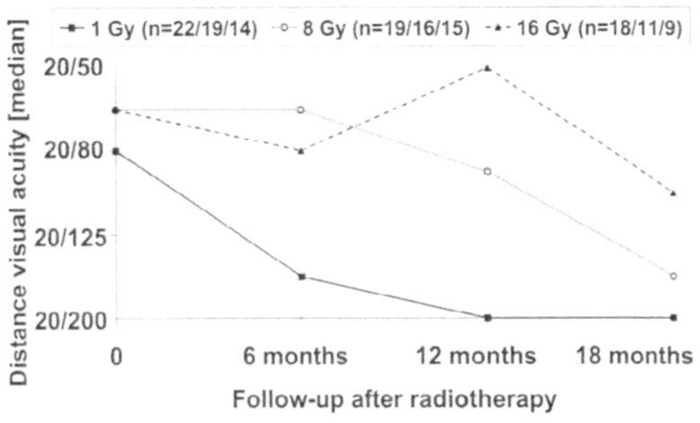

Fig. 20.2. Distance visual acuity of eyes with an initial acuity better than or equal to 20/100 after 6, 12, and 18 months in the 1-Gy control group (*solid line*) and the 8-Gy (*dotted line*) and 16-Gy (*broken line*) treatment groups

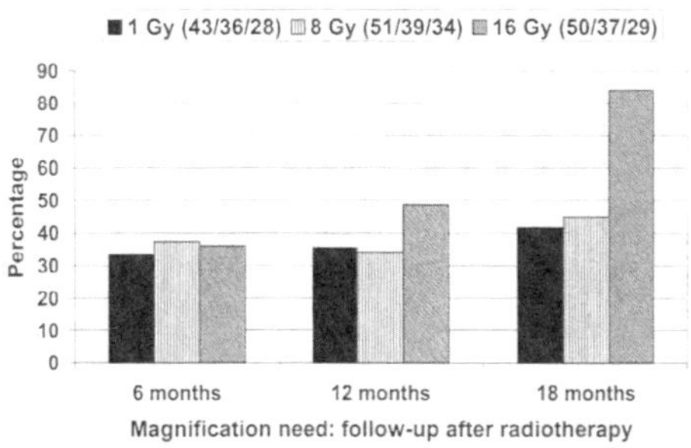

Fig. 20.3. Percentage of eyes with worsening in magnification need of two or more lines from baseline after 6, 12, and 18 months in the 1-Gy control group (*solid line*) and the 8-Gy (*dotted line*) and 16-Gy (*broken line*) treatment groups

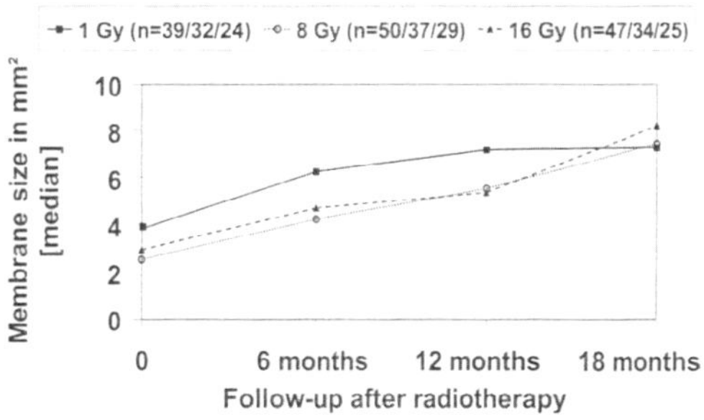

Fig. 20.4. Size of the subfoveal choroidal neovascularization in mm^2 after 6, 12, and 18 months in the 1-Gy control group (*solid line*) and the 8-Gy (*dotted line*) and 16-Gy (*broken line*) treatment groups

more often in the 1-Gy group than in the 8-Gy and 16-Gy groups after 6 months ($p<0.01$) and 12 months ($p<0.01$), but not after 18 (Fig. 20.1). A similar course could be observed in cases of afflicted eyes with a relatively good initial distance visual acuity of better than or equal to 20/100 (Fig. 20.2).

After 6, 12, and 18 months, magnification need worsened by two lines or more as follows: 1-Gy group 33.3%, 33.5%, and 41.7% respectively; 8-Gy group 37.3%, 34.2%, and 44.7%; 16-Gy group 36%, 48.6%, and 84%. The worsening in magnification need by two lines or more occurred without significant differences between the three groups (Fig. 20.3).

After 6, 12, and 18 months, membrane size increased continuously as follows: the 1-Gy group from 3.8 mm^2 to 6.2 mm^2, 7 mm^2, and 7.1 mm^2 respectively; the 8-Gy group from 2.6 mm^2 to 4.1 mm^2, 5.5 mm^2, and 7.2 mm^2; and the 16-Gy group went from 2.9 mm^2 to 4.6 mm^2, 5.3 mm^2, and 8 mm^2. The increase in membrane size occurred without significant differences between the three groups (Fig. 20.4).

20.4 Discussion

Today, the role of external beam radiation therapy for the treatment of CNV in AMD is still controversial (Finger and Chakravarthy 1998; Augsburger 1998). Prospective randomized double-blind studies investigating the effect of radiotherapy have not yet been realized. Creating such a study, we compared the effects of radiotherapy doses of 1 Gy (4×0.25 Gy), 8 Gy (4×2 Gy), and 16 Gy (4×4 Gy).

Compared with the 1-Gy group, we found a statistically significant, temporarily limited stabilization of distance visual acuity in the 8-Gy and 16-Gy groups after 6 months ($p<0.01$) and 12 months ($p<0.01$). A possible explanation for this positive result could be the anti-inflammatory effect of the doses of 8 Gy and 16 Gy, with better conservation of macular function. For this purpose, 8 Gy was as efficient as 16 Gy. The CNV size increased continuously in all three groups. This speaks against a sufficient antiangiogenic effect of the doses applied and was associated with an increase in the central scotoma leading to increased magnification need in all three groups. Patients with subfoveal CNV and paracentral fixation are actually still able to recognize isolated small letters but unable to read text of small size fluently due to the loss of their central visual field (Trauzettel-Klosinski 1997). This explains the discrepancy between our results for distance visual acuity and magnification need.

No treatment-related adverse effects could be observed thus far.

The temporary positive effect on distance visual acuity with doses of 8 Gy and 16 Gy should be considered encouraging if we consider the poor visual outcome associated with a diagnosis of CNV in AMD (Guyer et al. 1986). We are aware that we can speak only about stabilization and not improvementin vision. In addition, the insufficient antiangiogenic effect of a single series of radiotherapy, reflected by the continuous increase in CNV size, prevents long-term stabilization of vision. The risk of adverse effects impedes the application of continuously higher single doses during series of external beam radiation. Elderly patients like those in our collective with age-related arteriosclerotic vessels are more likely to develop complications. The Zürich study found radiation-induced retinopathy in four out of 16 patients treated with 36 Gy (18×2 Gy) for CNV in AMD (Thölen et al. 1998). On the other hand, the Graz study reported no effect on CNV in AMD after treatment with 25.2 Gy (14×1.8 Gy) (PRETTENHOFER at al. 1999). The therapeutic window for an antiangiogenic effect therefore seems to be small. Nevertheless, there is an anti-inflammatory effect with 8 Gy and 16 Gy as compared to 1 Gy leading to about 50% stabilization of distance visual acuity. As described elsewhere, these effects are probably restricted to a period of 6 to 12 months following treatment (KROTT et al. 1998; BERGINK et al. 1998). Therefore, several series of repeated low dose radiotherapy after intervals of 6 to 12 months should be taken into consideration.

References

Allen J, Sagerman R, Stuart M (1981) Irradiation decreases vascular prostacyclin formation with no concomitant effects on platelet thromboxane production. Lancet 2:1193–1196

Augsburger J (1998) Radiotherapy and the treatment of age-related macular degeneration. External beam radiation therapy is not effective in the treatment of age-related macular degeneration. Arch Ophthalmol 116:1509–1511

Bergink G, Hoyng C, van der Maazen R, Vingerling J, van Daal W, Deutman A (1998) A randomized controlled clinical trial on the efficacy of radiation therapy in the control of subfoveal choroidal neovascularization in age-related macular degeneration: Radiation versus observation. Graefes Arch Clin Exp Ophthalmol 236:321–325

Bicknell R, Harris A (1991) Novel growth regulatory factors and tumour angiogenesis. Eur J Cancer 27:781–785

Bischoff P, Niederberger H, Török B (1995) Simultaneous indocyanine green and fluorescein angiography. Retina 15:91–99

Finger P, Chakravarthy U (1998) Radiotherapy and the treatment of age-related macular degeneration. External beam radiation therapy is effective in the treatment of age-related macular degeneration. Arch Ophthalmol 116:1507–1509

Felten G (1968) Ueber die Behandlung der feuchten Maculadegeneration durch fraktionierte Röntgenbestrahlung des hinteren Augenpols. Dissertation, Universitäts-Augenklinik Hamburg-Eppendorf

Guyer D, Fine S, Maguire M, Hawkins B, Owen S, Murphy R (1986) Subfoveal choroidal neovascular membranes in age-related macular degeneration: Visual prognosis in eye with relatively good initial visual acuity. Arch Opthalmol 104:702–705

Haimovitz-Friedmann A, Vlodavsky I, Chaudhuri A, Witte L, Fuks Z (1991) Autocrine effects of fibroblast growth factor in repair of radiation damage in endothelial cells. Cancer Res 51:2552–2558

Krott R, Staar S, Müller R, Bartz-Schmidt K, Esser P, Heimann K (1998) External beam radiation in patients suffering from exudative age-related macular degeneration. Graefes Arch Clin Exp Ophthalmol 236:916–921

Lipowsky H, House S, Firnell J (1988) Leukocyte endothelial adhesion and microvascular hemodynamics. Adv Exp Med Biol 242:85–93

Macular Photocoagulation Study Group (1991) Subfoveal neovascular lesions in age-related macular degeneration: Guidelines for evaluation and treatment in the macular photocoagulation study. Arch Ophthalmol 109:1242–1257

Prettenhofer U, Mayer R, Stranzl H, Guss H, Wink A, Hackl A (1999) Radiotherapy in macular degeneration: Comparison of two different dose schedules. Radiother Oncol 53:7

Reinhold H, Hopewell W, Calvo W, Keyeux A, Reyners H (1988) Vasculoconnective tissue. In: Scherer E, Streffer C, Trott K (eds) Radiopathology of organs and tissues. Springer Verlag, New York, pp 244–268

Thölen A, Meister A, Bernasconi P, Messmer E (1998) Radiotherapie von subretinalen Neovaskularisationsmembranen bei altersabhängiger Makuladegeneration. Niedrig- versus hochdosierte Photonenbestrahlung. Ophthalmologe 95:691–698

Trauzettel-Klosinski S (1997) Lesefähigkeit bei altersabhängiger Makuladegeneration. In: Holz F, Pauleikhoff D (eds) Altersabhängige Makuladegeneration. Springer-Verlag, Heidelberg, pp 180–187

Special Radiotherapy Techniques

21 Brachytherapy for Macular Degeneration Associated with Subretinal Neovascularization

Paul T. Finger, Illka Immonen, Jorge Freire, and Gary Brown

CONTENTS

21.1 Introduction

Macular degeneration is the leading cause of severe irreversible blindness in the Western world (Bressler et al. 1988; Hyman et al. 1983). Most patients develop the "dry" form characterized by slowly progressive atrophy of the macular choroid and retina with mild to moderate loss of central vision. In contrast, a minority of patients develop the "wet" form of macular degeneration, which is characterized by the development of subretinal neovascularization, leakage, and scarring. Wet macular degeneration can be a rapid process destroying central vision in a matter of days, weeks, or months. Such subretinal neovascular events have been associated with age-related macular degeneration (ARMD), diabetes, high myopia, histoplasmosis, and laser photocoagulation. Clearly, the ability to control or stop neovascularization would be helpful in the management of these diseases.

Laser photocoagulation and photodynamic therapy (PDT) have been established as the only proven treatments for subretinal neovascularization associated with ARMD (Macular Photocoagulation Study Group 1994a,b; TAP Study Group 1999). Both treatments were tested by prospective, randomized clinical trials. Unfortunately, most eyes with neovascular ARMD have either occult membranes or hemorrhagic leakage, thereby making them ineligible (or likely to fail) such laser-based treatments. Yannuzzi pointed out that up to 70% of laser-photocoagulated macular neovascularization recurs within 5 years (Yannuzzi 1994). Neovascular fronds closed with PDT typically open within 3 months and must be retreated up to several times. Like laser photocoagulation, the success of each laser-activated PDT session is dependent on visualization of the subretinal neovascularization.

Radiation has been investigated as a method to control neovascularization associated with macular degeneration (Bergink et al. 1994, 1998; Berta et al. 1995; Brady et al. 1997; Chakravarthy et al. 1993; Finger et al. 1996, 1999; Hart et al. 1996; Sasai et al. 1997; Yonemoto et al. 1996). Multiple phase I clinical studies have investigated a range of radiation doses and most centers used external beam irradiation (EBRT) because it is widely available and inexpensive (Berson et al. 1996, 1999; Freire et al. 1996). A few centers have investigated temporary surgical implantation of radioactive materials for treatment of neovascular ARMD (Berta et al. 1995; Finger et al. 1996, 1999; Jaakola et al. 1998a,b). To date, Finger has reported on the use of palladium-103 (^{103}Pd) ophthalmic plaque radiotherapy, Jaakola and Freire on strontium-90 (^{90}Sr) applicators, and Berta on ruthenium-106 (^{106}Ru) applicators. All reports indicate that implant radiation therapy offers a method to irradiate the affected macula with less irradiation of most (ipsilateral and contralateral) normal ocular

P.T. Finger, MD
The New York AMDRT Center, 115 East 61st Street, New York City, New York 10021, USA
I. Immonen, MD
The University of Helsinki, Department of Ophthalmology, Haantimawinkatu 4C, Helsinki, Finland 00290
Jorge Freire, MD
Thomas Jefferson Medical School, Department of Radiation Oncology, 216 Summit Road, Mount Laurel, New Jersey 08054-4749, USA
G. Brown, MD
Wills Eye Hospital, Department of Ophthalmology, Ninth and Walnut Streets, Philadelphia, Pennsylvania, USA

structures, the sinuses, and brain (FINGER et al. 1996, 1999). While none of these groups have published results of prospective randomized clinical trials proving the efficacy of this approach to macular irradiation, no complications which might preclude it have been noted.

21.2 Radiation and Angiogenesis, Radiobiology

Radiation is known to induce acute vasculitis and edema followed by slowly progressive vascular closure which may take years to develop (BAKER and KROCHAK 1989; CHAKRAVARTHY et al. 1989a,b; LANGLEY et al. 1997; MAISON 1974). These effects are both dose- and dose rate-dependent (BARENDSEN 1982).

Radiation of a macula containing classic or occult subretinal neovascularization could affect angiogenesis directly by destroying neovascular endothelial cells and cytokine-producing macrophages or indirectly by affecting regulatory genes within cells which produce endothelial growth-regulating cytokines (Finger and Chakravarthy 1998). Widely employed to prevent scar formation, low doses have been used to inhibit recurrent cutaneous keloids and more recently were proven to prevent coronary artery stenosis (Teirstein et al. 1997). Similarly, Hart suggested that radiotherapy may inhibit the scar formation associated with end-stage exudative macular degeneration (Hart et al. 1995).

21.3 Patients and Methods

The majority of phase I clinical series employing radiation to treat subretinal neovascularization have used 4–6-MV EBRT because it is nonsurgical, widely available, and inexpensive. Unfortunately, a large number of fractions (days) are required to deliver the total dose (e.g., 200 cGy×10 working days). Also, this technique irradiates both eyes, the sinuses, and/or brain. Although not widely available, proton beam (charged particle external) irradiation has also been investigated and offers the advantages of being nonsurgical and unilateral. Usually, this technique employs one or two large doses and is more likely affected by eye movement.

Implant radiotherapy or brachytherapy involves placing a radiation source directly beneath the macula. ^{103}Pd and ^{106}Ru ophthalmic plaques or ^{90}Sr applicators have been used. Typically, implant brachytherapy allows for a relatively high dose of irradiation and relatively short duration (1–36 h). Both are monocular treatments which deliver almost no radiation to the fellow eye, sinuses, or brain. While the involved macula receives a larger dose with brachytherapy, all normal ocular structures outside the targeted zone receive less irradiation than with external beam or proton radiation therapy.

21.3.1 Case Selection

Patient-specific and disease-specific factors play a role in case selection. Informed consent involves a detailed explanation of the current methods of treatment available at each center. Our subjects were informed of the number of patients treated with each method and the implications. As it related to the ability to undergo surgery, their general medical condition was reviewed and discussed. In general, we have found that younger patients with monocular disease preferred to undergo brachytherapy. Many of our patients expressed concern over unnecessary (EBRT) irradiation to their normal ocular and intracranial structures. One ophthalmic exclusion factor was the proximity of exudative disease to the optic nerve. Due to perineural anatomy, it is difficult to place brachytherapy sources beneath subretinal neovascular membranes which touch the nerve head.

21.3.2 Preoperative Evaluation and Medical Clearance

Complete ophthalmic eye examination was performed on all patients prior to surgery. Refraction, pupillary, ocular motor, slit lamp examinations and Goldmann tonometry were performed. Direct, indirect, and contact lens ophthalmoscopy techniques were used, as necessary. Basal dimensions of the neovascular membranes were determined by ophthalmoscopy and fundus photography with angiography.

Although the retinal surface served as the initial prescription point for ^{103}Pd plaque radiotherapy, due to the small size of these lesions, all groups are currently using standard distances (1.5 mm–2 mm) from the inner scleral surface as the prescription point.

All patients were determined to represent good surgical and anesthesia risks by a complete medical history and physical examination.

21.3.3 Instrumentation

Brachytherapy of neovascular macular degeneration has involved the use of a variety of radionuclides, delivery systems, total doses, and dose rates (Table 21.1).

21.3.3.1 Palladium-103 Eye Plaques

Palladium-103 plaque assembly involved attaching radioactive seeds (Theragenics Corp., Buford, Georgia, USA) into a gold eye plaque (Trachsel Dental Studio Inc., Rochester, Minnesota, USA) with a thin layer of acrylic fixative (Fig. 21.1). A special 10-mm diameter gold eye plaque was constructed for this purpose. Dosimetric calculations for ^{103}Pd involved a number of assumptions. All seeds were calculated as point sources using the specific dose rate constant, which was aligned perpendicularly to the long axis of the seed. Attenuation related to the acrylic fixative was calculated to be 1.4 mm of water. Unlike the other devices described in this review, the gold of the eye plaque blocked more than 99.5% of radiation to the posterior and sides of the device. For juxtapapillary treatments, this effect shields the optic nerve and posterior orbital tissues.

Patients in the ^{103}Pd series were treated at a retinal dose rate of 35 cGy–56 cGy/hr for a mean treatment duration of 28 h, which achieved a retinal prescription dose of 1250 cGy–2362 cGy.

21.3.3.2 Strontium-90 Applicators

Specialized ^{90}Sr applicators were manufactured for each study. In general, 50% of beta particles are absorbed within 1.5 mm (in tissue) (Hokkanen et al. 1997).

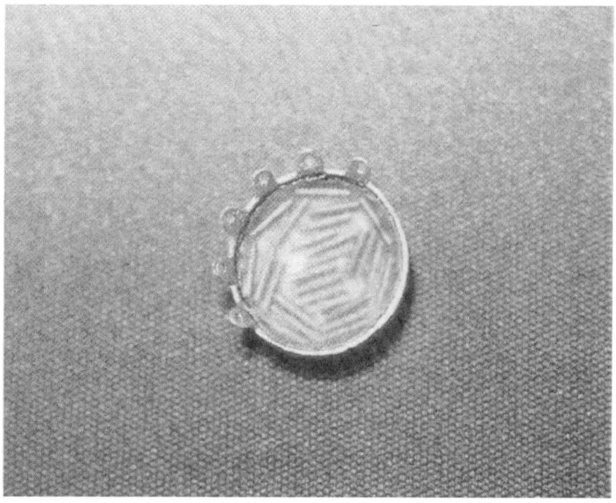

Fig. 21.1. A gold ^{103}Pd eye plaque loaded with seeds beneath acrylic fixative

Jaakola and colleagues' round applicator was constructed with an 8-mm active surface. It was calculated to deliver 15 Gy to a depth of 1.75 mm over 54 continuous minutes (Fig. 21.2).

The applicator used by Freire et al. was constructed as an 8-mm round concave ceramic disc. Treatments involved four to five applications of 65 s–100 s delivering either 10 Gy or 20 Gy to an intraocular distance of 1.5 mm (Fig. 21.3). The active component of the device is a 10-mCi (6-mm) ^{90}Sr button embedded in the head. The width of the metal ring surrounding the ^{90}Sr source is 1 mm.

The difference between these two methods is primarily the number of millicuries of ^{90}Sr contained in each applicator and therefore the resultant dose rate.

21.3.3.3 Radioactive Device Insertion

Implantation and brachytherapy were performed under general or local anesthesia for plaques and applicators, respectively. Indirect ophthalmoscopy was performed prior to surgery to assure that no changes occurred prior to treatment. A conjunctival peritomy was performed around the corneal scleral

Table 21.1. Characteristics of radioactive plaques used for neovascular macular degeneration

Author	Radionuclide	Prescription point (mm)	Treatment duration (h)	Radiation dose (Gy)	Radiation dose rate (cGy/h)
Finger et al	Palladium-103	2	28	12.5–23	35–56
Jaakola et al	Strontium-90	1.75	0.9	15	1.650
Freire et al	Strontium-90	1.5	0.1	10 or 20	10,000–20,000
Mean		1.75		16	

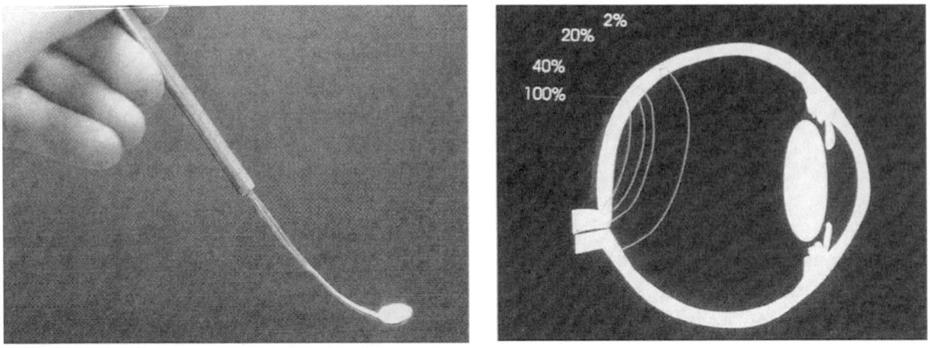

Fig. 21.2. *Left* Jaakola and colleagues' ^{90}Sr handheld applicator. *Right* the percent intraocular dose distribution with the applicator placed on the sclera beneath the macula

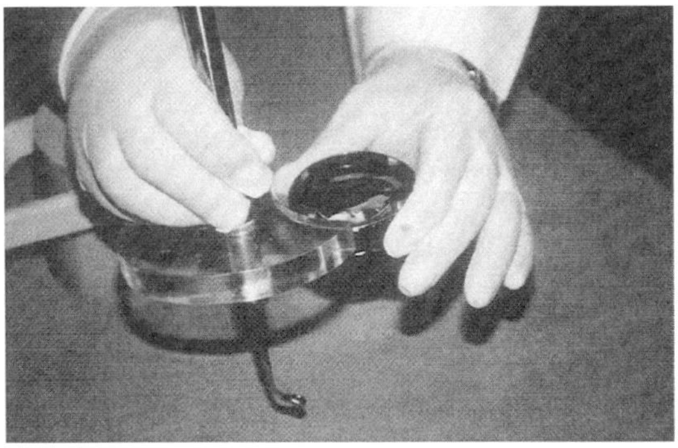

Fig. 21.3. Freire and colleagues' handheld ^{90}Sr applicator. The angle of the heel of the device is approximately 135° and a 6-mm acrylic shield is present along the midshaft to protect the treating physician from bremsstrahlung x-rays

limbus. A Stevens' scissors was then used to open Tenon's fascia. For ^{103}Pd plaque insertion, a line was drawn on the sclera perpendicular to the temporal limbus and toward the insertion of the lateral rectus muscle. Then the muscle was isolated, locked with a suture, transected, and allowed to retract. The episcleral line could now be extended posteriorly and used as a guide for plaque placement. The plaque was slid into place beneath the macula with its posterior edge against the optic nerve. Four episcleral sutures were placed through the suture eyelets to secure the plaque. Indirect ophthalmoscopy with scleral indentation was used to confirm the position of the plaque in relation to the macular target. Then the lateral rectus muscle was reattached. A lead shield was placed over the eye at the end of the surgery. Plaque removal was performed under local anesthesia without disturbing the lateral rectus muscle.

Strontium-90 applications were performed during one surgical procedure without disinsertion of the lateral rectus muscle. Following the administration of 4 cc of 2% bupivacaine with a 25-gauge retrobulbar needle (via the lower eyelid) to the affected eye, a 90° incision was made. It was found to reach the submacular sclera from a small incision through the superotemporal conjunctiva and Tenon's fascia at the limbus. The superior and lateral rectus muscles were secured (not disinserted) to allow for stabilization. Treatments required continuous ophthalmoscopic visualization of the applicator's indentation of the macula.

The presence and thickness of the inferior obliq- muscle was discounted by all investigators.

21.4 Results

After brachytherapy, all patients experienced the common side effects of surgery including edema, discharge, foreign body sensation, and transient diplopia. With long-term follow-up, a few scattered retinal hemorrhages (radiation retinopathy) have been noted in several patients.

21.4.1 Ruthenium-106

Radiotherapy of exudative AMD utilizing ^{106}Ru applicators was first described by Berta et al. (1995). Retinal doses in a relatively wide range (30 Gy–150 Gy) were employed. Total obstruction of the choroidal neovascular membrane and stable visual acuity were reported in nine of 13 irradiated patients.

21.4.2 Strontium-90

Jaakola et al. (1998) reported on 20 patients with recent subfoveal neovascular membranes. Visual acuity and fluorescein angiography was evaluated at 3, 6, and 12 months after treatment. Twelve untreated patients were followed as controls.

At 6 and 12 months, regression (decreased lesion size of choroidal neovascular membranes) was clearly present in 74% of patients. Visual acuity was within 2 lines of pretreatment evaluation in 55% at 6 months and 45% at 12 months (Table 21.2). The authors felt that decreases in the size of the neovascular membranes, diminished leakage, and resolution of exudates were related to the brachytherapy (Fig. 21.4).

Freire et al. (1996) reported on 22 patients. They found that 77% (17/22) were within two lines from baseline at 6 months after treatment, 64% (14/22) at 12 months, and 59% (13/22) at 24 months.

In no case did the choroidal neovascularization become totally eradicated, but most patients were felt to exhibit stabilization of their disease.

No radiation retinopathy or optic neuropathy was noted in either study.

21.4.3 Palladium-103

Finger et al. (1999) reported on the treatment of 23 patients with subretinal neovascularization associated with ARMD. Visual acuity was reported at 6-month intervals. At 6 months, 16% (three of 19), at 12 months 31% (four of 13), and at 24 months 22% (two of nine) had lost 3 or more lines of vision (Table 21.2).

By ophthalmoscopy and fluorescein angiography, 87% of patients were initially noted to be stabilized or improved (Fig. 21.5). One third of those patients went on to develop recurrent disease. At a mean 19 months of follow-up, 61% remained stable or improved. No radiation-related complications were noted.

21.5 Conclusion

All studies of brachytherapy for subretinal neovascularization have noted resolution of hemorrhages, exudates, and subretinal fluid. Despite these posi-

Table 21.2. Vision following brachytherapy of neovascular macular degeneration

Author	Radionuclide	Vision 6 months	Vision 12 months	Vision 18 months	Vision 24 months
Finger	Palladium-103	13/15 (87%)	6/8 (75%)	6/7 (86%)	3/4 (75%)
Immonen	Strontium-90	10/20 (50%)	9/20 (45%)	n/a	5/18 (28%)
Friere	Strontium-90	17/22 (77%)	14/22 (64%)	13/22 (59%)	n/a
Mean		40/57 (70%)	29/50 (58%)	19/29 (66%)	8/22 (36%)

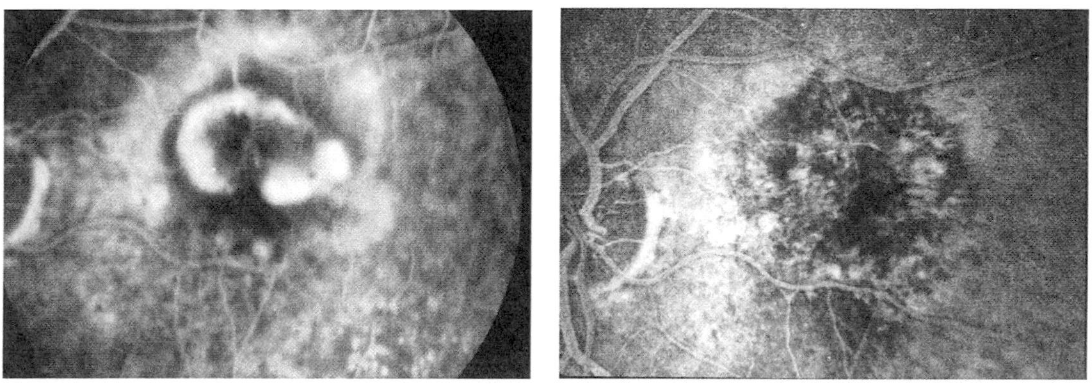

Fig. 21.4. Fluorescein angiography of a classic subfoveal neovascular membrane before (*left*) and after (*right*) ^{90}Sr radiotherapy demonstrates resolution of leakage and deceased chorioretinal blood flow

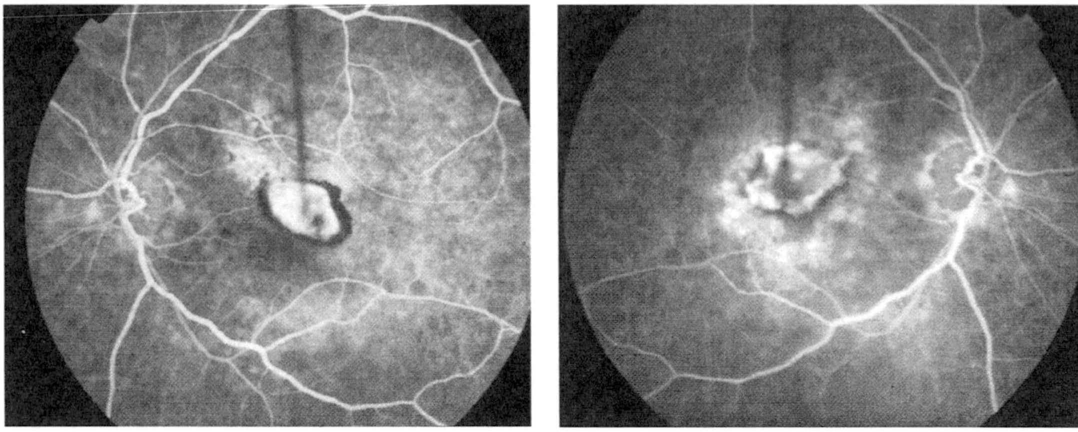

Fig. 21.5. Fluorescein angiography of a classic subfoveal neovascular membrane before (*left*) and after (*right*) ^{103}Pd radiotherapy demonstrates decreased leakage with less diminution of normal chorioretinal blood flow than with ^{90}Sr

tive findings, it has been difficult to assess the clinical effectiveness of brachytherapy. Difficulties inherent to the conclusion that radiation is helpful in the treatment of neovascular macular degeneration stem from the biology of the disease or diseases. It is accepted that patients with classic and recurrent subfoveal neovascularization lose vision more quickly than those with the occult form (GUYER et al. 1986; BRESSLER et al. 1982). Therefore, depending on the mixture of neovascular presentations included in each arm of a study makes it difficult to compare results. To complicate matters, untreated maculas can suffer intermittent choroidal hemorrhages with fluid and exudate deposition followed by reabsorption of these components. Therefore, depending upon the timing of treatment, it is difficult to tell whether the radiation is promoting resolution of these components or if these „effects“ would have occurred without treatment. These characteristics underscore the need for large prospective, controlled, randomized trials.

Certain conclusions can be made from this review. ^{103}Pd, ^{106}Ru, and ^{90}Sr can be used to deliver radiation to the macula. Brachytherapy provides a unilateral treatment with less irradiation of most normal ocular and intracranial structures. Compared to 6-MV photon external beam radiotherapy, it deposits more radiation within the targeted macula. Lastly, within the parameters mentioned in this review, low dose implant radiotherapy has been tolerated by eyes affected by subretinal neovascularization associated with ARMD. No complications which might preclude further investigation of these treatments have been noted.

Acknowledgement. This study was supported in part by The EyeCare Foundation, Inc., New York City, New York, USA (http:www.eyecarefoundation.org).

References

Baker DG, Krochak RJ (1989) The response of the microvascular system to radiation: A review. Cancer 7:287–294

Barendsen GW (1982) Dose fractionation, dose rate and the iso-effect relationships for normal tissue responses. Int J Radiat Oncol Biol Phys 8:1981–1997

Bergink GJ, Deutman AF, van den Broek JF et al (1994) Radiation therapy for subfoveal choroidal neovascular membranes in age-related macular degeneration. A pilot study. Graefes Arch Clin Exp Ophthalmol 232:591–598

Bergink GJ, Hoyng CB, van der Maazen RWM, Vingerling JR, van Daal WAJ, Deutman AF (1998) A randomized controlled clinical trial on the efficacy of radiation therapy in the control of subfoveal choroidal neovascularization in age-related macular degeneration – radiation versus observation. Graefes Arch Clin Exp Ophthalmol 236:321–325

Berson AM, Finger PT, Sherr DL, Emery R, Alfieri AA, Bosworth JL (1996) Radiation therapy for age-related macular degeneration: preliminary results of a potentially new treatment. Int J Radiation Oncol Biol Phys 36:861–865

Berson A, Finger PT, Chakravarthy U (1999) Radiation therapy for age-related macular degeneration. Sem Rad Oncol 9:155–162

Berta A, Vezendi L, Vamosi P (1995) Irradiation of macular subretinal neovascularization using ruthenium applicators. Szemeset (Hung J Ophthalmol) 132:67–75

Brady LW, Freire JE, Longton WA, Miyamoto CT, Augsburger JJ, Brown GC, Micaily B, Sagerman RH (1997) Radiation therapy for macular degeneration: Technical considerations and preliminary results. Int J Radiat Oncol Biol Phys 39:945–958

Bressler SB, Bressler NM, Fine SL et al (1982) Natural course of choroidal neovascular membranes within the foveal avascular zone in senile macular degeneration. Am J Ophthalmol 93:157–163

Bressler NM, Bressler SB, Fine SL (1998) Age-related macular degeneration. Surv Ophthalmol 32:375–413

Chakravarthy U, Biggart JH, Gardiner TA et al (1989a) Focal irradiation of perforating eye injuries. Curr Eye Res 8:1241–1250

Chakravarthy U, Gardiner TA, Archer DB, Maguire CJF (1989b) A light microscopic and autoradiographic study of non-irradiated and irradiated ocular wounds. Curr Eye Res 8:337–348

Chakravarthy U, Houston RF, Archer DB (1993) Treatment of age-related subfoveal neovascular membranes by teletherapy: A pilot study. Br J Ophthalmol 77:265–273

Finger PT, Berson A, Sherr DA, Riley R, Balkin RA, Bosworth JL (1996) Radiation therapy for subretinal neovascularization. Ophthalmology 103:878–889

Finger PT, Chakravarthy U (1998) External beam radiation therapy is effective in the treatment of age-related macular degeneration. Arch Ophthalmol 116:1507–1509

Finger PT, Berson A, Ng T, Szchecter A (1999) Ophthalmic plaque radiation therapy for age-related macular degeneration associated with subretinal neovascularization. Am J Ophthalmol 127:170–177

Freire J, Longton WA, Miyamoto CT, Brady LW, Augsburger J, Brown G, Micaily B, Unda R (1996) External radiotherapy in macular degeneration: Technique and preliminary subjective response. Int J Radiat Oncol Biol Phys 36:857–860

Guyer DR, Fine SL, Maguire MG et al (1986) Subfoveal choroidal neovascular membranes in age-related macular degeneration. Visual prognosis in eyes with relatively good initial visual acuity. Arch Ophthalmol 104:702–705

Hart PM, Archer DP, Chakravarthy V (1995) Asymmetry of disciform scarring disease when one eye is treated with radiotherapy. Br J Ophthalmol 79:562–568

Hart PM, Chakravarthy V, MacKenzie G, Archer DB, Houston RF (1996) Teletherapy for subfoveal CNVM of ARMD: Results of follow-up in a non-randomized study. Br J Ophthalmol 80:1046–1050

Hokkanen J, Heikkonen J, Holmberg P (1997) Theoretical Calculations of dose distributions for beta-ray eye applicators. Med Phys Feb; 24(2):211–3

Hyman LG, Lilienfeld AM, Ferris FL III, Fine SL (1983) Senile macular degeneration: A case controlled study. Am J Epidemiol 118:213–227

Jaakola A, Heikkonen J, Tomilla P, Laatikainen L, Immonen I (1998a) Strontium plaque irradiation of subfoveal neovascular membranes in age-related macular degeneration. Graefes Arch Clin Exp Ophthalmol 236:24–30

Jaakola A, Heikkonen J, Tarkkanen A, Immonen I (1998b) Visual function after strontium-90 plaque irradiation in patients with age-related subfoveal choriodal neovascularization. Acta Ophthalmol Scand 76:1–5

Langley RE, Bump EA, Quartuccio SG, Medeiros D, Braunhut SJ (1997) Radiation-induced apoptosis in microcascular endothelial cells. Br J Cancer 75:666–672

Macular Photocoagulation Study Group (1994a) Visual outcome after laser photocoagulation for subfoveal choroidal neovascularization secondary to age-related macular degeneration. The influence of initial lesion size and initial visual acuity. Arch Ophthalmol 112:480–488

Macular Photocoagulation Study Group (1994b) Persistent and recurrent neovascularization after laser photocoagulation for subfoveal choroidal neovascularization of age-related macular degeneration. Arch Ophthalmol 112:489–499

Maison JR (1974) The influence of radiation on blood vessels and microcirculation: III. Ultrastructure of the vessel wall. Curr Top Radiat Res 10:29–57

Sasai K, Murata R, Mandai M, Takahashi M, Ogura Y, Ngata Y, Nishimura Y, Hiraoka M (1997) Radiation therapy for ocular choroidal neovascularization (phase I/II study): preliminary report. Int J Radiat Oncol Biol Phys 39:173–178

TAP Study Group (1999) Photodynamic therapy of subfoveal choroidal neovascularization in age-related macular degeneration with verteporfin: One-year results of two randomized clinical trials – TAP report. Treatment of age-related macular degeneration with photodynamic therapy (TAP) study group. Arch Ophthalmol 117:1329–1345

Teirstein PS, Massullo V, Jani S, Popma JJ, Mintz GS, Russo RJ, Schatz RA, Guarneri EM, Steuterman S, Morris NB, Leon MB, Tripuraneni P (1997) Catheter-based radiotherapy to inhibit restenosis after coronary stenting. N Engl J Med 336(24):1697–1703

Yannuzzi LA (1994) A new standard of care for laser photocoagulation of subfoveal choroidal neovascularization secondary to age-related macular degeneration. Data revisited. Arch Ophthalmol 112:462–464

Yonemoto LT, Slater JD, Friedrichsen EJ, Loredo LN, Ing J, Archambreau JO, Tiechman S, Moyers MF, Blacharski PA, Slater JM (1996) Phase I/II study of proton beam irradiation for the treatment of subfoveal choroidal neovascularization in age-related macular degeneration: Treatment techniques and preliminary results. Int J Radiat Oncol Biol Phys 36:867–871

22 Proton Radiation Therapy of Age-Related Macular Degeneration

LES T. YONEMOTO, JERRY D. SLATER, PAUL BLACHARSKI, and JAMES M. SLATER

CONTENTS

22.1 Introduction

The rationale for radiation treatment of subfoveal choroidal neovascularization is the relative sensitivity of proliferating vascular cells to low doses of radiation, compared to the cells of the choroid and retina (DeGowin et al. 1974; Tannock and Hayashi 1972). Regression of choroidal neovascularization and stabilization of visual acuity was demonstrated with low-dose, fractionated, external beam photons (Chakravarthy et al. 1989, 1993). Other studies which followed also demonstrated promising early results with low-dose, fractionated irradiation (Bergink et al. 1994).

The goal of any therapy, including radiation therapy, is to enhance outcome by delivering the prescribed treatment while reducing the damage to normal tissue surrounding the target tissue. Proton therapy combined with three-dimensional (3D) treatment planning is used to improve precision in dose delivery to a specified target tissue while minimizing dose to normal tissue. The physical advantage of proton radiation therapy over x-ray and electron beam therapy owes to the fact that the maximum dose occurs at depth, rather than close to the surface (Fig. 22.1). This spares normal tissue to a far greater extent than is achievable with traditional radiation modalities.

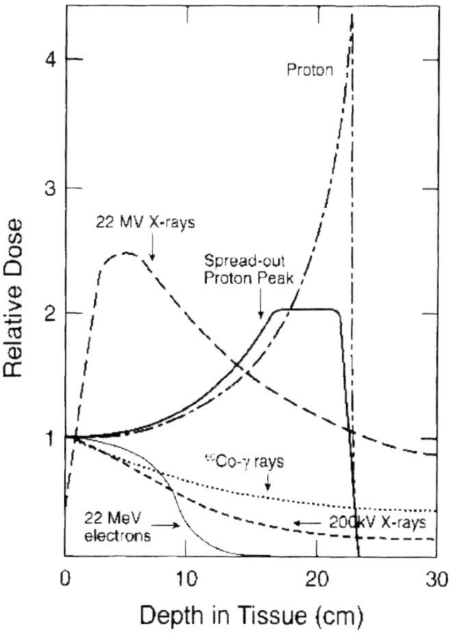

Fig. 22.1. Dose distribution of protons as a function of penetration depth in tissue compared with other forms of ionizing radiation

L.T. YONEMOTO, MD
J.D. SLATER, MD
Department of Radiation Medicine, Loma Linda University Medical Center, 11234 Anderson Street, Suite B121, Loma Linda, CA 92354, USA
P. BLACHARSKI, MD
Department of Ophthalmology, Loma Linda University Medical Center, 11234 Anderson Street, Loma Linda, CA 92354, USA
J.M. SLATER, MD, FACR
Department of Radiation Ophthalmology, Loma Linda University Medical Center, 11234 Anderson Street, Loma Linda, CA 92354, USA

22.2 Background of Proton Radiation Treatment

In the early 1930s, Ernest O. Lawrence invented the cyclotron, a circular particle accelerator that could accelerate charged particles such as protons to high energies. In the 1940s, several cyclotrons were built, including the 184-inch cyclotron at the University of California, Berkeley, and the much smaller 160-million electron volt (-MeV) Harvard cyclotron in 1948.

Robert R. Wilson (WILSON 1946) published the landmark paper that first suggested the medical application of protons. Because of the physician's inability to accurately define tumor and normal tissue boundaries using the imaging methods available at that time, however, protons were not immediately utilized for cancer treatment. However, orthogonal x-rays could localize pituitary tumors; accordingly, the first application of charged particle beams in humans occurred in 1954 at Berkeley (TOBIAS et al. 1956).

Clinical studies with protons were conducted at other research centers in the 1950s and 1960s. These included the Gustaf Werner Institute in Uppsala, Sweden, Harvard Cyclotron Laboratory in Cambridge, USA, the Physics Research Institute in Dubna, Russia, and the Institute for Experimental and Theoretical Physics in Moscow, Russia. Since 3D imaging was not available at that time, most of these patients had small pituitary tumors and arteriovenous malformations which could be localized with the help of orthogonal x-ray films.

In the early 1970s at Harvard, the proton beam was first used to treat uveal melanomas. A novel technique was employed to target the tumor and cause regression while preserving the eye (GRAGOUDAS et al. 1977). By 1987, over a thousand cases of uveal melaanoma had been treated.

Up to the end of the 1980s, all proton treatments had been delivered in physics laboratories using beams from accelerators that were designed for particle physics research, not for patient treatment. In 1985, an international group of physicists, physicians, and other scientists formed the Proton Therapy Cooperative Group, and plans were made to build the first medical proton facility at Loma Linda University Medical Center (LLUMC).

The proton treatment center at LLUMC was designed specifically for patient treatment and built in a hospital environment. Since treating the first patient in 1990, over 5000 persons have completed treatment: the facility currently treats more than 90 patients per day. It has four treatment rooms that operate simultaneously; this high treatment capacity has expanded the list of diseases and disease sites that can be treated with protons. One of the protocols developed was for treating the wet type of age-related macular degeneration (AMD).

22.3 Patients and Methods

The Institutional Review Board of LLUMC approved a study of the treatment of the wet type of AMD with proton therapy. This was a phase I/II dose escalation investigation designed to determine the optimum dose and technique with consideration for the toxicity and efficacy of the treatment.

Between March 1994 and August 1994, 21 patients received a dose of 8 GyE[1] in a single fraction. Before proceeding with escalation of the dose, the toxicity of this treatment phase was assessed and subsequently reported (YONEMOTO et al. 1996). No toxicity was seen; accordingly, the dose was escalated to the planned 14 GyE in a single fraction.

By January 1996, 27 patients had received doses of 14 GyE in single fractions. A statistically significant improved response was demonstrated with this dose (YONEMOTO et al. 2000). Toxicity and lesion control rates were judged sufficient to continue to use the dose of 14 GyE with intent to determine the characteristics of patients that would benefit from this therapy.

22.3.1 Patient Eligibility and Pretreatment Evaluation

Enrollment into the study required a diagnosis of wet-type AMD verified by fluorescein angiography within 2 weeks of treatment. Other eligibility requirements included progressive visual loss, age more than 50 years, and that laser photocoagulation was refused or not indicated by Macular Photocoagulation Study Group guidelines. Ineligibility criteria included prior laser photocoagulation in the treatment area, diabetes, and current corticosteroid therapy.

[1] GyE: Gray equivalent, the dose biologically equivalent to the same dose of cobalt-60 irradiation multiplied by a radiobiologic effectiveness (RBE) factor of 1.1.

All patients were evaluated prior to treatment. Evaluation included history and physical examination by the ophthalmologist and radiation oncologist; measurements of visual acuity, contrast sensitivity, and reading speed; fluorescein angiography; stereoscopic fundus photography; and ultrasonography to measure eyeball length.

22.3.2 Treatment Planning and Delivery

The LLUMC technique of 3D treatment planning and treatment has been described previously (YONEMOTO et al. 1996, 2000). Treatment planning parameters were based on lesion size, as determined by fluorescein angiography, and size of the eye as determined by ultrasound. A computer-generated model of the eye allowed the design of a stereotactic, lens-sparing technique. The specifications of beam-modifying devices were generated from the planning system; the devices were designed to contain the lesion within the 90% isodose line plus a 3-mm margin.

The energy of the LLUMC proton accelerator, a synchrotron, can be varied continuously from 70 MeV to 250 MeV. The protons generated from the synchrotron are switched dynamically between five clinical beam lines in four treatment rooms: three gantries, one fixed beam, and one eye beam. The treatment regimen for AMD uses the eye-beam nozzle, which delivers 100-MeV protons. All fields use apertures and a modulator to conform the beam to the target volume and spread out the Bragg peak sufficiently to provide a uniform dose over the range of the target volume depth.

Patients' individualized treatment programs began with fabrication of customized immobilization masks and bite blocks, which were employed at each treatment session. At treatment, each patient sat in a treatment chair and the head was immobilized by the face mask. Anesthetic drops were applied to the eye to permit placement of retractors that held the eyelid out of the beam line. The patient was asked to help the immobilization process by gazing at a positioning light. This lens-sparing setup was monitored by a remote closed circuit television system which enabled the radiation oncologist to detect any movement. Treatment could be interrupted instantly if the eye moved out of treatment position. Each patient was then treated to 8 GyE or 14 GyE in a single fraction. Treatment time was approximately 1 min for 8 GyE and 2 min for 14 GyE.

22.3.3 Follow-Up Evaluation

Follow-up data were gathered by means of history, physical examination, visual acuity measurements, and fluorescein angiography. Morbidity was defined as acute if it occurred within the first 3 months after treatment and as late if symptoms persisted or occurred 3 months or more after treatment. Morbidities were graded according to the Radiation Therapy Oncology Group (RTOG) system (LAWTON et al. 1991; PILEPICH et al. 1987) and the late effects of normal tissue (LENT) SOMA scale (PAVY et al. 1995). Follow-up examinations were performed every 3 months for the first 2 years and every 6 months thereafter. The study endpoints were cessation of growth of neovascular lesions, visual acuity, and treatment-related morbidity. Post-treatment status as determined by fluorescein angiography was defined as: (1) regression, if there was a 50% or more reduction in lesion size; (2) increased, if there was a 50% or more increase in size; and (3) stable, if the measured lesion size was within 50% of pretreatment lesion size, either larger or smaller. Post-treatment visual acuity as determined by follow-up examinations was defined as: (1) improved if improvement by more than 2 lines occurred; (2) decreased if a loss of more than 2 lines supervened; and (3) stable, if measured acuity was within 2 lines of pretreatment visual acuity.

The Kaplan-Meier (KAPLAN and MEIER 1958) product limit method was employed to determine actuarial lesion control and visual acuity. The log rank test was used for evaluating statistical inferences on actuarial curves, and a Cox regression model was used to examine the effects of clinical variables on lesion control, visual acuity, and morbidity.

22.4 Results

22.4.1 Treatment Response

The first patient group received 8 GyE in a single fraction. This regimen resulted in a good initial response, with follow-up ranging from 6 to 15 months (YONEMOTO et al. 1996). No treatment morbidity was seen on physical examination. Fluorescein angiography demonstrated lesion control in 53% of the group at 6 months; visual acuity was improved or stable after treatment in 74% at 6 months and in 58% at 11 months. Further follow-up revealed that the lesion control rate dropped to 36% at 21 months due to recurrence of the lesion.

In the second patient group, which received 14 GyE, a dose response was demonstrated: compared to the patients receiving 8 GyE, a significant improvement was found for lesion control (YONEMOTO at al. 2000). The actuarial lesion control rate at 21 months was 36% for patients treated with the single fraction of 8 GyE versus 89% for those treated with the 14-GyE fraction ($p=0.0001$).

Multivariate analysis of prognostic factors for lesion control included dose, initial lesion size, and initial visual acuity. The higher dose of 14 GyE ($p=0.0009$) and initial lesion size of less than 6 MPS standart disk areas ($p=0.05$) were significant for lesion control.

22.4.2 Visual Acuity

At 24 months, the mean loss of visual acuity for proton-treated eyes was zero. Multivariate analyses were performed on vision stabilization results at 18 months with respect to five factors: (1) initial visual acuity, (2) initial lesion size, (3) dose, (4) lesion status, and (5) late morbidity. The pretreatment parameters of visual acuity, lesion size, and dose did not demonstrate significance in terms of vision stabilization. Lesion status was a highly significant predictor of vision stabilization (79% and 40% for lesions that were stable/regressed and increased, respectively) in both univariate ($p=0.009$) and multivariate analyses ($p=0.004$); i.e., control of the lesion was associated significantly with vision stabilization.

22.4.3 Treatment Morbidity

Morbidity was evaluated at each follow-up examination; special attention was given to signs of radiation-induced cataract formation, keratitis, and retinopathy. According to RTOG criteria, there was no late morbidity. Seven (15%) patients had grade 1–2 (minor) late morbidity based on the (LENT) SOMA scale; no grade 3–4 late morbidity was observed. The findings for minor morbidity were analyzed with respect to initial lesion size and dose. Both larger lesion size ($p=0.022$) and higher dose ($p=0.003$) showed significance on univariate analysis. Minor morbidity was seen in 50% of lesions when the lesion size exceeded 6 MPS and was 8% for lesions less than 6 MPS. Minor morbidity was seen in 26% of patients receiving 14 GyE and 0% of those receiving 8 GyE. When minor morbidity was analyzed with respect to vision stabilization, no significant relationship was demonstrated ($p=0.59$). Vision stabilization was 66% for patients who had no minor morbidity and 71% for patients who did.

22.5 Discussion

Age-related macular degeneration is already a leading cause of adult blindness in the Western world. Given the increasing population of patients at risk, this health care problem surely will grow. Improvement over the standard therapy (laser photocoagulation) is needed inasmuch as an average of 3 lines of vision usually is lost immediately after that treatment. Laser photocoagulation is offered because the natural history of the disease demonstrates an average loss of visual acuity of 4 to 5 lines at 2 years after disease onset. However, many laser-eligible patients refuse therapy or it is not recommended due to the marginal benefit. In addition, only 20% of patients with the wet type of AMD are eligible for laser photocoagulation; the remaining 80% have no therapy that has been proven to be effective.

Our study took advantage of the unique characteristics of heavy charged particles. Protons in a homogenous medium follow a predetermined track, have little side scatter, and stop abruptly at any prescribed depth. The pattern of energy deposition is characterized by the Bragg peak, wherein the dose is at a minimum upon entry and reaches a maximum at the stopping region within the target volume (SLATER et al. 1988). The proton beam can be shaped to deliver a homogeneous dose of radiation to an irregular 3D volume. These capabilities make it possible to reduce the dose delivered to normal tissue by a factor of 20 (MOYERS 1999). This reduction of dose to normal tissues reduces the need to fractionate, as is required when x-ray therapy is used. Thus, an effective dose may be delivered in a single treatment, whereas 1 to 2 weeks are required to treat subfoveal choroidal neovascularization with x-ray therapy (BRADY 1996).

The pathophysiology of choroidal neovascularization is characterized by leakage from neovascular blood vessels in the subretinal space; this eventually causes scarring of the macula and severe loss of central vision (GASS 1967). Radiation therapy appears to effectively control the proliferative component of subfoveal choroidal neovascularization (ARCHAMBEAU et al. 1998).

Our phase I/II dose escalation study demonstrated that a statistically significant dose response exists in terms of controlling the subfoveal choroidal neovascularization lesion and that it was statistically significant in maintaining or improving visual acuity. The single dose of 14-GyE dose controlled the lesion in 89% of patients, compared to 36% of those treated with a dose of 8 GyE. Most human tissue has a dose response to radiation therapy; this study reveals that the higher dose (14 GyE) was more effective for controlling the neovascular process.

Toxicity (retinopathy) was seen in some patients treated with the higher dose (14 GyE) and having larger lesions. However, this retinopathy was scored as minor on the (LENT) SOMA scale and was not correlated with loss of visual acuity. Thus, these side effects were seen only on fluorescein angiography and were not "clinically apparent." In contrast, retinal changes induced by laser photocoagulation would be scored as a major side effect on the SOMA scale, in addition to producing an average loss of 3 lines on the eye chart.

In summary, this study demonstrated firstly that there is a clear, statistically significant dose response to this disease, secondly that the efficacy of proton radiation therapy is favorable when compared to historical data, and thirdly that toxicity was minor and not correlated with visual loss.

This study included patients whose lesions were not small enough or well enough defined for laser photocoagulation. Most patients(80%) with the wet type of AMD do not meet the criteria of the Macular Photocoagulation Study; for such patients, there is no treatment of proven efficacy. The natural histories of laser-ineligible eyes are assumed to be at least as poor as those of laser-eligible eyes, since their lesions are larger and less well defined. Some form of effective treatment is needed for these patients. The promising results seen in this study suggest that a treatment option may be available.

Further investigations and caution are warranted, however. The dose response observed in this study suggests that further dose escalation work should be done to determine the optimal patient characteristics, dose, fractionation, and radiotherapy technique. Then, laser photocoagulation might be compared with the optimal radiotherapeutic modality to determine whether findings such as ours do, in fact, obtain. For patients with laser-ineligible eyes and for whom no treatment exists to effect such a comparison, this study suggests that optimizing radiation therapy may be essential to improving the outcome of this devastating disease. Caution should be taken against comparing any form of radiation therapy in a phase III study until a phase I/II study has determined optimal dose, fractionation, and technique. Otherwise, a new treatment modality could be discredited.

Acknowledgments. The authors wish to thank William Preston, Ed.D. for editorial contributions and Sandra Teichman, RN, BSN. This work was supported in part by grants from The Hearst Foundation.

References

Archambeau JO, Mao XW, Yonemoto LT et al (1998) What is the role of radiation in the treatment of subfoveal membranes: review of radiobiologic, pathologic, and other considerations to initiate a multimodality discussion. Int J Radiat Oncol Biol Phys 40:1125–1136

Bergink GJ, Deutman AF, van den Broek JF et al (1994) Radiation therapy for subfoveal choroidal neovascular membranes in age-related macular degeneration. A pilot study. Graefes Arch Clin Exp Ophthalmol 232:591–598

Brady LW (1996) Radiotherapy in macular degeneration. Int J Radiat Oncol Biol Phys 36:963

Chakravarthy U, Gardiner TA, Archer DB et al (1989) A light microscopic and autoradiographic study of non-irradiated and irradiated ocular wounds. Curr Eye Res 8:337–348

Chakravarthy U, Houston RF, Archer DB (1993) Treatment of age-related subfoveal neovascular membranes by teletherapy: a pilot study. Br J Ophthalmol 77:265–273

DeGowin RL, Lewis LJ, Hoak JC et al (1974) Radiosensitivity of human endothelial cells in culture. J Lab Clin Med 84:42–48

Freund KB, Yannuzzi LA, Sorenson JA (1993) Age-related macular degeneration and choroidal neovascularization. Am J Ophthalmol 115:786–791

Gass JD (1967) Pathogenesis of disciform detachment of the neuroepithelium. Am J Ophthalmol 63 [Suppl]:1–139

Gragoudas ES, Goitein M, Koehler AM et al (1977) Proton irradiation of small choroidal malignant melanomas, Am J Ophthalmol 83:665–73

Kaplan EL, Meier P (1958) Nonparametric estimation from incomplete observations. Am J Stat Assoc 53:447–457

Lawton CA, Won M, Pilepich MV et al (1991) Long-term treatment sequelae following external beam irradiation for adenocarcinoma of the prostate: Analysis of RTOG studies 7506 and 7706. Int J Radiat Oncol Biol Phys 21:935–939

Macular Photocoagulation Study Group (1990) Krypton laser photocoagulation for neovascular lesions of age-related macular degeneration. Results of a randomized clinical trial. Arch Ophthalmol 108:816–824

Macular Photocoagulation Study Group (1991). Laser photocoagulation of subfoveal neovascular lesions in age-related macular degeneration. Results of a randomized clinical trial. Arch Ophthalmol 109:1220–1231

Moyers MF, Galindo RA, Yonemoto LT et al (1999) Treatment of macular degeneration with proton beams. Med Phys 26:777–782

National Society to Prevent Blindness (1980) Vision problems in the U.S., statistical analysis. The National Society to Prevent Blindness, Operational Research Department

Pavy JJ, Denekamp J, Letschert J et al (1995) EORTC Late Effects Working Group. Late effects toxicity scoring: the SOMA scale. Radiother Oncol 35:11–15

Pilepich MV, Asbell SO, Krall JM et al (1987) Correlation of radiotherapeutic parameters and treatment related morbidity – analysis of RTOG Study 77-06. Int J Radiat Oncol Biol Phys 13:1007–1012

Slater JM, Miller DW, Archambeau JO (1988) Development of a hospital-based proton beam treatment center. Int J Radiat Oncol Biol Phys 14:761–775

Tannock IF, Hayashi S (1972) The proliferation of capillary endothelial cells. Cancer Res 32:77–82

Tobias CA, Roberts JE, Lawrence JCH, et al (1956) Irradiation hypophysectomy and related studies using 340-MeV protons and 190-MeV deuterons. Peaceful Uses of Atomic Energy 10:93–106

Wilson RR (1946) Radiological use of fast protons. Radiology 47:487–91

Yonemoto LT, Slater JD, Friedrichsen EJ et al (1996) Phase I/II study of proton beam irradiation for the treatment of subfoveal choroidal neovascularization in age-related macular degeneration: Treatment techniques and preliminary results. Int J Radiat Oncol Biol Phys 36:867–871

Yonemoto LT, Slater JD, Blacharski PB et al (2000) Dose response in the treatment of subfoveal choroidal neovascularization in age-related macular degeneration: Results of a phase I/II dose-escalation study using proton radiotherapy. J Radiosurg 3:47–54

23 Various Therapeutic Regimens for Proton Beam Irradiation of Neovascular Membranes in Age-Related Macular Degeneration

Emmanuel Egger, L. Zografos, A. Schalenbourg, and G. Goitein

CONTENTS

23.1 Introduction

Age-related macular degeneration (AMD) is the leading cause of legal blindness in elderly people in industrialized nations. In Western Europe (with 320 million habitants), 16% of the population is aged above 60 years. The prevalence of AMD increases with age, from 11% of persons between 65 and 74 years to 28% of those aged over 75 years (Bergink et al. 1994).

The most severe cases of AMD are associated with serous retinal detachment of the central macula (the wet or exudative type of AMD) caused by the presence of subfoveal choroidal neovascular membranes (CNVM). About 10% to 30% of AMD patients are subject to this type of the disease. For a long time, the only accepted and proven treatment was the ablation of the new blood vessels with laser photocoagulation (Macular Photocoagulation Study Group 1993). This treatment limits disease progression but is associated with immediate loss of central vision. Furthermore, it never produces visual improvement when the CNVM is located in the fovea. For these reasons, laser treatment is often refused by patients who prefer to follow the natural course of the disease and hope that an effective treatment associated with less morbidity will become available before they lose even more vision.

In the last decade, interferon alfa-2a was used for the treatment of AMD in a large prospective randomized placebo-controlled study. (Pharmacological Therapy for Macular Degeneration Study Group 1997). Forty-five ophthalmic centers participated in this study worldwide. The conclusion was that interferon alfa-2a provides no benefit for CNVM secondary to AMD.

More recently, photodynamic therapy has been recognized as an effective treatment for classic subfoveal CNVM (TAP Study group 1999). However, for cases of occult CNVM, there is still no proven effective treatment.

In Switzerland, Bangerter treated AMD with external beam irradiation beginning in 1953 (Bangerter and Jäger 1996). It is his opinion that more than one irradiation course is often necessary to control the formation of new CNVM. His first course of irradiation consisted of seven fractions of 150 cGy followed months or years later, if necessary, by a second course of five fractions of 150 cGy. Occasionally, a third course of 5×70 cGy was applied. Bangerter generally did not apply radiotherapy alone but in combination with an individually adjusted retrobulbar injection therapy (Teichmann 1997). He reported permanent improvement of vision over a period of 12 years in 37% of patients and preservation of initial status in 43%.

In 1993, Chakravarthy reported using low dose irradiation for the treatment of CNVM secondary to AMD (Chakravarthy et al. 1993). Her results were encouraging, with up to 77% of patients experiencing stabilization or improvement in visual acuity. Triggered by this report and considering our experience treating choroidal hemangioma, in which we demonstrated that 22 CGE (cobalt Gray equivalent dose,

E. Egger, PhD
Division of Radiation Medicine, Paul Scherrer Institute, 5232 Villigen-PSI, Switzerland
L. Zografos, MD
A. Schalenbourg, MD
Hôpital Ophthalmique Jules Gonin, Avenue de France 15, 1004 Lausanne, Switzerland
G. Goitein, MD
Division of Radiation Medicine, Paul Scherrer Institute, 5232 Villigen-PSI, Switzerland

a radiobiologic effectiveness (RBE) factor of 1.1) induced resorption of the hemangioma, allowing reattachment of the retina and improvement in visual acuity without significant morbidity, we initiated a proton beam treatment program for patients whose CNVM was progressing despite all conventional therapy. (Zografos et al. 1998).

23.2 Patients and Methods

We treated 42 eyes in 39 patients (18 women and 21 men) presenting with AMD associated with CNVM with proton beam radiotherapy between 1992 and 1999. Mean age was 74 years (range 48–86 years). The size of treated lesions as measured from the treatment plan was between 4 and 14 mm, with a mean of 7.3 mm. Pretreatment visual acuity ranged from 1/200 to 9/10. Seven eyes had been treated with laser photocoagulation before being referred to our center. All 31 patients treated before 1997 and two treated in 1998 received doses of 18 CGE (28 cases), 19 CGE (three), or 20 CGE (two). All were treated with one frontal irradiation field in four fractions within 4 days. To avoid irradiation of the lens, each patient's eye was fixed on a light diode placed so that the patient looked upward (Fig. 23.1). This technique is similar to that used for uveal melanoma (Egger et al. 1993) except that tantalum clips were not used to delimit the border of the target volume.

Nine patients treated between 1997 and 1999 were treated with a two-field technique. The aim was to increase the dose to the CNV without exceeding the tolerance dose of the optic disc and the optic nerve which are known to be lower than 22 CGE from our experience with choroidal hemangioma (Zografos et al. 1998). To allow very precise irradiation, tantalum clips were fixed around the target lesion. Two irradiation fields were used, one covering the whole target with a safety margin of 2 mm and the second outlined in such a way that the optic disc and nerve were completely spared. The total dose applied to part of the target volume was 36 CGE in one case and 40 CGE in eight. In none of the cases did the optic disc receive more than half the total dose. In these cases, the positioning technique was exactly the same as for the treatment of uveal melanoma and choroidal hemangioma (Egger et al. 1993; Zografos et al. 1998).

Before initiating treatment, a custom bite block and thermoplastic head mask were manufactured for each patient. Individual treatment plans were designed in order to define a custom aperture (see below). After completion of the individual head fixation mask, finalization of the treatment plan, and manufacturing of the aperture, the first treatment was given. Before entering the treatment room, anesthetic drops were inserted into the eye to be treated. The patient was seated on a stereotactic chair with the head mask fixed on a frame. The patient then brought his or her face into the mask and bit the block. Once the appropriate sitting position was found, patient motion was restricted by applying gentle pressure to the back of the head using a foam pad and drop weight. Upper and lower eyelid retractors were placed onto the eye to be treated. The patient's individual collimator was placed on the beam line. The patient was then asked to gaze at a yellow light mounted on a coordinate system surrounding the beam line. This resulted in a 25° upward rotation of the eye. A light field simulating the proton beam was turned on. The chair was then moved with the patient still gazing at the fixation light in order to place the eye in position according to the beam's eye view. The position of the iris relative to the irradiation field was used as a reference. The edge of the light field was designed to match the 50% isodose at the edges of the proton field. After proper positioning of the eye, a camera was focused on the eye to display the pupil on monitors inside and outside the treatment room. A last control of the correct positioning of the eye using the light field was done and the position of the pupil delineated on the monitor. The pupil appeared magnified 40 times on the monitor, so any movement of the eye could be detected immediately. If the patient moved the eye during irradiation, delivery of the proton beam could be stopped immediately. The irradiation lasted approximately 5 s.

The patients who received tantalum clips prior to irradiation were positioned using axial and lateral x-ray pictures showing the clips. A reference x-ray picture provided by the treatment planning program allowed for detection of positioning errors of 0.1 mm. Only after all positioning errors were corrected (when the position of the tantalum clips was within 0.2 mm of that on the x-ray reference picture) was the first field applied. The collimator was then exchanged and the position of the eye checked with the marks on the monitor. If the eye was not within the marks, x-ray pictures were taken again and the positioning procedure repeated before applying the second field.

23.2.1 Treatment planning

Individual treatment plans were designed for each patient using the EYEPLAN treatment planning software developed at the Harvard Medical School (GOITEIN and MILLER 1983) and further improved at the Clatterbridge Centre of Oncology (SHEEN 1993). In a first step, a model of the eye was built using ultrasound measurement of the eye length as reference. Then, based on eye fundus photographs and fluorescein angiography, the base of the lesion was modeled with the treatment-planning software. The thickness of the lesion is entered based on B-scan ultrasound measurement of the lesion. Once the eye and the lesion were modeled, a treatment position was sought that allowed irradiation of the target volume while sparing the lens, if possible. A position with a view angle of 25° upward was chosen for the first 31 patients treated without clip surgery before treatment. The nine patients with clips were treated with a view angle of 25° in the nasal direction. This direction was also chosen for the two patients treated without clips in 1999. The target volume was moved into the isocenter, and a collimator shaped to target volume surrounded by a safety margin of 4 mm was manufactured individually for the patients treated without clip surgery. A typical case treated with one single field is illustrated in Figs. 23.1–23.3. Figure 23.1 shows a beam's eye view of the eye in the treatment position, while a fundus view with the CNVM covering the macula and the isodose distribution is shown in Fig. 23.2. A plane through the eye showing the dose to the lens can be seen in Fig. 23.3. A typical case treated with two fields is illustrated in Figs. 23.4–23.9. Figures 23.4–23.6 illustrate the first field covering the whole CNVM with a margin of 2 mm, while Figs. 23.7–23.9 demonstrate how additional doses were applied to the CNVM while the optic disc and nerve were spared further irradiation.

Patients treated with two fields and a higher total dose had clip surgery prior to proton radiotherapy. The treatment plan was similar to those of patients without clip surgery. In addition to the fundus pictures and fluorescein angiography, the target volume was also delineated according to the position of the tantalum clips. The first field covered the whole target volume surrounded by a 2-mm safety margin, similar to the field used for the treatment of uveal melanoma. A second field was delineated to deliver an additional dose to the target volume while ensuring that the optic disc and nerve received no irradiation, i.e., the size of the collimator for the second field was reduced on the side of the optic disc.

These patients were positioned using the tantalum clips visible on axial and lateral x-ray pictures as a reference. The treatment planning software delivers reference x-ray pictures allowing detection of positioning errors of 0.1 mm or more. The sharp falloff of the proton beam in the lateral penumbra, combined with the high positioning precision achieved with the tantalum clips, allows precise sparing of the optic disc.

23.2.2 Dosimetry

The range and the modulation of the 70-MeV proton beam were adapted for each patient. Before each irradiation, a depth–dose distribution curve was measured using a Markus type ionization chamber and Perspex phantom to verify that range and modulation had been adjusted correctly.

23.3 Results

Follow-up time ranged from no follow-up at all to 5 years and 3 months. Three months after treatment, visual acuity in the group of patients treated with one field increased for three, was stable for seven, and decreased for 17 and six patients had no follow-up examination. At 1 year, two patients had better vision and 21 had worse vision than before treatment, while no data was available for 19 patients. Evolution of the size of CNVM depended on the initial size. Lesions with an initial size less than or equal to 5 mm showed a decrease in 60% of cases, while lesions initially larger than 5 mm regressed in 84% of cases. The exudation showed similar behavior: a decrease in 56% of the lesions less than 5 mm and a decrease in 84% of the larger lesions.

23.4 Discussion

In the last decade there has been increasing interest in the use of radiation therapy for wet-type macular degeneration. The main goal of using radiation is to induce regression and/or promote inactivation of

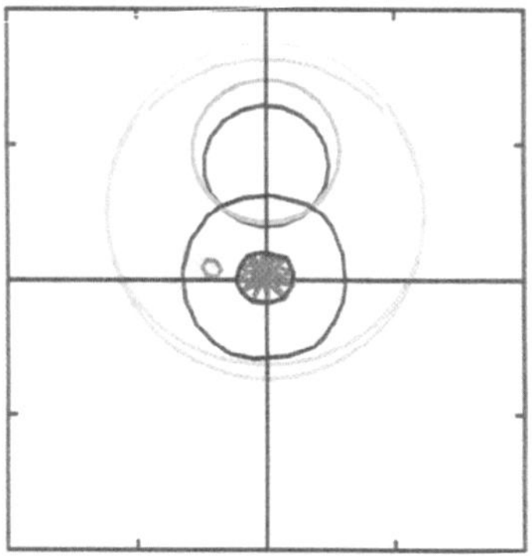

Fig. 23.1. Beam's eye view of a typical case treated with a single field

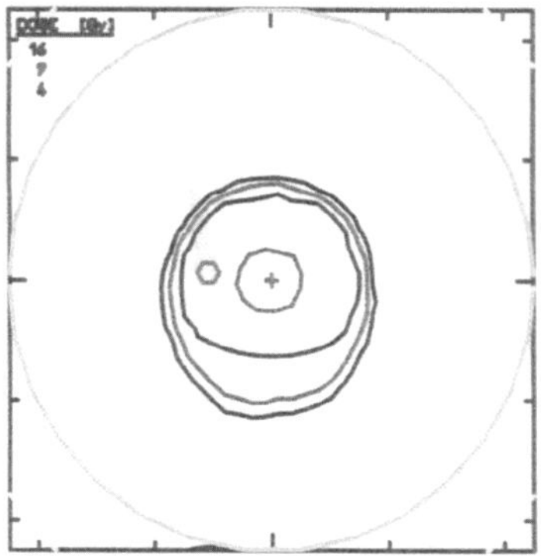

Fig. 23.2. Eye fundus view of the single field. Note the CNVM surrounding the macula (*cross*) and the 90%, 50%, and 20% isodoses. The optic disc (*left*) is within the 90% isodose

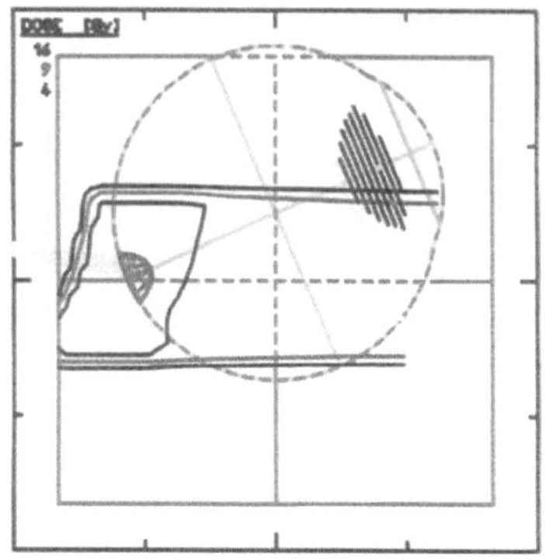

Fig. 23.3. Plane through the eye showing the CNVM and part of the optic nerve within the 90% isodose. Part of the lens is also in the treatment field

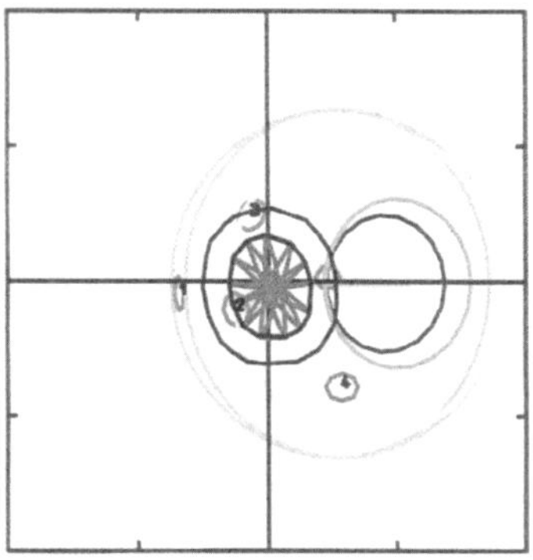

Fig. 23.4. Beam's eye view of a typical case treated with two fields. This view shows the first field with the collimator allowing irradiation of the total target volume

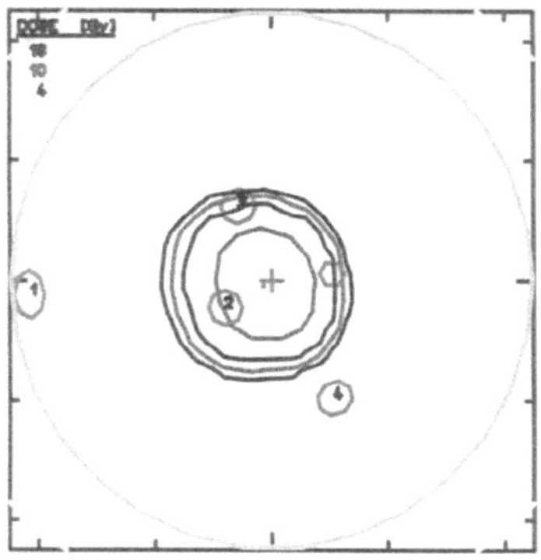

Fig. 23.5. Eye fundus view of the large field with the isodose distribution. Note the *clips* numbered *2*, *3*, and *4* which delimit the border of the CNVM. The optic nerve abuts the CNVM on the right side

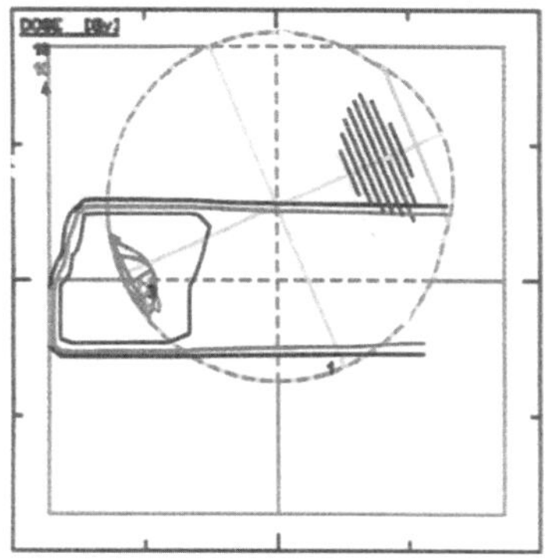

Fig. 23.6. Plane through the eye with isodose distribution. Note that the dose to the lens is less here, compared to the CNVM irradiated without clip positioning

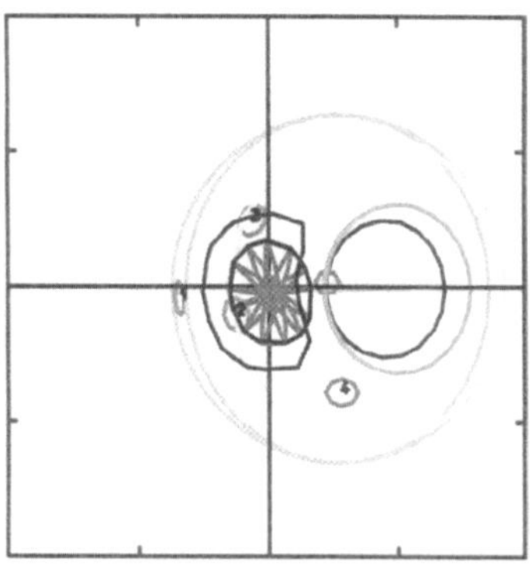

Fig. 23.7. Beam's eye view showing the second field. Note that the size of the collimator was reduced on the optic nerve side to avoid further irradiation of the optic disc and nerve

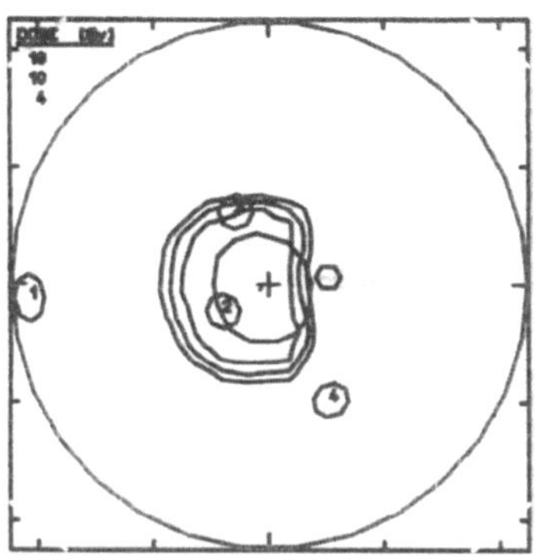

Fig. 23.8. Eye fundus view of the small field with the isodose distribution

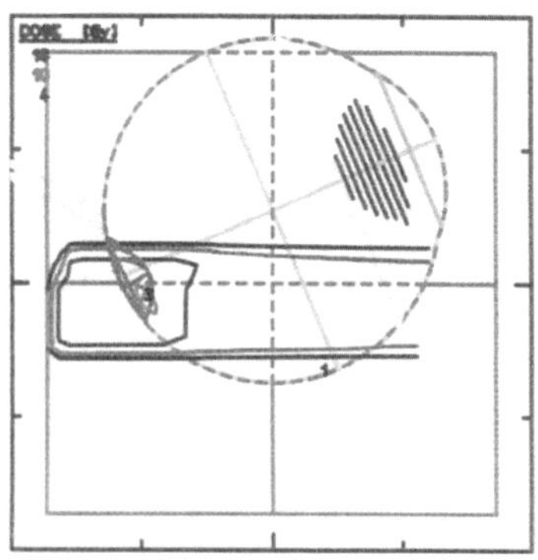

Fig. 23.9. Plane through the eye and isodose distribution of the small field. The optic nerve and lens are spared from any irradiation

the subretinal neovasculature that results in reabsorption of subretinal fluid and lipid deposits. This reduces the risk of further leakage, bleeding, and subretinal fibrosis. The beneficial effects are expected to be translated into stabilization of visual acuity, prevention of progression of AMD, possibly regression of the size of the CNVM, and an increase in visual acuity when subfoveal bleeding, exudates, and retinal detachment are resorbed.

Many reports on this subject have been published in recent years. While some authors show benefits to stabilization or even improvement of vision (Bergink et al. 1995; Brady et al. 1997), others found no long-term benefits (Bergink et al. 1998; Prettenhofer et al. 1998;, RAD Study 1999; Stalmans et al. 1997). It is interesting to note that Bergink found a positive effect in the short term (Bergink et al. 1995) but concluded that radiation therapy would not prevent visual loss in *all* patients over the long term (Bergink et al. 1998).

Comparison of the different studies is difficult if not impossible because different doses and fractionation schemes are used. Photons were employed by Spaide et al. (1998) and Freire et al. (1996), electrons by Valanconny et al. (2000), protons by Yonemoto et al. (1996), Moyers et al. (1999), and brachytherapy was used with palladium-103 (Finger et al. 1996) and strontium-90 (Jaakkola et al. 1999) episcleral plaques. As a consequence, some eyes received irradiation of the whole posterior pole while others treated with strontium plaques and proton beams had a circumscribed irradiation limited to the target volume. Mazal and coworkers (Mazal et al. 1998) studied the dose distribution within treated and contralateral eyes from different treatment techniques such as lateral irradiation with photons, electrons, and protons and frontal irradiation with protons. They concluded that frontal irradiation using a proton beam was the technique best allowing sparing of the structures located outside the target volume. However, as long as the total dose is below the tolerance limit of these structures, due to the age of the patients (who will not have to worry about radiation-induced cancers), to our understanding there is still no proven benefit in using circumscribed irradiation. In the literature on radiotherapy of AMD, one finds plenty of fractionation schemes (Archambeau et al. 1998) varying from a single fraction (Yonemoto et al. 1996; Char et al. 1999) to ten fractions within 2 weeks (Sasai et al. 1997). The total dose applied also varies widely between 8 Gy and 40 Gy (Hart et al. 1997; Mauget-Faysse et al. 2000; Ries 1994; Bergink et al. 1995). Some authors suggest that a higher dose correlates with a greater reduction in CNV size (Sasai 1997). This is consistent with our own observation. Applying higher doses to the CNVM argues for circumscribed irradiation, since higher doses are more likely to produce radiation-induced retinopathy or even optic neuropathy followed by loss of vision.

With the recognition of photodynamic therapy for the treatment of classic subfoveal CNVM in AMD, radiotherapy might only play a role in the treatment of occult CNVM in the future (Chang et al. 1995). In conclusion, the following questions still remain unanswered:

1. Would patients with occult CNV benefit from radiotherapy?
2. What kind of radiotherapy should be applied: diffuse or circumscribed ?
3. How many fractions should be given?
4. What dose per fraction should be delivered?
5. Should radiotherapy be applied alone or combined with other treatments?
6. If applied with other treatments, which treatments should they be?

In view of these questions, we strongly recommend further research to be conducted to define the role of irradiation in the treatment of AMD.

References

Bangerter A, Jäger T (1996) Forty years' experience with a special, non-tumorous application of radiotherapy for the eye. Eur J Med Res 1:582–588

Goitein M, Miller T (1983) Planning proton therapy of the eye. Med Phys 10:275–283

Archambeau JO, Mao XW, Yonemoto LT et al (1998) What is the role of radiation in the treatment of subfoveal membranes: Review of radiobiologic, pathologic, and other considerations to initiate a multimodality discussion. Int J Radiat Oncol Biol Phys 40:1125–1136

Brady LW, Freire JE, Longton WA et al (1997) Radiotherapy in macular degeneration: Technical considerations and preliminary results. Int J Radiat Oncol Biol Phys 39:945–948

Bergink GJ, Deutman AF, van den Broek JFCM et al (1994) Radiation therapy for subfoveal choroidal neovascular membranes in age-related macular degeneration – a pilot study. Graefes Arch Clin Exp Ophthalmol 232:591–598

Bergink GJ, Deutman AF, Van den Broek JE et al (1995) Radiation therapy for age-related subfoveal choroidal neovascular membranes – a pilot sudy. Doc Ophthalmol 90:67–74

Bergink GJ, Hoyng CB, Van der Maazen RWM et al (1998) A randomized controlled clinical trial on the efficacy of radiation therapy in the control of subfoveal choroidal neovascularization in age-related macular degeneration: Radiation versus observation. Graefes Arch Clin Exp Ophthalmol 236:321–325

Chakravarty U, Houston R, Archer D (1993) Treatment of age-related subfoveal neovascular membranes by teletherapy: A pilot study. Br J Ophthalmol 77: 265–273
Chang BM, Yannuzzi LA, Ladas ID et al (1995) Choroidal neovascularization in second eyes of patients with unilateral exudative age-related macular degeneration. Ophthalmology 102:1380–1386
Char DH, Irvine AI, Posner MD et al (1999) Randomized trial of radiation for age-related macular degeneration. Am J Ophthalmol 127:574–578
Egger E, Zografos L, Perret C et al (1993) Proton beam irradiation of choroidal melanomas at the PSI: Technique and results. In: Alberti WE, Sagerman RH (eds) Radiotherapy of intraocular and orbital tumors. Springer-Verlag, Berlin. pp 57–72
Finger PT, Berson A, Sherr D et al (1996) Radiation therapy for subretinal neovascularization. Ophthalmology 103:878–889
Freire J, Longton WA, Miyamoto CT et al (1996) External radiotherapy in macular degeneration: Technique and preliminary subjective response. Int J Radiat Oncol Biol Phys 36:857–860
Hart PM, Archer DB, Chakravarty U (1997) Teletherapy in the management of patients with age-related macular degeneration complicated by subfoveal neovascularization: An overview. In: Wiegel T, Bornfeld N, Foerster MH, Hinkelbein W (eds) Radiotherapy of ocular disease. Front Radiat Ther Oncol 30:229–237
Jaakkola A, Heikkonen J, Tarkkanen et al (1999) Visual function after strontium-90 plaque irradiation in patients with age-related subfoveal choroidal neovascularization. Acta Ophthalmol Scand 77:57–61
Macular Photocoagulation Study Group (1993) Laser photocoagulation of subfoveal neovascular lesions of age-related macular degeneration. Updated findings from two clinical trials. Arch Ophthalmol 111:1200–1209
Mauget-Faysse M, Coquard R, Francais-Maury C et al (2000) Radiotherapy for age-related macular degeneration: Risk factors of complications, prevention, and treatment of side effects. J Fr Ophthalmol 23:127–137
Mazal A, Schwartz L, Lacroix F et al (1998) A preliminary comparative treatment planning study for radiotherapy of age-related maculopathy. Radiother Oncol 47:91–98
Moyers MF, Galindo RA, Yonemoto LT et al (1999) Treatment of macular degeneration with proton beam. Med Phys 26:777–782
Neovaskularisation bei altersbedingter Makuladegeneration. Ergebnisse einer prospektiven Studie an 40 Patienten. Strahlenther Onkol 174:613–617
Pharmacological Therapy for Macular Degeneration Study Group. (1997) Interferon alfa-2a is ineffective for patients with choroidal neovascularization secondary to age-ralated marcular degeneration. Results of a prospective randomized placebo-controlled clinical trial. Arch Ophthalmol 115:865–872
Prettenhofer U, Haas A, Mayer R et al (1998) Photonentherapie der subfovealen choroidalen Neovaskularisation bei altersabhängiger Makuladegeneration. Strahlenther Onkol 174:613–617
RAD Study (1999) A prospective, randomized, double-masked trial on radiation therapy for neovascular age-related macular degeneration (RAD study). Radiation therapy for age-related macular degeneration. Opthtalmology 106:2239–2247
Ries G (1994) Niedrigdosierte perkutane Radiotherapie der senilen Makuladegeneration. Strahlenther Onkol 170:243–244
Sasai K, Murata R, Mandai M et al (1997) Radiation therapy for ocular choroidal neovascularization (phase I/II study): Preliminary report. Int J Radiat Oncol Biol Phys 39:173–178
Sheen M (1995) EYEPLAN proton therapy planning program. Clatterbridge Centre for Oncology, Internal Report
Paide RF, Guyer DR, McCormick et al (1998) External beam radiation therapy for choroidal neovascularization. Ophthalmology 105:24–30
Stalmans P, Leys A, Van Limbergen E (1997) External beam radiotherapy (20 Gy, 2 Gy fractions) fails to control the growth of choroidal neovascularization in age-related macular degeneration: A review of 111 cases. Retina 17:481–492
Teichmann KD (1997) Treatment of macular degeneration, according to Bangerter. Eur J Med Res 2:445–454
Treatment of Age-Related Macular Degeneration with Photodynamic Therapy (TAP) Study Group. (1999) Photodynamic therapy of subfoveal neovascularization in age-related macular degeneration with verteporfin: One-year results of two randomized clinical trials. Arch Ophthalmol 117:1329–1345
Valanconny C, Koenig F, Benchaboune M et al (2000) Complications of radiotherapy in patients with age-related macular degeneration (AMD). A study of 48 cases. J Fr Ophthalmol 23:151–157
Yonemoto LT Slater JD, Friedrichsen EJ et al (1996) Phase I/II study of proton beam irradiation for the treatment of subfoveal choroidal neovascularization in age-related macular degeneration: Treatment technique and preliminary results. Int J Radiat Oncol Biol Phys 36:867–871
Zografos L, Egger E, Bercher L et al (1998) Proton beam irradiation of choroidal hemangiomas. Am J Ophthalmol 126:261–268

24 Radiation Therapy for Age-Related Macular Degeneration

W. CHRIS SHEILS, S. YOUNG LEE, and DENNIS M. MARCUS

CONTENTS

24.1 Introduction

Age-related macular degeneration (AMD) is the leading cause of irreversible blindness in people over the age of 65 in the United States (KLEIN et al. 1992a, 1997; NATIONAL ADVISORY EYE COUNCIL 1998; TIELSCH 1995; VINGERLING et al. 1995). It has been estimated that nearly 6.3 million Americans will be diagnosed with AMD by the year 2030. With increased longevity, AMD will continue to represent a growing public health problem affecting the lives of millions.

AMD can be categorized into non-neovascular (nonexudative or „dry“) and neovascular (exudative or „wet“) forms. Although only a small proportion of cases progress to neovascular AMD, nearly 90% of blindness secondary to AMD is related to the choroidal neovascularization (CNV) found in wet AMD. Standard macular laser photocoagulation as described in the Macular Photocoagulation Study (MPS) until recently has been the only well-accepted method of treating juxtafoveal, extrafoveal (MACULAR PHOTOCOAGULATION STUDY GROUP 1982, 1991a, 1994a), and small subfoveal neovascular lesions (MACULAR PHOTOCOAGULATION STUDY GROUP 1991b, 1993, 1994b). However, laser photocoagulation by nature is destructive not only to the neovascularization but also to the retina. In addition, the majority of patients with CNV do not meet MPS guidelines for standard laser therapy, leaving many patients with untreatable severe visual loss (FREUND et al. 1993; MOISSEIEV et al. 1995).

<The visual impact of CNV in the growing elderly population has sparked great interest in finding alternative therapies for treating the ingrowth of new vessels before severe visual loss takes place. Radiation therapy, a treatment with known antiangiogenic properties, has been investigated as a modality to prevent visual loss in exudative AMD. Although the outlook is promising, conclusions from the majority of reports studying radiotherapy have been limited by short follow-up, retrospective data collection, and absence of appropriate randomized control groups. This chapter outlines the scientific and clinical rationales, clinical experience, and future of radiation therapy in the treatment of CNV complicating AMD.

24.2 Clinical Features and Classification

The macula is the highly specialized region of the retina with the greatest concentration of photoreceptors which provide central vision and high-resolution visual acuity. Clinically, the macula is a circular area 5–6 mm in diameter centered on the fovea and nestled between the vascular arcades of the retina. Anatomically, the macula is defined as the region of the retina with two or more layers of ganglion cells (GASS 1997).The fovea rests at the center of the macula and is 1.5–2.0 mm in size and located

W.C. SHEILS, MD, FACR; S.Y. LEE, MD; D.M. MARCUS, MD
Georgia Radiation Therapy Center, Medical College of Georgia, Building HK-112, Augusta, GA 30912-3965, USA

approximately 4 mm temporally and 0.8 mm inferiorly to the center of the optic disc (Fig. 24.1). Since the macula facilitates central vision, advanced AMD often leads to irreversible loss of the ability to read, drive, and even recognize faces. Fortunately, even patients with extensive macular degeneration in both eyes can often maintain enough peripheral vision to perform many daily activities (Fine et al. 2000).

AMD can be divided into early and late stages. The early stage involves minimal visual acuity loss. Large soft drusen and pigmentary abnormalities in the macula occur in the early stage (Fig. 24.2). Drusen are extracellular deposits and acellular debris accumulating below the basement membrane of the retinal pigment epithelium (Bressler et al. 1994).Clinically, drusen show great variation in size, color, shape, number, borders, and elevation. Most people older than 50 have at least one small drusen (less than or equal to 63 μm) in one or both eyes (Klein et al. 1992b). Eyes with large drusen (greater than 63 μm) have a greater risk of developing late AMD (Klein et al. 1997).

The late stage of AMD can be further divided into atrophic or „dry" and neovascular or „wet" forms (Fig. 24.3). The dry form typically involves atrophic changes without leakage of blood or serum in the deeper choriocapillaris, retinal pigment epithelium, or the overlying photoreceptor elements (rods and cones). In contrast, the neovascular form involves CNV and detachment (serous or hemorrhagic) of retinal pigment epithelium. CNV represents the ingrowth of new vessels through the deeper layers of the retina (Fig. 24.4). Unfortunately, these are abnormal vessels with the propensity to leak and cause fibrovascular scarring in the macula. As a result, severe visual loss most commonly occurs in the neovascular form of the disorder. Even patients with the atrophic form may suffer from fluctuating vision, reading difficulty secondary to limited area of good central vision, and limited vision at night. Hence, loss of vision can occur in either form of AMD (Fine et al. 2000).

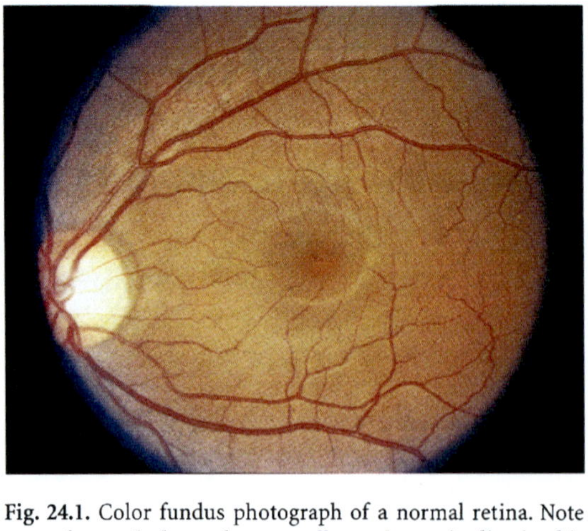

Fig. 24.1. Color fundus photograph of a normal retina. Note normal macula located temporally to the optic disc in this right eye

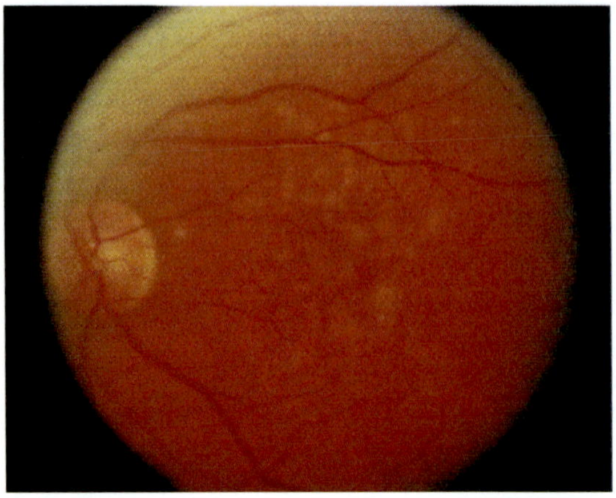

Fig. 24.2. Color fundus photograph showing soft drusen in the macula (left eye)

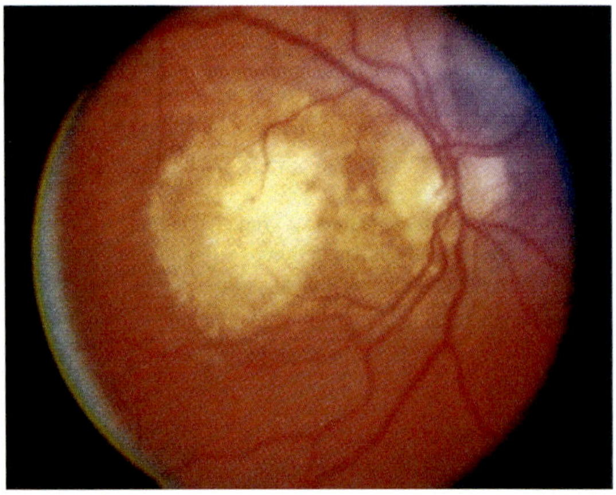

Fig. 24.3. Large disciform scarring of the central macula in a patient with end-stage wet AMD

The CNV found in AMD can be categorized on fluorescein angiogram as classic, occult, or mixed. The classic type is manifest in early phases of the angiogram by a well-defined area of hyperfluorescence. Significant dye leakage occurs in the later phases as the dye pools in the subretinal space. A lacy pattern of vessels may be seen in the early phase frames, but not always. In contrast, occult CNV is characterized by ill-defined, diffuse hyperfluorescence (Figs. 24.5, 24.6). Occult CNV can occur as fibrovascular pigment epithelial detachments (PED) and late-phase leakage of undetermined source. The fibrovascular PED shows

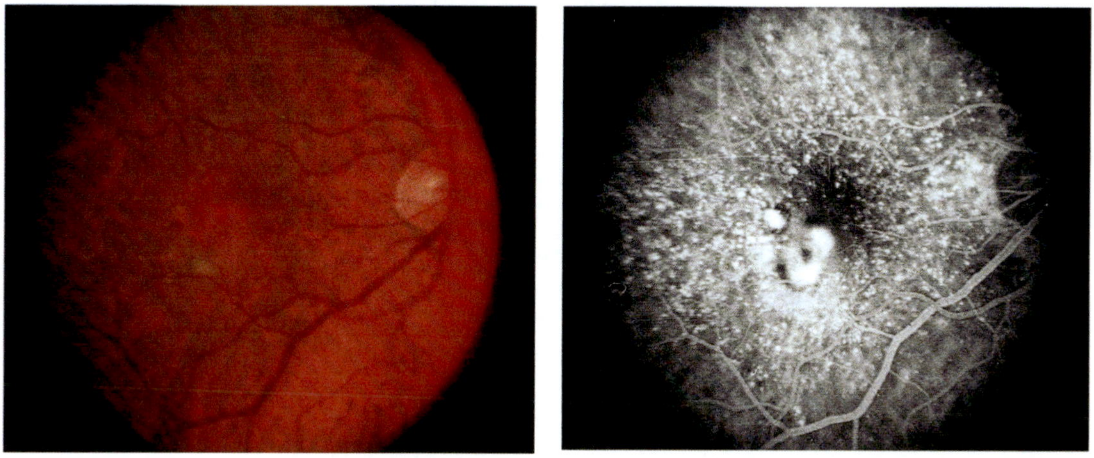

A B

Fig. 24.4A,B. Classic CNV. **A** Fundus photograph demonstrating subtle subretinal fluid just inferotemporally to the fovea in a patient with wet AMD. **B** Fluorescein angiography demonstrates classic CNV noted as white hyperfluorescence of fluorescein dye

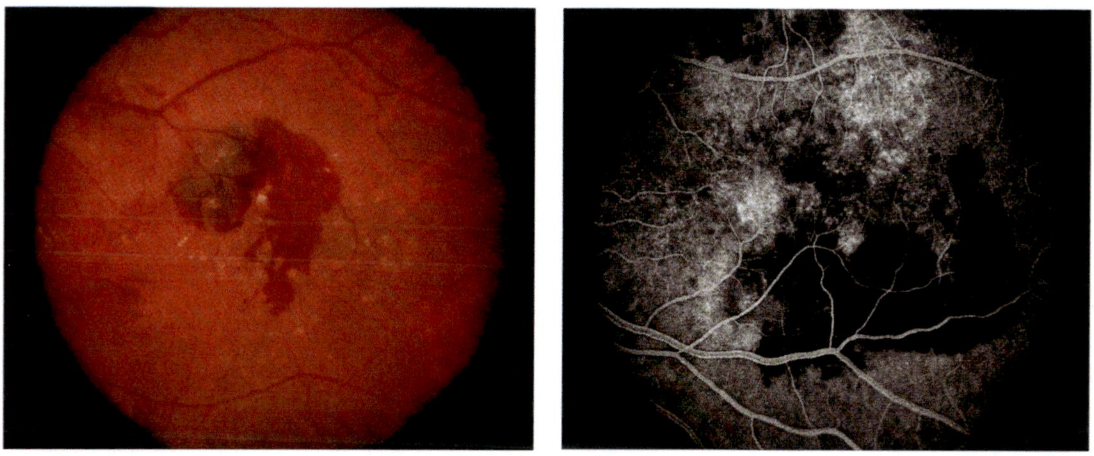

A B

Fig. 24.5A,B. Occult subfoveal CNV. **A** Color fundus photograph demonstrating elevated choroidal neovascular membrane obscured by submacular hemorrhage. **B** Midphase fluorescein angiogram shows large areas of hyperfluorescence with poorly delineated boundaries and leakage of undetermined source

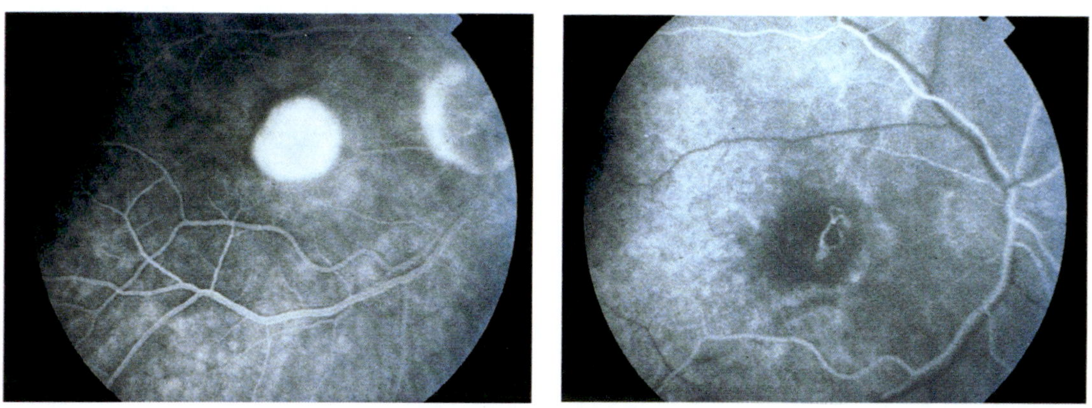

A B

Fig. 24.6. A Pretreatment late-phase fluorescein angiograms of subfoveal CNV. After a single dose of proton beam irradiation (14 Gy), CNV regression occurs at **B** 9 months after treatment. (Photographs courtesy of Eric J. Fredrichsen, MD and Loma Linda University Medical Center, Loma Linda, Calif., USA)

an irregular elevation of the retinal pigment epithelium with stippled hyperfluorescent dots in the early phase and persistence of staining with late leakage. In late leakage of undetermined source, angiography shows speckled hyperfluorescence without well-defined areas of hyperfluorescence in the early phases. Hence, occult CNV can be very difficult to treat, as its boundaries often cannot be precisely determined.

24.3 Treatment of Choroidal Neovascularization in AMD

24.3.1 Laser Photocoagulation Therapy

The MPS group published more than two dozen reports examining the potential benefit of laser photocoagulation treatment of neovascular lesions in AMD. The MPS randomized affected eyes to either laser treatment or observation. Their results led to the recommendation of laser photocoagulation for eligible eyes with extrafoveal (200 μm or more from the center of the macula), juxtafoveal (more than 1 μm but less than 200 μm from the foveal center), and subfoveal (directly beneath the fovea) CNV (Macular Photocoagulation Study Group 1992, 1993, 1994).Laser photocoagulation by the MPS guidelines constitutes the only treatment for AMD with proven long-term benefit. Unfortunately, standard laser photocoagulation has several limitations: most neovascular lesions are poorly delineated by fluorescein and ineligible for laser treatment, approximately half of treated lesions will recur within 2 years, and in addition, laser treatment causes an immediate reduction in central vision, particularly in cases of subfoveal CNV.

24.3.2 Photodynamic Therapy

Photodynamic therapy (PDT) represents a new treatment modality for AMD that relies on selective photochemical injury to the vessel walls of CNV. Photoreactive compounds injected intravenously into the patient accumulate in proliferating tissues. When these molecules are activated by light from a nonthermal laser at the appropriate wavelength, localized production of reactive oxygen species selectively destroy the new blood vessels (Miller et al. 1995). In clinical trials, PDT with verteporfin as the photosensitizer delayed or prevented loss of vision in patients with predominantly classic neovascular lesions at 1-year follow-up (Treatment of Age-Related Macular Degeneration with Photodynamic Therapy Study Group 1999).Most patients require an average of 3.4 treatments in the first year, as leakage from CNV often reoccurs despite initial closure of the CNV. While PDT with verteporfin represents a major advance in treatment of exudative AMD, visual improvement is rare and only patients with predominantly classic (not occult) CNV benefit.

24.3.3 Submacular Surgery

Subretinal surgery has been examined as an alternative therapy for CNV, particularly subfoveal CNV not amenable to laser photocoagulation. The Submacular Surgery Trials (SST) represent randomized clinical trials designed to evaluate submacular surgery in eyes with subfoveal CNV. Although no outcomes have been published by the SST group, the benefit of submacular surgery for subfoveal CNV appears most likely to be palliative. Currently, there is no evidence that submacular surgery is better than observation for subfoveal CNV.

24.3.4 Thalidomide

Although thalidomide has been described as teratogenic in pregnant mothers, the drug has known antiangiogenic properties which may be effective in treating AMD. Experiments with animal models of corneal angiogenesis showed that oral thalidomide inhibited growth factor-induced blood vessel development (D'Amato et al. 1994). A randomized, double-masked clinical trial is currently underway to examine thalidomide's ability to inhibit untreatable subfoveal CNV and recurrent extrafoveal CNV.

24.3.5 Treatments on the Horizon

Advances in microsurgical technique have led to experimentation with *retinal translocation*. This procedure involves moving functional sensory retina away from subfoveal areas of CNV so that laser photocoagulation can safely destroy new blood vessels without destroying the overlying retina. Transpupillary thermotherapy (TTT) has recently been explored as a novel treatment of occult CNV in AMD. Using a diode laser or TTT to heat occult subfoveal CNV lesions has shown promising results in one clinical study (REICHEL et al. 1999). A multicenter randomized study examining the effect of TTT on occult CNV has been initiated. Advances in molecular genetics have led to identification of the genes responsible for some forms of AMD. Several groups are studying the potential of *gene therapy* to reverse the progression of the disorder (BENNET and MAGUIRE 1999). Perhaps one of the most intriguing approaches for the future is the prophylactic treatment of nonexudative AMD. The National Eye Institute has funded a clinical trial to evaluate the effect of low-intensity laser as prophylaxis in high risk patients with numerous large drusen in both eyes (CHOROIDAL NEOVASCULAR PREVENTION TRIAL RESEARCH GROUP 1998; FIGUEROA et al. 1994; FRENNESSON and NILSSON 1998; HO et al. 1980; LITTLE et al. 1997).

24.4 Rationale for Radiation Therapy

24.4.1 Clinical Need

Prior to the first MPS reports published in 1982, the prevailing notion for AMD was that nothing could be done to preserve central vision once the exudative process was underway (FINE 1980).The MPS demonstrated in a prospective, multicenter, randomized clinical trial that laser photocoagulation decreased the risk of severe visual acuity loss (defined as loss of six lines of vision) in patients with extrafoveal classic CNV (located 200–2500 μm from the foveal center) or juxtafoveal classic CNV (located between 1 and 199 μm from the foveal center) compared to observation alone (MACULAR PHOTOCOAGULATION STUDY GROUP 1982, 1991a, 1994a).The MPS has also reported findings from randomized trials of laser treatment for subfoveal neovascular lesions secondary to AMD (MACULAR PHOTOCOAGULATION STUDY GROUP 1991b, 1993, 1994b). At 2-year follow-up, laser-treated patients with subfoveal CNV fared better than controls in terms of reading ability and central contrast sensitivity (MACULAR PHOTOCOAGULATION STUDY GROUP 1991b, 1993, 1994b). In eyes with recurrent subfoveal CNV at the periphery of an earlier laser scar, the benefits of laser treatment were similarly demonstrated (MACULAR PHOTOCOAGULATION STUDY GROUP 1991c). Despite the long-term benefits of laser treatment of subfoveal lesions in the context of the MPS, the management of subfoveal CNV in AMD remains controversial, especially in light of the recent approval of PDT with verteporfin. Standard laser treatment results in immediate visual loss after foveal ablation (YANUZZI 1994). Alternative, less destructive therapies for subfoveal CNV are therefore essential. Although PDT provides ophthalmologists with a less destructive beneficial treatment, it has not been shown helpful for patients with occult CNV. In addition, as only a minority of PDT-treated eyes demonstrate visual improvement, investigation of additional therapies is necessary to optimize outcomes.

24.4.2 Scientific Rationale

24.4.2.1 Experimental Support: In Vitro and In Vivo Studies

Radiation therapy has been investigated as an alternative treatment for exudative AMD because of the known radiosensitivity of vascular endothelial cells. Ionizing radiation has been used to inhibit cellular proliferation in neoplasia (Arlett and Harcourt 1980).The radiosensitivity of capillary endothelium has long been recognized, with increased susceptibility in young or new vessels with proliferating endothelial cells. In vitro studies have shown that low-dose radiation inhibits neovascularization (Bicknell and Harris 1991; Zhan et al. 1993). Single radiation doses of 8.7 Gy prevent endothelial cell division (Johnson et al. 1982). In particular, a single dose of 5 Gy arrests division in 99% of cultured retinal endothelial cells (Chakravarthy and McQuaid 1989). In vivo studies have also supported the radiosensitivity of endothelium. Radiation at single doses from 1.7 to 15 Gy inhibits survival of subcutaneous endothelium in wound healing models (Reinhold and Buisman 1973; Van den Brenk 1959). Similarly, Chakravarthy and coworkers demonstrated in an animal model that the neovascular component of healing ocular wounds is significantly reduced by radiation doses exceeding 9.5 Gy (Chakravarthy et al. 1989a, b). Animals receiving radiation demonstrated choriocapillaris occlusion with sparing of larger choroidal vessels, thus further supporting a role for radiotherapy in CNV (Amoaku et al. 1992; Irvine et al. 1981; Irvine and Wood 1987; Midena et al. 1996).

24.4.2.2 Clinical Support

24.4.2.2.1

RADIOSENSITIVITY OF NEOPLASIA AND VASCULAR TUMORS

In malignant ocular disease, ionizing radiation not only inhibits neoplastic cells but also damages the malignant blood supply. This vascular susceptibility has been demonstrated after proton beam irradiation (SAORNIL et al. 1992) or iodine-125 brachytherapy (SAORNIL et al. 1997) for ocular melanoma. Enucleated eyes with melanoma treated with proton beam irradiation or iodine-125 brachytherapy are more likely than nonirradiated eyes (SAORNIL et al. 1992) to show vascular changes such as endothelial edema, decreased lumen size, endothelial basement membrane thickening, and vessel thrombosis. Radiation therapy has also been used to inhibit benign vascular ocular and nonocular tumors. The proliferating vascular tumor choroidal hemangioma has shown susceptibility to external beam irradiation at doses of 12 Gy to 40 Gy in standard fractions of less than 2 Gy (MADREPERLA et al. 1997; PLOWMAN and HARNETT 1988; SCOTT et al. 1991). Radiation-induced complications were not observed after follow-up at 1–7 years (MADREPERLA et al. 1997). Similarly, proton beam irradiation (30 Gy in four fractions) (HANNOUCHE et al. 1997) and plaque brachytherapy (50 Gy) (MADREPERLA et al. 1997) have been shown to be safe and effective for the treatment of choroidal hemangioma.

24.4.2.2.2

OCULAR RADIATION TOXICITY

An understanding of the safety window for radiation therapy is important for employing radiation therapy in the treatment of CNV. Surrounding normal retina and choroid appear relatively radioresistant, compared with normal endothelium or the proliferating endothelium of CNV (EGBERT et al. 1980; MAGUIRE and SCHACHAT 1994; NAKISSA et al. 1983; ROSS et al. 1973). Radiotherapy of various periorbital tumors with a cumulative exposure of less than 25 Gy (in standard fractions of approximately 2 Gy) does not result in significant ocular toxicity (CHAN and SHUKOVSKY 1976; PARSONS et al. 1983). However, external beam irradiation in fraction sizes greater than 2.5 Gy may predispose to ocular toxicity, especially with total doses exceeding 45 Gy (ARISTIZABAL 1997; BROWN et al. 1982a; HARRIS and LEVENE 1976; PARSONS et al. 1994). The toxic effects on the eye of various radiation doses and fractions are summarized in Table 24.1. The main factors influencing the development of radiation retinopathy and optic neuropathy include total dose delivered, daily fraction size, pre-existing microangiopathy or diabetes, previous or concurrent chemotherapy, and irradiation field design. In particular, patients with diabetes or pre-existing microangiopathy and those receiving chemotherapy have a decreased threshold for radiation toxicity, in some cases with total doses as low as 15 Gy (BROWN et al. 1982a, b; LOPEZ et al. 1991; PARSONS et al. 1983; VIEBAN et al. 1991; VOLGER et al. 1990; YOUNG et al. 1992).

Table 24.1. Ocular radiation toxicity

Tissue	Side effects	Dose (Gy)
Cornea	Keratitis, edema, ulcer, perforation	30–50
Conjunctiva	Conjunctivitis	55–75
Lacrimal system	Atrophy, stenosis	50–65
Lens	Radiation cataract	2
Retina	Radiation retinopathy	50
Optic nerve	Optic neuropathy	55

24.5 Radiation Therapy for AMD – Clinical Experience

24.5.1 Nonrandomized Clinical Studies

The antiangiogenic properties of ionizing radiation led CHAKRAVARTHY and coworkers (1993) to investigate low-dose external beam irradiation for the treatment of CNV complicating AMD. Since their first report in 1993, more than 2000 patients worldwide have received various forms of radiation for this disease (Figs. 24.7–24.9). Nonrandomized, uncontrolled studies (BERGINK et al. 1995; BERSON et al. 1996; CHAKRAVARTHY et al. 1993; FINGER et al. 1996; FREIRE et al. 1996; HART et al. 1995, 1996; POSTGENS et al. 1997; SPAIDE et al. 1998; STALMANS et al. 1997; YONEMOTO et al. 1996) indicate that radiation therapy for CNV does not demonstrate significant short-term side effects, cause immediate visual loss, or require complete angiographic visualization. The majority of these uncontrolled, nonrandomized studies have utilized external beam irradiation using standard fractions of approximately 2 Gy to a total of 10 Gy–20 Gy. Some investigators reported minimal or no effect from therapeutic external beam irradiation (POST-

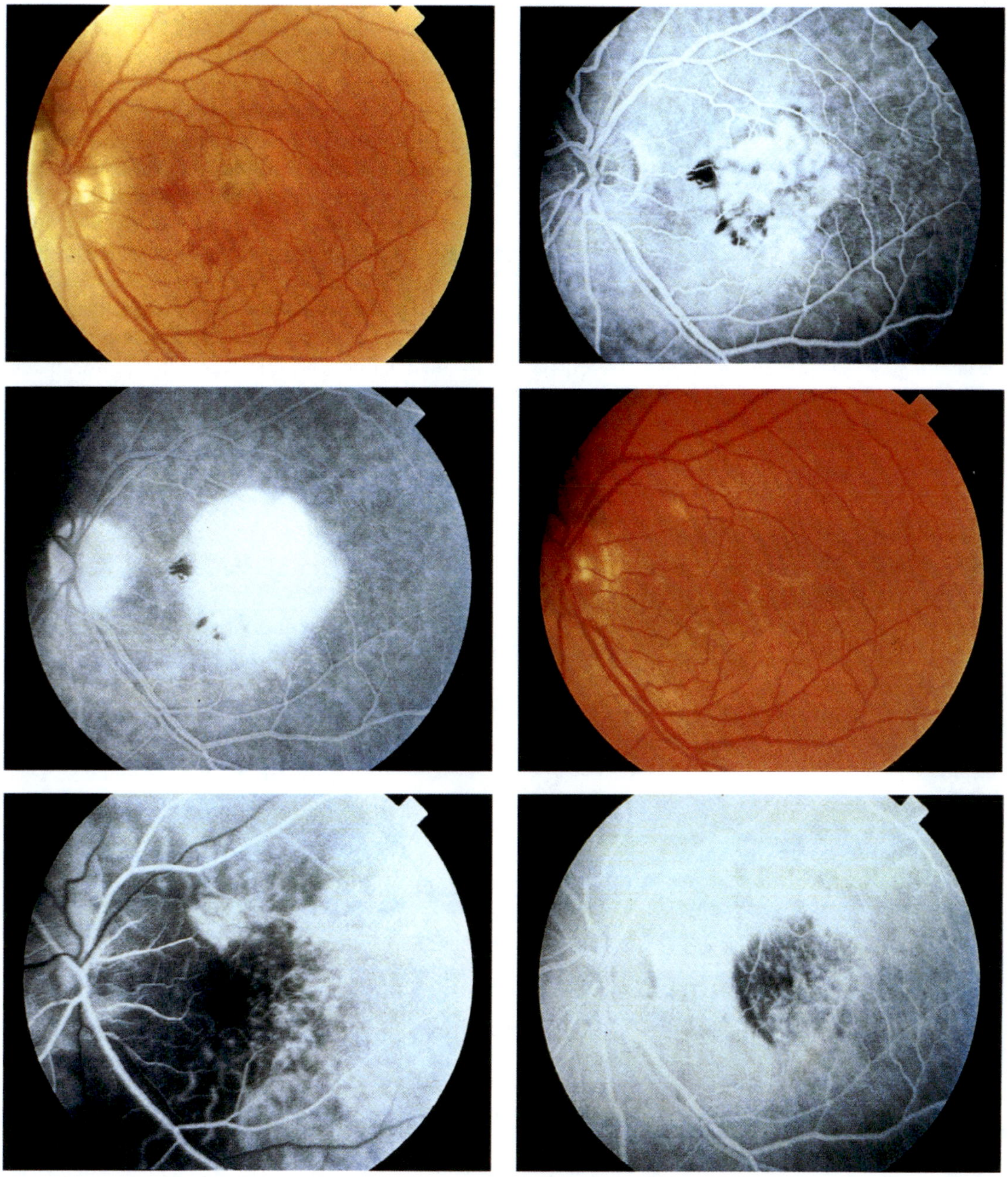

Fig. 24.7. A Pretreatment fundus photograph. **B** Arteriovenous-phase and **C** late-phase fluorescein angiograms of subfoveal CNV. **D-F** After a single dose of proton beam irradiation (14 Gy), CNV regression occurs at 9 months after treatment. (Photographs courtesy of Eric J. Fredrichsen, MD and Loma Linda University Medical Center, Loma Linda, Calif., USA)

GENS et al. 1997; SPAIDE et al. 1998; STALMANS et al. 1997), while others showed moderate benefit with standard fractions (CHAKRAVARTHY et al. 1993; BERGINK et al. 1995; BERSON et al. 1996; FINGER et al. 1996; FREIRE et al. 1996; HART et al. 1995, 1996). Although these results appear promising, conclusions from the majority of radiotherapy studies are limited by short follow-up, small numbers of cases, retrospective data collection, absence of standardized visual acuity measurement, lack of strict angiographic and visual entry criteria, and absence of appropriate randomized control groups (BERGINK et al. 1995; BERSON et al. 1996; CHAKRAVARTHY et al. 1993; FINGER et al. 1996; FREIRE et al. 1996; HART

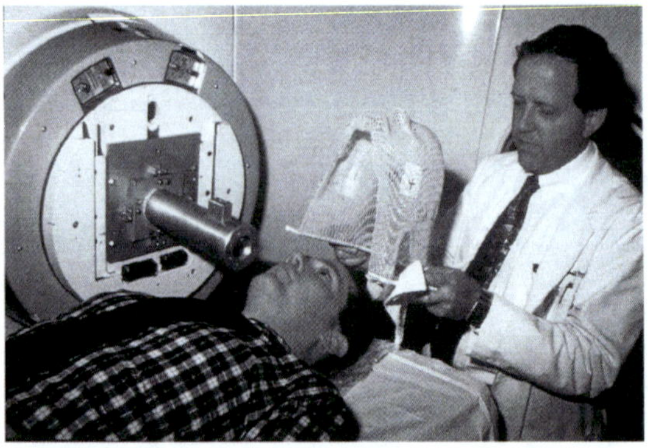

Fig. 24.8. The patient is positioned in a custom-fit Aquaplast face mask for external beam irradiation. The linear accelerator is positioned on the patient's right side for treatment of the right macula. The lateral beam is angled 15° posteriorly to avoid the contralateral retina

A

B

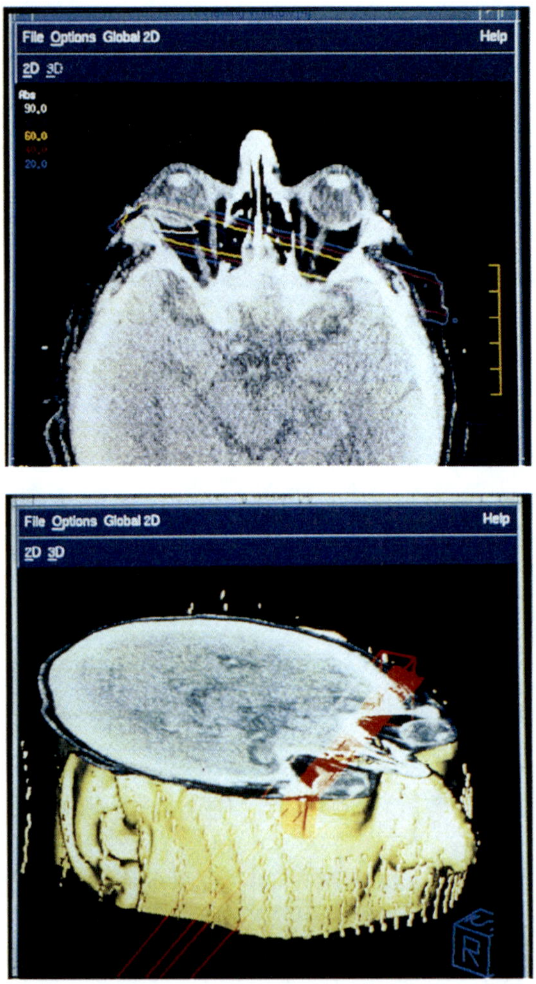

Fig. 24.9. A Standard two-dimensional CT scan is used to display calculated isodose distribution for external beam irradiation. B Three-dimensional reconstruction showing the beam path

et al. 1995, 1996; Postgens et al. 1997; Spaide et al. 1998; Stalmans et al. 1997; Yonemoto et al. 1996).

Similarly, higher fractions and doses of external beam irradiation (Bergink et al. 1995) and other modalities such as brachytherapy (Finger et al. 1996) or proton beam irradiation (Yonemoto et al. 1996) have also been examined. Nonstandard fractions of external beam irradiation (6-Gy–8-Gy fractions) (Bergink et al. 1995) and proton beam irradiation (8-Gy and 14-Gy fractions) (Yonemoto et al. 1996) have been proposed as beneficial therapy in uncontrolled, nonrandomized studies. Some evidence of angiographic regression of CNV has been observed with higher fractions, especially after proton beam irradiation. However, the fractions used are not conventional and may result in increased risk of long-term side effects and ocular toxicity.

24.5.2 Randomized Clinical Studies

Two published randomized studies comparing radiation to observation have employed higher, nonstandard fractions (Bergink et al. 1998; Char et al. 1999). Bergink and coworkers (1998) randomized 74 patients with classic, mixed, or occult subfoveal CNV to observation versus external beam irradiation. This study utilized six nonstandard fractions of 4 Gy (total 24 Gy). At 1-year follow-up, 52% of the observation group versus 32% of the irradiated group had lost three or more lines of visual acuity (p=0.03), with loss of six or more lines in 41% of the observation group versus 9% of the radiation group (p=0.002). While radiotherapy appeared to have a stabilizing effect, a significant proportion of irradiated eyes lost visual acuity and irradiated eyes demonstrated progressive growth of CNV (Bergink et al. 1998). In addition, Char and coworkers (1999) reported a small randomized trial of 27 eyes with classic and subfoveal CNV. These patients were randomized to observation versus external beam irradiation with a single fraction of 7.5 Gy. Irradiated eyes demonstrated a loss of 1.9 lines of visual acuity compared to 5.5 lines in observed eyes (p =0.046). Similarly to Bergink and coworkers (1998), Char and coworkers found no difference in angiographic progression between irradiated and observed eyes (Char et al. 1999). Holz and coworkers recently discussed the absence of treatment benefit in a randomized, multicenter radiotherapy trial (Radiation Therapy for Age-Related Macular Degeneration Study Group 1999). Two hundred five patients were randomly assigned to treatment with eight fractions of 2-Gy external beam irradiation or to control with eight fractions of 0 Gy. At 1-year follow-up, 51.1% of treated patients and 52.6% of control subjects had lost 3 or more lines (p =0.88) (Table 24.2).

Additional randomized clinical trials are ongoing in the United States and United Kingdom. We are performing a prospective, double-masked, randomized study evaluating the efficacy of low-dose external beam irradiation (14 Gy, seven fractions of 2 Gy). Preliminary data indicate no significant benefit or harm from low-dose irradiation in patients with CNV ineligible for standard laser treatment (Marcus et al. 1996). In the United Kingdom, Chakravarthy and coworkers have been performing a prospective, single-masked clinical trial evaluating 12 Gy (standard fraction size) of external beam irradiation in the treatment of subfoveal CNV with a classic component. Two hundred patients with classic or mixed occult and classic CNV have enrolled and results are anticipated (personal communication, U. Chakravarthy). In addition, Fine, Maguire, and Marcus have initiated a multicenter, national, randomized pilot trial (AMD Radiotherapy Trial) investigating external beam irradiation for subfoveal CNV at 20 Gy in five fractions of 4 Gy.

24.6 Radiotherapy Techniques

Historically, radiation has been widely used for a number of benign conditions such as heterotopic bone formation, keloids, hemangiomas, and hyperthyroid ophthalmopathy. More recently, interest has led to the study of radiation as a treatment modality for AMD.

A pilot study was published in 1993 by Chakravarthy et al. (1993) at the Royal Victoria Hospital, Belfast, Northern Ireland. In this study, a total of 19 patients were treated using two different fractionation schemes. The first 11 received 10 Gy delivered in 2-Gy fractions over 7 days. The next eight patients received 15 Gy delivered in 3-Gy fractions over 7 days. A custom-made Perspex beam direction shield was made for each patient. All treatment was delivered through a single lateral port, with treatment prescribed to the 90% isodose. Since this effort, a number of institutions have published studies using different techniques and dose regimes.

Bergink et al. (1994) at the Institute of Ophthalmology in Nijmegen, The Netherlands, published a pilot study in 1994. Forty patients were placed in four groups of ten each. All were treated using a lens-sparing technique. A photon beam energy of 16 MV was used. Two treatment beams, one placed cranially at 30° to the optical axis and one caudally at 30°, were directed to a 1-cm^2 area of the macula. Each group was treated with a different fractionation scheme: ten patients received 8 Gy in one fraction, ten received 12 Gy in two fractions of 6 Gy, ten received 18 Gy in three fractions of 6 Gy, and ten received 24 Gy in four fractions of 6 Gy. At the time of publishing, the authors noted that no side effects from the radiation therapy were seen, although the possibility of future cataract development remained.

Finger et al. (1996) in the Department of Ophthalmology at the New York Eye and Ear Infirmary, New York, published a study in 1996. They described a number of treatment techniques, including both external beam therapy and brachytherapy. A total of 137 patients were treated, although the analysis was restricted to patients treated with 4-MV or 6-MV external beam radiation, or palladium-103 plaque brachytherapy for a total of 81 patients. Dose to the retina was 1200–1500 cGy. All plaque brachytherapy was given in a single treatment beginning at insertion and continuing to the point of prescribed dose delivery. Retinal dose rate ranged from 35–56 cGy per hour, treatment time from 24–43 h, maximum dose to the overlying retina of 1000–1500 cGy. External

Table 24.2. Summary of published randomized clinical trials

CNV type	Patients (n)	Randomization	Dose/fraction	Follow-up (months)	Visual results
Bergink et al. (1998),	74	EBR vs. observation	24 Gy/6 Gy	12	52.2% Obs vs. 32% EBR subfoveal lost 3 or more lines of VA (p=0.03)
Char et al. (1999),	27	EBR vs. observation	750 cGy/single	17	Five of 13 Obs vs. 10 of subfoveal 14 EBR lost <3 lines of VA
RAD group (1999),	205	EBR vs. observation	16 Gy/8 Gy	12	52.6% Obs vs. 51.1% subfoveal EBR lost 3 or more lines of VA (p=0.88

EBR, external beam radiation; Obs, observation group; VA, visual acuity

therapy was delivered through a single angled lateral port. Prescription volume included the entire ipsilateral posterior pole.

Proton beam irradiation for AMD has been reported by Yonemoto and associates (1996). Twenty-one patients received 8 cobalt Gray equivalents (CGE) in a single fraction. Fluorescein angiography and stereofundus color photography were used to define the subfoveal CNV. Three-dimensional treatment planning was used along with complex positioning including treatment chair, head immobilization device, bite block, eyelid retractors, and alignment camera. Distance from beam nozzle to eye was determined by the camera with less than a 1-mm depth of field. The treatment chair was positioned to assure that the center of the isodose distribution was on the macula. Light field projection through the proton beam aperture was used to confirm beam placement at the temporal conjunctiva, sparing lashes and limbus. Patients gazed at a red blinking fixation light to assure proper alignment.

The Medical College of Georgia, USA, has been conducting a prospective randomized study of the use of radiation in the treatment of AMD. Their treatment technique employs a 6-mv X-ray beam with a small field defined by an extended collimator, resulting in a semicircular field of 3.0×1.5 cm (3.0 cm diameter, 1.5 cm radius). With the patient in the supine position, lateral lasers are used to align the tragus on each side of the head. Over the patient's face, an Aquaplast positioning mask is molded from which material in the area of the treated eye is removed to allow the patient to stare at a fixed point. On the patient's skin, reference marks near each lateral canthus are carefully applied by the physician, followed by placement of small radio-opaque markers over the ink marks. Lateral radio-opaque markers are placed on the mask as additional reference points. A dedicated CT simulator is used to scan the patient in the positioning mask. The physician selects the appropriate CT slice for treatment planning, during which careful attention is paid to ensure that the treatment beam encompasses the macula. The resulting field is a single lateral port, usually angled 15° anteriorly to posteriorly to the coronal plane. The patient is placed on the treatment couch in the supine position with the mask in place. The treatment field is set based on the CT simulation. Initially, a 5×5 cm double exposure port film is taken and checked against the position of the markers. The contralateral reference marker on the mask is then repositioned, based on the CT-simulation, to coincide with the central axis of the exit beam of the treatment field using the extended collimator. The patient is instructed to look at a fixed spot on the ceiling before treatment and the physician directs final positioning, cephalocaudad according to the position of the central field axis in relation to the center of the patient's pupil. The final field position is marked on the mask and a verification film is taken during the first treatment.

Initially, 1400 cGy in seven evenly divided fractions was delivered. Along with the conventional fractionation of 200 cGy per treatment, this dose was selected as a baseline for initial evaluation. A dose of 2000 cGy in five evenly divided fractions is now being used for evaluation.

24.7 Summary

Recent breakthroughs in the treatment of CNV provide hope for the millions of patients suffering from neovascular AMD. PDT has extended the group of eyes that can benefit from some form of treatment. However, clinical trials have demonstrated PDT as beneficial only in patients with predominantly classic CNV. Hence, the quest for an effective treatment of subfoveal and occult CNV continues. In addition, investigation of potential adjuvant therapies to PDT may optimize visual outcomes.

Radiotherapy remains controversial as a potential treatment for exudative AMD. Although safe, low doses with standard fractions of external beam irradiation do not show visual acuity improvement or fluorescein angiographic regression, nonstandard fractions and higher total doses may have a more substantial effect. Therefore, radiotherapy remains a potential experimental option as a primary or even as an adjunctive modality in treating classic, occult, or subfoveal CNV. It is hoped that ongoing and future randomized trials will provide useful information in determining a therapeutic window for radiotherapy.

References

Amoaku WM et al (1992) Late ultrastructural changes in the retina of the rat following low-dose x-irradiation. Graefes Arch Clin Exp Ophthalmol 230:569–574

Aristizabal S, Caldwell WL, Avilla J (1977) The relationship of time dose fractionation factors to complications in the treatment of pituitary tumors by irradiation. Int J Radiat Oncol Biol Phys 2:667–673

Arlett C, Harcourt S (1980) Survey of radiosensitivity in a variety of human cell strains. Cancer Res 40:926–932

Bennet J, Maguire AM (1999) Gene therapy. In: Berger JW, Fine

SL, Maguire MG (eds) Age-related macular degeneration. Mosby, St Louis, pp 395–412

Bergink G, Deutman A, Van den Broek J, Van Daal W, Van der Maazen R (1994) Radiation therapy for subfoveal choroidal neovascular membranes in age-related macular degeneration a pilot study. Graefes Arch Clin Exp Ophthalmol 232: 591–598

Bergink GJ, Deutman AF, Van den Broek JECM et al (1995) Radiation therapy for age-related subfoveal choroidal neovascular membranes. Doc Ophthalmol 90:67–74

Bergink GJ, Hoyng CB, Van der Maazen RWM et al (1998) A randomized controlled clinical trial on the efficacy of radiation therapy in the control of subfoveal choroidal neovascularization in age-related macular degeneration: Radiation versus observation. Graefes Arch Clin Exp Ophthalmol 236:321–325

Berson AM, Finger PT, Sherr DL et al (1996) Radiotherapy for age-related macular degeneration: Preliminary results of a potentially new treatment. Int J Radiat Oncol Biol Phys 36:861–865

Bicknell R, Harris AL (1991) Novel growth regulatory factors and tumour angiogenesis. Eur J Cancer 27:781–785

Bressler NM, Silva JC, Bressler SB, Fine SL, Green WR (1994) Clinicopathological correlation of drusen and retinal pigment epithelial abnormalities in age-related macular degeneration. Retina 14:130–142

Brown GC et al (1982a) Radiation retinopathy. Ophthalmology 89:1494–1501

Brown GC et al (1982b) Radiation optic neuropathy. Ophthalmology 89:1489–1493

Chakravarthy U, McQuaid M (1989) Radiosensitivity of retinal capillary endothelial cells and pericytes. Paper presented at the 30th meeting of the Association for Eye Research, Montpellier, France

Chakravarthy U et al (1989a) Focal irradiation of perforating eye injuries with iodine-125 plaques. Curr Eye Res 8:1241–1250

Chakravarthy U et al (1989b) A light microscopic and autoradiographic study of irradiated ocular wounds, Curr Eye Res 8:337–347

Chakravarthy U, Houston RF, Archer DB (1993) Treatment of age-related subfoveal neovascular membranes by teletherapy: a pilot study. Br J Ophthalmol 77:265–273

Chan RC, Shukovsky LJ (1976) Effects of irradiation on the eye. Radiology 120:673–675

Char DH, Irvine A, Posner MD et al (1999) Randomized trial of radiation for age-related macular degeneration. Am J Ophthalmol 127:574–578

Choroidal Neovascular Prevention Trial Research Group (1998) Laser treatment in eyes with large drusen: short-term effects seen in a pilot randomized clinical trial. Ophthalmology 105:11–23

D'Amato RJ et al (1994) Thalidomide is an inhibitor of angiogenesis. Proc Natl Acad Sci U S A 91:4082–4085

Egbert PR et al (1980) Posterior ocular abnormalities after irradiation for retinoblastoma: a histopathological study. Br J Ophthalmol 64:660–665

Figueroa MS, Regueras A, Bertrand J (1994) Laser photocoagulation to treat macular soft drusen in age-related macular degeneration. Retina 14:391–396

Fine SL (1980) The Macular Photocoagulation Study. Editorial. Arch Ophthalmol 98:832

Fine SL, Berger JW, Maguire MG, Ho AC (2000) Drug therapy: age-related macular degeneration. N Engl J Med 342:483–492

Finger PT, Berson A, Sherr D et al (1996) Radiation therapy for subretinal neovascularization. Ophthalmology 103:878–889

Freire J, Longton WA, Miyamoto CT et al (1996) External radiotherapy in macular degeneration: technique and preliminary subjective response. Int J Radiat Oncol Biol Phys 36:857–860

Frennesson C, Nilsson SEG (1998) Prophylactic laser treatment in early age-related maculopathy reduced the incidence of exudative complications. Br J Ophthalmol 82:1169–1174

Freund KB, Yannuzzi LA, Sorenson JA (1993) Age-related macular degeneration and choroidal neovascularization. Am J Ophthalmol 115:786–791

Gass JDM (1997) Stereoscopic atlas of macular diseases: Diagnosis and treatment. Fourth ed. Mosby, St. Louis

Hannouche D et al (1997) Efficacy of proton therapy in circumscribed choroidal hemangiomas associated with serous retinal detachment. Ophthalmology 104:1780–1784

Harris JR, Levene MB (1976) Visual complications following irradiation for pituitary adenomas and craniopharyngiomas. Radiology 120:167–171

Hart PM, Archer DB, Chakravarthy U (1995) Asymmetry of disciform scarring in bilateral disease when one eye is treated with radiotherapy. Br J Ophthalmol 79:562–568

Hart PM et al (1996) Teletherapy for subfoveal choroidal neovascularization of age-related macular degeneration: Results of follow-up in a non-randomized study. Br J Ophthalmol 80:1046–1050

Ho AC, Maguire MG, Yoken J et al (1980) Laser-induced drusen reduction improves visual function at 1 year. Ophthalmology 106:1367–1374

Irvine AR, Wood IS (1987) Radiation retinopathy as an experimental model for ischemic proliferative retinopathy and rubeosis iridis. Am J Ophthalmol 103:790–797

Irvine AR et al (1981) Radiation retinopathy: An experimental model for the ischemic-proliferative retinopathies. Trans Am Ophthalmol Soc 79:103–122

Johnson LK, Longnecker JP, Fajardo LF (1982) Differential radiation response of cultured endothelial cells and smooth myocytes. Anal Quant Cytol 4:188–198

Klein R, Klein BEF, Linton KLP (1992a) Prevalence of age-related maculopathy: The Beaver Dam Eye Study. Ophthalmology 99:933–943

Klein R, Klein BEK, Linton KLP (1992b) Prevalence of age-related maculopathy: The Beaver Dam Eye Study. Ophthalmology 99:933–945

Klein R, Klein BEF, Jensen SE et al (1997) The five-year incidence and progression of age-related maculopathy, the Beaver Dam Study. Ophthalmology 104:7–21

Little HL, Showman JM, Brown BW (1997) A pilot randomized controlled study on the effect of laser photocoagulation of confluent soft macular drusen. Ophthalmology 104:623–31

Lopez PF et al (1991) Bone marrow transplant retinopathy. Am J Ophthalmol 112:635–646

Macular Photocoagulation Study Group (1982) Argon laser photocoagulation for senile macular degeneration: Results of a randomized clinical trial. Arch Ophthalmol 100:912–918

Macular Photocoagulation Study Group (1991a) Argon laser photocoagulation for neovascular maculopathy after five years: Results from randomized clinical trials. Arch Ophthalmol 109:1109–1114

Macular Photocoagulation Study Group (1991b) Laser photocoagulation of subfoveal neovascular lesions in age-related macular degeneration. Arch Ophthalmol 109:1220–1231
Macular Photocoagulation Study Group (1991c) Laser photocoagulation of subfoveal neovascular lesions in age-related macular degeneration: Results of a randomized clinical trial. Arch Ophthalmol 109:1232–1241
Macular Photocoagulation Study Group (1992) Argon laser photocoagulation for neovascular maculopathy: five-year results from randomized clinical trials. Arch Ophthalmol 109:1109–1114,1991. [Erratum, Arch Ophthalmol 110:761, 1992]
Macular Photocoagulation Study Group (1993) Laser photocoagulation of subfoveal neovascular lesions in age-related macular degeneration: updated findings from two clinical trials. Arch Ophthalmol 111:1200–1209
Macular Photocoagulation Study Group (1994a) Laser photocoagulation for juxtafoveal choroidal neovascularization: five-year results from randomized clinical trials. Arch Ophthalmol 112:500–509
Macular Photocoagulation Study Group (1994b) Visual outcome after laser photocoagulation for subfoveal choroidal neovascularization secondary to age-related macular degeneration: the influence of initial lesion size and initial visual acuity. Arch Ophthalmol 112: 480–488
Madreperla SA et al (1997) Choroidal hemangiomas: visual and anatomic results of treatment by photocoagulation or radiation therapy. Ophthalmology 104:1773–1779
Maguire AM, Schachat AP (1994) Radiation retinopathy. In: Ryan SJ (ed) Retina. Mosby Year Book, St. Louis
Marcus D, Sheils C, Burch S et al (1996) The radiation of age-related macular degeneration (ROARMD) study. Invest Ophthalmol Vis Sci 37 [Suppl]:abstract 1016
Midena E et al (1996) The effect of external eye irradiation on choroidal circulation. Ophthalmology 103:1651–1660
Miller JW, Walsh AW, Kramer M et al (1995) Photodynamic therapy of experimental choroidal neovascularization using lipoprotein-delivered benzoporphyrin. Arch Ophthalmol 113:810–818
Moisseiev J et al (1995) The impact of the Macular Photocoagulation Study results on the treatment of exudative age-related macular degeneration. Arch Ophthalmol 113:185–189
Nakissa N et al (1983) Ocular and orbital complications following radiation therapy of paranasal sinus malignancies and review of literature. Cancer 51:980–986
National Advisory Eye Council (1998) Vision research, a national plan: 1994–1998. Publication NIH 93-3186. National Institutes of Health, Bethesda
Parsons JT et al (1983) The effects of irradiation on the eye and optic nerve. Int J Radiat Oncol Biol Phys :609–622
Parsons JT et al (1994) Radiation retinopathy after external-beam irradiation: Analysis of time-dose factors. Int J Radiat Oncology Biol Phys 30:765–773
Plowman PN, Harnett AN (1988) Radiotherapy in benign orbital disease. I. Complicated ocular angiomas. Br J Ophthalmol 72:286–288
Postgens H, Bodanowitz S, Kroll P (1997) Low-dose radiation therapy for age-related macular degeneration. Graefes Arch Clin Exp Ophthalmol 235:656–661
Radiation Therapy for Age-related Macular Degeneration (RAD) Study Group (1999) A prospective, randomized, double-masked trial on radiation therapy for neovascular age-related macular degeneration (RAD Study). Ophthalmology 106:2239–2247
Reichel E, Berrocal A, Ip M, Kroll A, Desai V, Duker J, Puliafito C (1999) Transpupillary thermotherapy of occult subfoveal choroidal neovascularization in patients with age-related macular degeneration. Ophthalmology 106:1908–1914
Reinhold HS, Buisman GH (1973) Radiosensitivity of capillary endothelium. Br J Radiol 46:54–57
Ross HS, Rosenberg S, Friedman AH (1973) Delayed radiation necrosis of the optic nerve. Am J Ophthalmol 76:683–686
Saornil MA et al (1992) Histopathology of proton beam irradiated versus enucleated uveal melanomas. Arch Ophthalmol 110:1112–1118
Saornil MA et al (1997) Histopathologic study of eyes after iodine-125 episcleral plaque irradiation for uveal melanoma. Arch Ophthalmol 115:1395–1400
Scott TA et al (1991) Low dose ocular irradiation for diffuse choroidal hemangiomas associated with bullous nonhegmatogenous retinal detachment. Retina 11:389–393
Spaide RF, Guyer DR, McCormick B et al (1998) External beam radiation therapy for choroidal neovascularization. Ophthalmology 105:24–30
Stalmans P, Leys A, Van Limbergen E (1997) External beam radiotherapy (20 Gy, 2 Gy fractions) fails to control the growth of choroidal neovascularization in age-related macular degeneration: a review of 111 cases. Retina 17: 481–492
Tielsch JA (1995) Vision problem in the U.S. A report on blindness and vision impairment in adults aged 40 and older. Prevent Blindness Inc., Schaumburg, pp 1–20
Treatment of Age-Related Macular Degeneration with Photodynamic Therapy (TAP) Study Group (1999) Photodynamic therapy of subfoveal choroidal neovascularization in age-related macular degeneration with verteporin: One-year results of two randomized clinical trials – TAP report. Arch Ophthalmol 117:1329–1345
Van den Brenk HAS (1959) The effect of ionizing radiation on capillary sprouting and vascular remodeling in the regenerating repair blastema observed in the rabbit ear chamber. Am J Roentgenol 81:859–884
Vieban M, Barricks ME, Osterloh MD (1991) Synergism between diabetic and radiation retinopathy: case report and review. Br J Ophthalmol 75:629–632
Vingerling JR, Dielemans I, Hofman A et al (1995) The prevalence of age-related maculopathy in the Rotterdam Study. Ophthalmology 102(2):205–210
Volger WR et al (1990) Ophthalmological and other toxicities related to cytosine arabinoside and total body irradiation as preparative regimen for bone marrow transplantation. Bone Marrow Transplant 6:405–409
Yanuzzi LA (1994) A new standard of care for laser photocoagulation of subfoveal choroidal neovascularization secondary to age-related macular degeneration. Arch Ophthalmol 112:462–464
Yonemoto LT, Slater JD, Friedrichsen EJ (1996) Phase I/II study of proton beam irradiation for the treatment of subfoveal choroidal neovascularization in age-related macular degeneration: treatment techniques and preliminary results. Int J Radiat Oncol Biol Phys 36:867–871
Young W et al (1992) Radiation-induced optic neuropathy: correlation of MRI imaging and radiation dosimetry. Radiology 185:904–907
Zhan Q, Carrier F, Fornace AJ Jr (1993) Induction of cellular p53 activity by DNA-damaging agents and growth arrest. Mol Cell Biol 13:4242–4250

Subject Index

List of Contributors

WINFRIED E. ALBERTI, MD
Professor, Department of Radiotherapy and Radiooncology
University Hospital Hamburg
Martinistrasse 52
20246 Hamburg
Germany

KAH-GUAN AU EONG, MBBS, MMed (Ophth), FRCS (Edin), FRCS (Glasg), DRCO, FAMS
Clinical Fellow in Diseases and Surgery
of the Vitreous and Retina
The Wilmer Ophthalmological Institute
The Johns Hopkins University School of Medicine
The Johns Hopkins Hospital
Maumenee 7th Floor
600 North Wolfe Street
Baltimore, MD 21287-9277
USA
and
Consultant Ophthalmologist
Department of Ophthalmology
Tan Tock Seng Hospital
11 Jalan Tan Tock Seng
Singapore 308433
Singapore
and
Adjunct Associate Scientist
Singapore Eye Research Institute
500 Dover Road
Singapore Polytechnic Workshop 2 (W212)
Singapore 139651
Singapore

CAREN BELLMANN, MD
Department of Ophthalmology
University Hospital Heidelberg
Im Neuenheimer Feld 400
69120 Heidelberg
Germany

G.J. BERGINK, MD
University Hospital Rotterdam
Park Arenberg 54a
3731 ET De Bilt
The Netherlands

PETER BISCHOFF, MD
Department of Ophthalmology
Kantonsspital
9007 St. Gallen
Switzerland

PAUL BLACHARSKI, MD
Department of Radiation Ophthalmology
Loma Linda University Medical Center
11234 Anderson Street
Loma Linda, CA 92354
USA

LUTHER W. BRADY, MD
Hylda Cohn/American Cancer Society
Professor of Clinical Oncology, and
Professor, Department of Radiation Oncology
Hahnemann University Hospital
Broad & Vine Sts., Mail Stop 200
Philadelphia, PA 19102
USA

GARY BROWN, MD
Wills Eye Hospital
Department of Ophthalmology
9th and Waltnut Streets
Philadelphia, PA
USA

USHA CHAKRAVARTHY, MD
Professor of Vision Science/Consultant Ophthalmologist
The Royal Group of Hospitals and Dental Hospital
Health and Social Services Trust
Grosvenor Road
Belfast BT12 6BA
Northern Ireland, UK

RÉGIS COQUARD, MD
Clinique St-Jean
69003 Lyon
France

PETER COSSMANN
Department of Medical Physics Radiation
Inselspital
3010 Bern
Switzerland

J. DEBUS, MD
Department of Radiotherapy
University Hospital Heidelberg
Im Neuenheimer Feld 400
69120 Heidelberg
Germany

Eugene de Juan, Jr., MD
Joseph E. Green Professor of Ophthalmology
The Wilmer Ophthalmological Institute
The Johns Hopkins University School of Medicine
The Johns Hopkins Hospital
Maumenee 719
600 NorthWolfe Street
Baltimore, MD 21287-9277
USA

A.F. Deutmann, MD
Professor and Chairman, Institute of Ophthalmology
University Hospital Nijmegen
P.O. Box 9101
6500 Nijmegen
The Netherlands

Emmanuel Egger, PhD
Radiation Medicine
Paul Scherrer Institute
5232 Villigen-PSI
Switzerland

Katrin Engelmann, MD
Professor, Department of Ophthalmology
University of Hamburg
Martinistrasse 52
20246 Hamburg
Germany

Rita Engenhart-Cabillic, MD
Department of Radiotherapy
University Hospital Heidelberg
Im Neuenheimer Feld 400
69120 Heidelberg
Germany

Paul T. Finger, MD
The New York AMDRT Center
115 E. 61st Street
New York City
NY 10021
USA

Jorge Freire, MD
Thomas Jefferson University
Department of Radiation Oncology
Philadelphia, PA 19107
USA

Gildo Y. Fujii, MD
Research Fellow in Diseases and Surgery
of the Vitreous and Retina
The Wilmer Ophthalmological Institute
The Johns Hopkins University School of Medicine
The Johns Hopkins Hospital
Maumenee 7th Floor
600 North Wolfe Street
Baltimore, MD 21287-9277
USA

Jean-Pierre Gerard, MD
Professor, Service de Radiothérapie
Centre Hospitalier Lyon-Sud
69003 Lyon
France

Heinrich Gerding, MD
Professor, Klinik und Poliklinik für Augenheilkunde
Universität Münster
Domagkstrasse 15
48129 Münster
Germany

G. Goitein, MD
Division of Radiation Medicine
Paul Scherer Institute
5323 Villingen-PSI
Switzerland

Sri Gorty, MD
Department of Radiation Oncology
State University of New York
Upstate Medical University
750 East Adams Street
Syracuse, NY 13210
USA

Andrea Hassenstein, MD
Department of Ophthalmology
University of Hamburg
Martinistrasse 52
20246 Hamburg
Germany

K. Heimann, MD
Department of Ophthalmology
University Cologne
Josef-Stelzmann-Strasse 9
50933 Köln
Germany

Ulrike Höller, MD
Department of Radiotherapy and Radiooncology
University Hospital Hamburg
Martinistrasse 52
20246 Hamburg
Germany

Frank G. Holz, MD
Department of Ophthalmology
University Hospital Heidelberg
Im Neuenheimer Feld 400
69120 Heidelberg
Germany

C.B. Hoyng, MD
Institute of Ophthalmology
P.O. Box 9101
6500 Nijmegen
The Netherlands

Illka Immonen, MD
The University of Helsiniki
Department of Ophthalmology
Haantimawinkatu 4C
Helsinki 00290
Finland

Susan B. Klein, MD
Indiana University Cyclotron Facility
2401 Milo B Sampson Lane
Bloomington, IN 47408
USA

M. Kocher, MD
Department of Radiation Oncology
University Cologne
Josef-Stelzmann-Strasse 9
50933 Köln
Germany

G. Kovács, MD
Clinic for Radiation Therapy (Radio-oncology)
University Hospital Kiel
Arnold-Heller-Strasse 9
24105 Kiel
Germany

N. Kovács, MD
Department of Ophthalmology and Orbital Centre
University Hospital Kiel
Arnold-Heller-Strasse 9
24105 Kiel
Germany

K. Krause, PhD
Professor, Klinik und Poliklinik für Augenheilkunde
Universität Münster
Domagkstrasse 15
48129 Münster
Germany

R. Krott, MD
Department of Ophthalmology
University of Cologne
Josef-Stelzmann-Strasse 9
50933 Köln
Germany

John E. Lahaniatis, MD
Department of Radiation Oncology
MCP Hahnemann University
Broad & Vine Sts., Mail Stop 200
Philadelphia, PA 19102
USA

S. Young Lee, MD
Georgia Radiation Therapy Center
Medical College of Georgia
Building HK-112
Augusta, GA 30912-3965
USA

Dennis M. Marcus, MD
Georgia Radiation Therapy Center
Medical College of Georgia
Building HK-112
Augusta, GA 30912-3965
USA

Philippe Martin, MD
Clinique St-Jean
69003 Lyon
France

Martine Mauget-Faÿsse, MD
Ophthalmologiste, Attachée des Hôpitaux de Lyon
Centre d'Imagerie et de Laser
14, Rue Rabelais
69003 Lyon
France

Bizhan Micaily, MD
Department of Radiation Oncology
MCP Hahnemann University
Broad & Vine Sts., Mail Stop 200
Philadelphia, PA 19102
USA

Curtis T. Miyamoto, MD
Department of Radiation Oncology
MCP Hahnemann University
Broad & Vine Sts., Mail Stop 200
Philadelphia, PA 19102
USA

R.-P. Mueller, MD
Professor, Department of Radiation Oncology
University of Cologne
Josef-Stelzmann-Strasse 9
50933 Köln
Germany

Hugo Niederberger, MD
Department of Ophthalmology
Kantonsspital
9007 St. Gallen
Switzerland

Peter Niehoff, MD
Clinic for Radiation Therapy (Radio-oncology)
University Hospital Kiel
Arnold-Heller-Strasse 9
24105 Kiel
Germany

Dante J. Pieramici, MD
Assistant Professor of Opthalmology
The Wilmer Ophthalmological Institute
The Johns Hopkins University School of Medicine
The Johns Hopkins Hospital
Maumenee 719
600 North Wolfe Street
Baltimore, MD 21287-9277
USA

GISBERT RICHARD, MD
Professor
Augenklinik und Poliklinik
University Hospital Eppendorf
Martinistrasse 52
20246 Hamburg
Germany

GERHARD RIES, MD
Professor, Department of Radiation Oncology
Kantonsspital
9007 St. Gallen
Switzerland

ROBERT H. SAGERMAN, MD, FACR
Professor, Department of Radiation Oncology
State University of New York
Upstate Medical University
750 East Adams Street
Syracuse, NY 13210
USA

A. SCHALENBOURG, MD
Hôpital Ophthalmique Jules Gouin
Avenue France 15
1004 Lausanne
Switzerland

FLORIAN SCHÜTT, MD
Department of Ophthalmology
University Hospital Heidelberg
Im Neuenheimer Feld 400
69120 Heidelberg
Germany

R. SCHWARTZ, MD
Augenklinik und Poliklinik
University Hospital Eppendorf
Martinistrasse 52
20246 Hamburg
Germany

W. CHRIS SHEILS, MD, FACR
Georgia Radiation Therapy Center
Medical College of Georgia
Building HK-112
Augusta, GA 30912-3965
USA

JAMES M. SLATER, MD, FACR
Department of Radiation Ophthalmology
Loma Linda University Medical Center
11234 Anderson Street
Loma Linda, CA 92354
USA

JERRY D. SLATER, MD
Department of Radiation Medicine
Loma Linda University Medical Center
11234 Anderson Street
Loma Linda, CA 92354
USA

SUSANNE STAAR, MD
Department of Radiation Oncology
University of Cologne
Josef-Stelzmann-Strasse 9
50933 Köln
Germany

S. TANERI, MD
Klinik und Poliklinik für Augenheilkunde
Universität Münster
Domagkstrasse 15
48129 Münster
Germany

C. E. UHLIG, MD
Klinik und Poliklinik für Augenheilkunde
Universität Münster
Domagkstrasse 15
48129 Münster
Germany

KRISTINA UNNEBRINK, MD
Department of Biostatistics
University Hospital Heidelberg
Im Neuenheimer Feld 400
69120 Heidelberg
Germany

CHRISTOPHE VALMAGGIA, MD
Department of Ophthalmology
Kantonsspital
9007 St. Gallen
Switzerland

MONIKA VALTINK
Dipl.-Ing. (FH) Biotechnologie
Department of Ophthalmology
University of Hamburg
Martinistrasse 52
20246 Hamburg
Germany

W.A.J. VAN DAAL, MD
Institute of Radiotherapy
University Hospital Nijmegen
P.O. Box 9101
6500 Nijmegen
The Netherlands

R.W.M. VAN DER MAAZEN, MD
Institute of Radiotherapy
University Hospital Nijmegen
P.O. Box 9101
6500 Nijmegen
The Netherlands

J.R. VINGERLING, MD
Institute of Ophthalmology
University Hospital Rotterdam
Rotterdam
The Netherlands

M. Wannenmacher
Professor, Department of Radiotherapy
University Hospital Heidelberg
Im Neuenheimer Feld 400
69120 Heidelberg
Germany

Judith Weichel
Veterinary Surgeon, Department of Ophthalmology
University of Hamburg
Martinistrasse 52
20246 Hamburg
Germany

Theodore E. Yaeger, MD
Department of Radiation Oncology
Halifax Medical Center
Daytona Beach, FL 32115
USA

Les T. Yonemoto, MD
Department of Radiation Medicine
Loma Linda University Medical Center
11234 Anderson Street
Loma Linda, CA 92354
USA

L. Zografos, MD
Hôpital Ophthalmique Jules Gouin
Avenue France 15
1004 Lausanne
Switzerland

Jan Zurdel, MD
Augenklinik und Poliklinik
University Hospital Eppendorf
Martinistrasse 52
20246 Hamburg
Germany

Medical Radiology
Diagnostic Imaging and Radiation Oncology

Titles in the series already published

Radiation Oncology

Lung Cancer
Edited by C.W. Scarantino

Innovations in Radiation Oncology
Edited by H.R. Withers and L.J. Peters

Radiation Therapy of Head and Neck Cancer
Edited by G.E. Laramore

Gastrointestinal Cancer – Radiation Therapy
Edited by R.R. Dobelbower, Jr.

Radiation Exposure and Occupational Risks
Edited by E. Scherer, C. Streffer, and K.-R. Trott

Radiation Therapy of Benign Diseases - A Clinical Guide
S.E. Order and S.S. Donaldson

Interventional Radiation Therapy Techniques - Brachytherapy
Edited by R. Sauer

Radiopathology of Organs and Tissues
Edited by E. Scherer, C. Streffer, and K.-R. Trott

Concomitant Continuous Infusion Chemotherapy and Radiation
Edited by M. Rotman and C.J. Rosenthal

Intraoperative Radiotherapy – Clinical Experiences and Results
Edited by F.A. Calvo, M. Santos, and L.W. Brady

Radiotherapy of Intraocular and Orbital Tumors
Edited by W.E. Alberti and R.H. Sagerman

Interstitial and Intracavitary Thermoradiotherapy
Edited by M.H. Seegenschmiedt and R. Sauer

Non-Disseminated Breast Cancer
Controversial Issues in Management
Edited by G.H. Fletcher and S.H. Levitt

Current Topics in Clinical Radiobiology of Tumors
Edited by H.-P. Beck-Bornholdt

Practical Approaches to Cancer Invasion and Metastases
A Compendium of Radiation Oncologists' Responses to 40 Histories
Edited by A.R. Kagan with the Assistance of R.J. Steckel

Radiation Therapy in Pediatric Oncology
Edited by J.R. Cassady

Radiation Therapy Physics
Edited by A.R. Smith

Late Sequelae in Oncology
Edited by J. Dunst and R. Sauer

Mediastinal Tumors. Update 1995
Edited by D.E. Wood and C.R. Thomas, Jr.

Thermoradiotherapy and Thermochemotherapy

Volume 1:
Biology, Physiology, and Physics

Volume 2:
Clinical Applications
Edited by M.H. Seegenschmiedt, P. Fessenden, and C.C. Vernon

Carcinoma of the Prostate
Innovations in Management
Edited by Z. Petrovich, L. Baert, and L.W. Brady

Radiation Oncology of Gynecological Cancers
Edited by H.W. Vahrson

Carcinoma of the Bladder
Innovations in Management
Edited by Z. Petrovich, L. Baert, and L.W. Brady

Blood Perfusion and Microenvironment of Human Tumors
Implications for Clinical Radiooncology
Edited by M. Molls and P. Vaupel

Radiation Therapy of Benign Diseases. A Clinical Guide
2nd Revised Edition
S.E. Order and S.S. Donaldson

Carcinoma of the Kidney and Testis, and Rare Urologic Malignancies
Innovations in Management
Edited by Z. Petrovich, L. Baert, and L.W. Brady

Progress and Perspectives in the Treatment of Lung Cancer
Edited by P. Van Houtte, J. Klastersky, and P. Rocmans

Combined Modality Therapy of Central Nervous System Tumors
Edited by Z. Petrovich, L. W. Brady, M. L. Apuzzo, and M. Bamberg

Age-Related Macular Degeneration
Current Treatment Concepts
Edited by W. A. Alberti, G. Richard, and R. H. Sagerman

Springer

Medical Radiology
Diagnostic Imaging and Radiation Oncology

Titles in the series already published

Diagnostic Imaging

Innovations in Diagnostic Imaging
Edited by J.H. Anderson

Radiology of the Upper Urinary Tract
Edited by E.K. Lang

The Thymus - Diagnostic Imaging, Functions, and Pathologic Anatomy
Edited by E. Walter, E. Willich, and W.R. Webb

Interventional Neuroradiology
Edited by A. Valavanis

Radiology of the Pancreas
Edited by A.L. Baert, co-edited by G. Delorme

Radiology of the Lower Urinary Tract
Edited by E.K. Lang

Magnetic Resonance Angiography
Edited by I.P. Arlart, G.M. Bongartz, and G. Marchal

Contrast-Enhanced MRI of the Breast
S. Heywang-Köbrunner and R. Beck

Spiral CT of the Chest
Edited by M. Rémy-Jardin and J. Rémy

Radiological Diagnosis of Breast Diseases
Edited by M. Friedrich and E.A. Sickles

Radiology of the Trauma
Edited by M. Heller and A. Fink

Biliary Tract Radiology
Edited by P. Rossi

Radiological Imaging of Sports Injuries
Edited by C. Masciocchi

Modern Imaging of the Alimentary Tube
Edited by A. R. Margulis

Diagnosis and Therapy of Spinal Tumors
Edited by P. R. Algra, J. Valk, and J. J. Heimans

Interventional Magnetic Resonance Imaging
Edited by J. F. Debatin and G. Adam

Abdominal and Pelvic MRI
Edited by A. Heuck and M. Reiser

Orthopedic Imaging
Techniques and Applications
Edited by A.M. Davies and H. Pettersson

Radiology of the Female Pelvic Organs
Edited by E.K.Lang

Magnetic Resonance of the Heart and Great Vessels
Clinical Applications
Edited by J. Bogaert, A. J. Duerinckx, and F. E. Rademakers

Modern Head and Neck Imaging
Edited by S. K. Mukherji and J. A. Castelijns

Radiological Imaging of Endocrine Diseases
Edited by J. N. Bruneton in collaboration with B. Padovani and M.-Y. Mourou

Trends in Contrast Media
Edited by H. S. Thomsen, R. N. Muller, and R. F. Mattrey

Functional MRI
Edited by C. T. W. Moonen and P. A. Bandettini

Radiology of the Pancreas
2nd Revised Edition
Edited by A. L. Baert
Co-edited by G. Delorme and L. Van Hoe

Emergency Pediatric Radiology
Edited by H. Carty

Spiral CT of the Abdomen
Edited by F. Terrier, M. Grossholz, and C. D. Becker

Liver Malignancies
Diagnostic and Interventional Radiology
Edited by C. Bartolozzi and R. Lencioni

Medical Imaging of the Spleen
Edited by A. M. De Schepper and F. Vanhoenacker

Radiology of Peripheral Vascular Diseases
Edited by E. Zeitler

Diagnostic Nuclear Medicine
Edited by C. Schiepers

Radiology of Blunt Trauma of the Chest
P. Schnyder and M. Wintermark

Portal Hypertension
Diagnostic Imaging-Guided Therapy
Edited by P. Rossi
Co-edited by P. Ricci and L. Broglia

Virtual Endoscopy and Related 3D Techniques
Edited by P. Rogalla, J. Terwisscha Van Scheltinga, and B. Hamm

Recent Advances in Diagnostic Neuroradiology
Edited by Ph. Demaerel

Transfontanellar Doppler Imaging in Neonates
A. Couture and C. Veyrac

Springer

FSC
www.fsc.org
MIX
Papier | Fördert gute Waldnutzung
FSC® C083411

Kolibri 360 GmbH
Ferdinand-Jühlke-Straße 7
99095 Erfurt, Deutschland
produktsicherheit@kolibri360.de